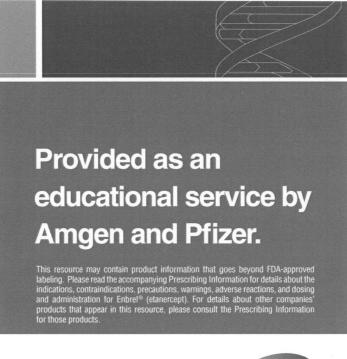

Provided as an educational service by Amgen and Pfizer.

This resource may contain product information that goes beyond FDA-approved labeling. Please read the accompanying Prescribing Information for details about the indications, contraindications, precautions, warnings, adverse reactions, and dosing and administration for Enbrel® (etanercept). For details about other companies' products that appear in this resource, please consult the Prescribing Information for those products.

Therapeutic Strategies

RHEUMATOLOGY

Therapeutic Strategies

RHEUMATOLOGY

Edited by

Michael Doherty

CLINICAL PUBLISHING

OXFORD

Clinical Publishing
an imprint of Atlas Medical Publishing Ltd

Oxford Centre for Innovation
Mill Street, Oxford OX2 0JX, UK
Tel: +44 1865 811116
Fax: +44 1865 251550
Email: info@clinicalpublishing.co.uk
Web: www.clinicalpublishing.co.uk

Distributed in USA and Canada by:
Clinical Publishing
30 Amberwood Parkway
Ashland OH 44805 USA

Tel: 800-247-6553 (toll free within U.S. and Canada)
Fax: 419-281-6883
Email: order@bookmasters.com

Distributed in UK and Rest of World by:
Marston Book Services Ltd
PO Box 269
Abingdon
Oxon OX14 4YN UK

Tel: +44 1235 465500
Fax: +44 1235 465555
Email: trade.orders@marston.co.uk

A catalogue record for this book is available from the British Library

ISBN-13   978 1 84692 026 4
ISBN e-book   978 1 84692 611 2

The publisher makes no representation, express or implied, that the dosages in this
book are correct. Readers must therefore always check the product information and
clinical procedures with the most up-to-date published product information and
data sheets provided by the manufacturers and the most recent codes of conduct
and safety regulations. The authors and the publisher do not accept any liability for
any errors in the text or for the misuse or misapplication of material in this work

Typeset by Prepress Projects Ltd, Perth, UK
Printed by Marston Book Services Ltd, Abingdon, Oxon, UK

Cover image courtesy of Dr Adrian Jones and Dr Michael Doherty, Nottingham City Hospital, Nottingham,
UK

Contents

Editor and Contributors   vii

Acknowledgement   ix

1   Early arthritis   1
Jackie Nam, Edith Villeneuve, Paul Emery

2   Established rheumatoid arthritis   17
Pieternella J. Barendregt, J. Mieke W. Hazes

3   Beyond anti-TNF: other biological drugs in inflammatory arthritis   35
Peter C. Taylor

4   Pharmacogenetics of inflammatory arthritis   51
Judith A. M. Wessels, Tom W. J. Huizinga, Henk-Jan Guchelaar

5   Psoriatic arthritis   71
Eliza Pontifex, Oliver Fitzgerald

6   Therapy of ankylosing spondylitis   85
Jurgen Braun

7   Systemic lupus erythematosus   101
Tim Y.-T. Lu, Jose M. Pego-Reigosa, David A. Isenberg

8   Antiphospholipid syndrome   117
Ann Scott-Russell, Christopher J. Edwards, Graham R. V. Hughes

9   Progress in the therapy of systemic sclerosis   129
Emma C. Derrett-Smith, Christopher P. Denton

10   Inflammatory myositis   139
David L. Scott

11   Disease-modifying drugs in osteoarthritis   151
Alexandra N. Colebatch, Nigel K. Arden

12   Management of gout   163
        Edward Roddy, Michael Doherty

13   Osteoporosis   179
        Ira Pande

Abbreviations   195

Index   201

Editor

MICHAEL DOHERTY, MA, MD, FRCP, Professor of Rheumatology, Academic Rheumatology, Nottingham City Hospital, Nottingham, UK

Contributors

NIGEL K. ARDEN, MBBS, MSc, MD, FRCP, MRC Epidemiology Resource Centre, University of Southampton, Southampton General Hospital, Southampton, UK

PIETERNELLA J. BARENDREGT, MD, Department of Rheumatology, Erasmus Medical Center, Rotterdam, The Netherlands

JURGEN BRAUN, Professor, Ruhrgebiet Rheumatology Centre, Herne, Germany

ERNEST CHOY, MD, FRCP, Senior Lecturer, Consultant Rheumatologist, Sir Alfred Baring Garrod Clinical Trials Unit, Academic Department of Rheumatology, Kings College Hospital, Weston Education Centre, London, UK

ALEXANDRA N. COLEBATCH, MBBS, BSc(Hons), DOccMED, MRCP, (UK), MRC Epidemiology Resource Centre, University of Southampton, Southampton General Hospital, Southampton, UK

CHRIS DENTON, Centre for Rheumatology and Connective Tissue Disease, Royal Free & UCL School of Medicine, London, UK

EMMA DERRETT-SMITH, BSc, MRCP, Centre for Rheumatology and Connective Tissue Disease, Royal Free & UCL School of Medicine, London, UK

CHRISTOPHER J. EDWARDS, BSc, MBBS, MD, FRCP, Consultant, Department of Rheumatology, Southampton University Hospitals NHS Trust, Southampton General Hospital, Southampton, UK

PAUL EMERY, MD, FRCP, Arc Professor of Rheumatology, Clinical Director, Rheumatology, Leeds Teaching Hospitals Trust, Leeds General Infirmary, Leeds, UK

OLIVER FITZGERALD, MD, FRCPI, FRCP(UK), Newman Clinical Research Professor, Department of Rheumatology, St. Vincents University Hospital, Dublin, Ireland

HENK-JAN GUCHELAAR, PharmD, PhD, Department of Rheumatology, Leiden University Medical Center, Leiden, The Netherlands

J. MIEKE W. HAZES, MD, PhD, Professor, Department of Rheumatology, Erasmus Medical Center, Rotterdam, The Netherlands

GRAHAM R.V. HUGHES, MD, FRCP, Consultant Rheumatologist, The London Lupus Centre, London Bridge Hospital, London, UK

TOM W.J. HUIZINGA, MD, PhD, Department of Rheumatology, Leiden University Medical Center, Leiden, The Netherlands

DAVID ISENBERG, MD, FRCP, Professor, Director, Centre for Rheumatology, Division of Medicine, University College London, London, UK

TIM Y-T LU, FRACP, Centre for Rheumatology, University College London, London, UK

JACKIE L. NAM, MBBCh, FCP, Academic Unit of Musculoskeletal Disease, Chapel Allerton Hospital, Leeds, UK

IRA PANDE, MD, FRCP, PhD, Consultant Rheumatologist, Nottingham University Hospitals, Nottingham, UK

JOSE M PEGO-REIGOSA, MD, PhD, Hospital do Meixoeiro (Complexo Hospitalario Universitario de Vigo), Rheumatology Section, Vigo (Pontevedra), Spain

ELIZA PONTIFEX, MBBS, FRACP, Department of Rheumatology, St. Vincents University Hospital, Dublin, Rep. Ireland

EDWARD RODDY, DM, MRCP, Clinical Lecturer and Consultant Rheumatologist, Staffordshire Rheumatology Centre, Arthritis Research Campaign National Primary Care Research Centre, Primary Care Sciences, Keele University, Keele, UK

DAVID L SCOTT, BSc, MD, FRCP, Professor of Clinical Rheumatology, Department of Rheumatology, King's College London, London, UK

ANN SCOTT-RUSSELL, MBBS, BMedSci, Specialist registrar, Rheumatology department, Southampton University Hospitals NHS Trust, Southampton, UK

PETER C TAYLOR, MA, BM, BCh, PhD, FRCP, Professor of Experimental Rheumatology and Head of Clinical Trials, Kennedy Institute of Rheumatology Division, Imperial College London, London, UK

EDITH VILLENEUVE, MD, FRCPC, Academic Unit of Musculoskeletal Disease, Chapel Allerton Hospital, Leeds, UK

JUDITH AM WESSELS, PharmD, PhD, Department of Clinical Pharmacy and Toxicology, Leiden University Medical Center, Leiden, The Netherlands

Acknowledgement

The editor and publisher acknowledge the part played in the development of this book by Dr Christopher Deighton, Consultant Rheumatologist at the Derbyshire Royal Infirmary, who conceived the project and recruited the contributors.

1

Early arthritis

Jackie Nam, Edith Villeneuve, Paul Emery

INTRODUCTION

Rheumatoid arthritis (RA) is the most common type of inflammatory arthritis, affecting about 1% of the population. It typically presents between the ages of 40 and 50 years, affecting twice as many women as men. Untreated, it results in joint destruction, functional impairment and increased mortality [1]. In recent years, with the availability of effective therapies and the use of early intensive treatment strategies, disease outcomes have improved considerably [2–6]. Studies confirm that all therapies – monotherapy, combination therapies with disease-modifying antirheumatic drugs (DMARDs) and the newer biological agents – work better in early disease than in established RA. Further improvements are achieved with regular monitoring of disease activity and escalation of therapy if optimal disease control is not obtained. The goal of treatment is no longer simply symptom control but early suppression of inflammation and aiming for remission (a low disease activity state that, if sustained, is neither damaging nor disabling) [7].

Although rheumatologists agree that these patients should be seen and treated at the earliest opportunity and optimal disease control should be achieved, a number of issues remain. These include the choice of initial therapy, patient criteria for combination therapy and the use and timing of the newer biological agents [8]. Treating patients with early undifferentiated inflammatory arthritis and preventing the development of RA is another therapeutic strategy under investigation.

THE RATIONALE FOR EARLY THERAPY [9]

Joint damage occurs early in the inflammatory process. There is evidence that radiographic damage [10], loss of bone mineral density [11–13] and loss of function [14] occur early. Radiological outcome studies have shown that 70% of patients with recent-onset RA develop bone erosions within the first 3 years [15]. Furthermore, within 3 months of disease onset, 25% of patients have erosions evident on radiographs [16]. Presence of these early erosions predicts the future development of radiographic lesions. Newer imaging techniques, such as magnetic resonance imaging (MRI) and ultrasound, have confirmed evidence of damage within weeks of onset of symptoms [17, 18]. These lesions also correlate reliably with later radiographic erosions [19].

Further evidence suggests that the disease process exists in the preclinical stage, i.e. before the symptoms of RA. Rheumatoid factor (RF) [20] and anti-cyclic citrullinated peptide (anti-CCP) antibodies [21, 22] have been found in patients with RA years before the onset of symptoms. Raised levels of highly sensitive C-reactive protein (CRP) have also been shown before onset of clinical disease [23]. Complementary to the serological changes, arthroscopy and imaging with ultrasound and MRI help to detect synovitis in clinically normal joints of patients with early RA [24].

Moreover, there is evidence that very early RA may be an immunopathologically distinct phase compared with later disease [25, 26]. Treatment during this period is believed to optimize outcomes in terms of achieving remission and halting disease progression as measured by disease activity and radiographic progression [27]. This suggests that there may be a 'window of opportunity', a period early in the course of the disease when the disease process can be modified or perhaps even reversed with a complete return to normality.

Several studies have tested this very early window of opportunity and suggest that early treatment has a greater effect on disease progression than treatment later on. There is good evidence that patients with recent-onset polyarthritis who receive earlier DMARD treatment have better outcomes with regards to radiographic progression, function and ability to work than those in whom DMARD treatment is delayed by a few months [16, 28–31]. Disease duration at the time of DMARD initiation was shown to be the main predictor of response to treatment in the meta-analysis of 14 randomized controlled trials by Anderson *et al.* [32]. The best response was seen in those with less than 1 year of symptoms at commencement of therapy. Another meta-analysis of 12 studies examined the effect of early DMARD therapy on the long-term radiographic progression in patients with early RA (less than 2 years at presentation). Six were open-label extensions of randomized controlled trials in which patients initially on placebo later started DMARD therapy, and six were observational cohort studies. The average delay between early and late therapy was 9 months. After a median of 3 years of observation, those patients who received early treatment had 33% less radiological progression than those with delayed treatment [33].

In a case–control parallel-group study, clinical and radiological outcomes were significantly better at 3 years in one group of 20 patients with RA who started DMARD therapy 3 months after disease onset (very early) than in a second group of 20 patients with a median disease duration of 12 months at treatment start (early). Remission was achieved in 50% in the very early group compared with only 15% in the early group. The major differences between the two groups occurred within the first year, and especially during the first 3 months of treatment. An unblinded study of a single dose of glucocorticosteroid in 63 patients with mild early inflammatory arthritis (median duration 20 weeks) also found that the strongest predictor of disease remission at 6 months was a disease duration of less than 12 weeks at time of therapy [34].

These studies highlight the need to identify and treat patients with early RA as soon as possible. Early intervention may induce remission, whereas delayed therapy can result in irreversible damage.

ACHIEVING TIGHT CONTROL

Optimal therapeutic response may be achieved by a combination of early therapy and 'tight control' of disease activity. In practice, tight control for RA means that therapy is increased if disease activity is not suppressed below a predefined level (ideally remission).

In the TICORA ('Tight Control for Rheumatoid Arthritis') study [35], 110 patients with RA of less than 5 years' duration were randomly assigned to an intensive treatment in order to reach a low disease activity state, defined as an original disease activity score (DAS) of less than 2.4, or to regular clinical care. Patients in the tight control group were examined monthly and DMARD therapy was escalated, according to a predefined strategy, if the DAS was above 2.4. Those in the routine care group were seen every 3 months without formal assessment or feedback on disease activity scores, and therapy was adjusted according to the clinical judgement of the rheumatologist. After 18 months of follow-up, the intensive-treatment group had a significantly higher rate of remission (DAS < 1.6, 65%

vs. 16%; $P < 0.001$) and developed less radiographic damage than the control group. In the intensive-treatment group there was also a higher treatment retention rate, a lower rate of discontinuation owing to side-effects and lower costs per patient (based on lower admission costs) than in the routine care group over the 18 months of observation. Of note, however, more intra-articular steroids were used in the intensive-treatment group.

The CAMERA (Computer-Assisted Management of Early Rheumatoid Arthritis) trial [36] also showed intensive treatment and monitoring to be more beneficial than routine care. A total of 299 patients with early RA were randomized to intensive treatment or routine treatment, with oral methotrexate (MTX). If necessary, therapy was changed to subcutaneous MTX and ciclosporin was added to achieve disease control. Patients in the intensive-treatment group were seen more frequently in clinics, and dosages were adjusted based on predefined criteria and tailored to achieve remission using a computer-assisted programme. At 2 years, results showed that more patients in the intensive-management group achieved sustained remission for at least 3 months than in the routine care group (50% vs. 37%; $P < 0.03$). Median area under the curve for all clinical variables (erythrocyte sedimentation rate [ESR], early morning stiffness, visual analogue scale for pain, visual analogue scale for general well-being, number of swollen joints and number of tender joints) were significantly better in the intensive-management group than in the routine care group. Patients in the intensive-management group also used less non-steroidal anti-inflammatory drugs (NSAIDs) than the routine care group.

Further trials have also shown better outcomes where intensive care was based on regular monitoring of disease activity and treatment to target [6, 37].

Regular monitoring of disease activity and adverse events, therefore, should guide decisions on choice and changes in treatment strategies. This includes both traditional DMARDs and biologicals. Monitoring of disease activity should include tender and swollen joint count, patient's and physician's global assessment, ESR and CRP [38]. Arthritis activity should be assessed at 1- to 3-month intervals, aiming for 'remission' or 'low disease activity' as defined by available scores [39–42]. Structural damage should be assessed using radiographs and may be done every 6–12 months during the first few years. Functional assessment (e.g. the Health Assessment Questionnaire [HAQ]) can be used to complement the disease activity and structural damage monitoring.

THERAPEUTIC OPTIONS

GLUCOCORTICOIDS

Several randomized controlled trials and systematic reviews have shown that systemic low-dose glucocorticoids, typically prednisolone ≤10mg/day, were effective in relieving short-term signs and symptoms in patients with established RA [43–45]. Furthermore, despite controversial data [46, 47], several studies have shown that glucocorticoids – either alone or in combination with other DMARD therapy – are effective in slowing radiographic progression in early and established RA [2, 3, 48–52].

In a recent randomized controlled trial, 45 patients with RA and symptom duration of less than 1 year were randomized to receive MTX alone, MTX plus intravenous (i.v.) methylprednisolone (MP) 1g, or MTX plus infliximab (3mg/kg) infusions on day 0 and weeks 2, 6, 14, 22, 38 and 46. At week 22 the clinical response rates, according to the American College of Rheumatology 20% improvement criteria (ACR20), the ACR50 and ACR70, were significantly higher in both groups receiving i.v. MP and infliximab than those receiving MTX. At week 52, remission was achieved in 40% of patients in the MTX group and in 70% of the patients in the i.v. MP or infliximab group. HAQ scores improved significantly over time in all groups, with patients receiving i.v. MP showing a significantly greater improvement than patients receiving MTX alone. The combination therapy groups also showed a greater reduction in MRI-detected synovitis and bone oedema. The progression of MRI-detected erosions, however, was greater in patients treated with MTX plus i.v. MP than in those who received MTX plus infliximab [53].

The use of intra-articular steroids has also been shown to be of benefit. From the 2-year follow-up data of the Ciclosporin–Methotrexate Steroid Treatment in Rheumatoid Arthritis (CIMESTRA) study [54], betamethasone injections resulted in 50% of patients achieving remission (DAS28 < 2.6), and 70% of patients had no progression in the Sharp–van der Heijde scores.

Concerns are often raised about the side-effects of glucocorticoids. Evidence suggests the side-effect profile depends on the dose used and the disease which is being treated. A review of the published literature has shown that in RA, low doses of glucocorticoids may have very few side-effects [55]. Those known to occur in other diseases treated with higher doses of glucocorticoids may not occur when low-dose glucocorticoids are used to treat RA. These include increased cardiovascular risk [56, 57], lipid abnormalities [58] and osteoporosis [59].

Newer glucocorticoids and glucocorticoid analogues that will target inflammatory tissues or specific gene activations are under investigation to obtain the anti-inflammatory effect of the drug with minimal or no increased risk of adverse reactions [60].

DISEASE-MODIFYING ANTIRHEUMATIC DRUGS

Disease-modifying antirheumatic drugs have an effect on the disease process within weeks to months of commencing treatment. Methotrexate, sulfasalazine (SSZ) and leflunomide [61] are commonly used DMARDs. They have been shown to improve clinical outcomes and to delay radiological progression. Less commonly used agents include azathioprine, gold and ciclosporin. Among the DMARDs, MTX is considered the anchor drug and is generally used first in patients at risk of developing persistent or erosive disease because of its relatively beneficial safety profile [62], clinical and radiological efficacy [63, 64], and its beneficial properties in treatment combinations with biological agents [4, 5, 65]. Leflunomide and SSZ have similar clinical efficacy and are considered the best alternatives.

Despite early treatment, substantial structural damage may still occur in some early patients with RA treated with DMARDs alone [66]. In a cohort of patients with very early RA, with symptom duration of less than 3 months, 64% developed erosive disease by 3 years.

COMBINATION DISEASE-MODIFYING ANTIRHEUMATIC DRUG THERAPY [67]

Another therapeutic strategy in the treatment of RA is the early use of combination therapy with conventional DMARDs. Most of the evidence is based on studies of patients with early or established RA and has been extrapolated to the management of early arthritis.

Several studies have addressed the issue of whether initial combination therapy of early RA confers benefit over more conservative strategies. In the COBRA (Combination Therapy in Early Rheumatoid Arthritis) trial, a combination of MTX (7.5 mg weekly), SSZ (2 g/day) and prednisolone (starting with 60 mg/day and tapering over 6 months) resulted in long-term effects on radiographic progression, compared with SSZ monotherapy in 155 patients with RA of duration under 2 years [2, 68]. These results were consistent with those from the FIN-RACo (Finnish Rheumatoid Arthritis – Combination Therapy) study, in which 197 patients with onset of RA within 2 years were randomly assigned to receive either a four-drug regimen with MTX, SSZ, hydroxychloroquine (HCQ) and prednisolone (maximum doses: 15 mg/week, 2 g/day, 300 mg/week and 10 mg/day, respectively) or a single DMARD [3, 69, 70] for 2 years. After 18 months, a greater proportion of the combination group was less likely to have radiographic progression, and the work disability rate was lower than for patients on monotherapy. In neither study was there an arm with DMARD monotherapy plus steroids. Although, in the latter study, steroid was permitted in the single-treatment group; this was introduced later, at up to 93 weeks from baseline. The effects achieved in the combination treatment arms may therefore be attributed, at least in part, to the use of steroids rather than the combination of DMARDs alone.

To establish whether a combination of SSZ and MTX may be superior to either drug alone in patients with early RA with suboptimal response to SSZ, the MASCOT (Methotrexate and Sulfasalazine Combination Therapy) study, a randomized controlled study of step-up DMARD treatment, was designed by Capell and colleagues [71]. At 6 months, 191 of 687 (28%) patients had a DAS < 2.4 on SSZ alone. Of the remaining patients, 165 took part in the second phase of the study and were randomized to receive SSZ alone, MTX alone or a combination of the two. The DAS at 18 months was significantly lower in those who received combination treatment than in those who received either SSZ or MTX; monotherapy arms did not differ. Clinical improvement, as measured by the European League Against Rheumatism (EULAR) and ACR scores, favoured combination therapy. In the combination group, SSZ-only and MTX-only groups, the ACR20 responses were 48%, 32% and 33% respectively, the ACR50 responses were 25%, 10% and 7%, respectively, and the ACR70 responses were 13%, 7% and 4%, respectively. No increase in toxicity was seen. These results provide evidence for the use of this combination in patients inadequately treated with monotherapy.

Early parallel triple therapy has been compared with step-up therapy within an intensive disease management regimen. Ninety-six patients with early RA (mean disease duration 11.5 months) were randomized to receive step-up therapy (with SSZ monotherapy, then sequentially adding MTX and HCQ) or parallel triple therapy (SSZ/MTX/HCQ) [72]. Patients were assessed monthly for 12 months. If their disease activity score in 28 joints (DAS28) was ≥3.2, the dosage of DMARDs was increased according to protocol, and swollen joints were injected with triamcinolone acetonide. Both groups showed substantial improvements in disease activity and functional outcome. At 12 months, the mean decrease in the DAS28 score was 4.0 (step-up therapy group) versus 3.3 (parallel therapy group) ($P = 0.163$). No significant differences in the percentages of patients with DAS28 remission (step-up therapy group 45% vs. parallel triple therapy group 33%), or ACR20 (77% vs. 76%, respectively), ACR50 (60% vs. 51%, respectively) or ACR70 (30% vs. 20%, respectively) responses were seen. Radiological progression was similar in both groups. This study shows that control of disease activity can be achieved using conventional DMARDs as part of an intensive disease management strategy. Within this setting, step-up therapy is as effective as parallel triple therapy.

Similar benefits of the more intensive approach over 'conservative' treatment have been demonstrated by some studies [73]. However, others comparing MTX/SSZ combination with single agents [74, 75] were unable to identify better outcomes for any treatment arm over the other. Results from the Behandel Strategieën (BeSt) study demonstrated that after a failure of MTX 25 mg/week, adding SSZ to MTX resulted in an original DAS of 2.4 or less in only 22% of patients. An equally low response was obtained when switching from MTX to SSZ [76].

Taken together, some benefit is seen with the use of combination DMARD therapy with or without steroids, at least for the clinical course. The COBRA [2] and FIN-RACo [69] trials also reported radiographic benefits in the more intensive-treatment groups. However, not all of the studies compared radiographic progression, and in others deterioration still occurred with respect to radiological scores.

BIOLOGICAL THERAPY [77]

An alternative approach to managing patients with early arthritis is to target the subgroup of patients with very early synovitis who are at high risk of developing RA with potent anti-inflammatory therapy. Tumour necrosis factor alpha (TNF-α) is a cytokine that is central to the inflammatory cascade. It has pleiotropic effects driving the immune response, with powerful modulatory effects on many aspects of cellular and humoral immunity [78, 79], and has an important role in persistence of early RA [80].

The concept that intensive interventions early in the course of persistent arthritis may improve clinical activity and profoundly affect long-term radiographic progression is supported by several recent randomized controlled trials with anti-TNF agents in early RA (Table 1.1). In patients with a disease duration of less than 3 years, the use of a TNF blocking drug (adalimumab, etanercept or infliximab) – especially in combination with MTX – revealed an increased rate of clinical remission and slowing of radiographic progression compared with MTX monotherapy [5, 65, 81, 82]. These data are consistent with those from several randomized controlled trials in established RA [4, 83, 84]. In addition, at least for infliximab, it has been demonstrated that, even in cases in which clinical activity was not optimally suppressed ('poor response'), radiographic progression appeared to be significantly retarded in comparison with MTX [85].

PREMIER (a trial of lifestyle interventions for blood pressure control) examined the efficacy of adalimumab and MTX combination therapy compared with adalimumab or MTX alone. Rapidly, clinical response was achieved with adalimumab, and the combination therapy group achieved the highest proportion of responses [65]. The ERA trial compared etanercept at two different doses or MTX as monotherapy. Patients receiving etanercept monotherapy also had a more rapid clinical response [82]. The ASPIRE (Active-Controlled Study of Patients Receiving Infliximab for Treatment of Rheumatoid Arthritis of Early Onset) trial assessed the efficacy of infliximab at different doses with MTX versus MTX alone in MTX-naive patients with early RA. Patients treated with infliximab and MTX had a more rapid clinical improvement in terms of their HAQ scores and achieved higher 1-year clinical responses and remission rates (defined by a DAS28 score < 2.6) and less radiographic progression [86].

In the Combination of Methotrexate and Etanercept (COMET) study, the first major study looking at remission as the primary end-point in patients with early RA, patients with symptom duration of less than or equal to 2 years were randomized to MTX or MTX and etanercept. At week 52, remission as defined by a DAS28 < 2.6 was achieved in 48.4% with MTX plus etanercept versus 25.9% with MTX alone (P < 0.001) (Figure 1.1). Radiographic progression at week 52 was also significantly lower in the group receiving combination therapy (Figure 1.2). No differences were seen between the two groups in terms of serious adverse events, serious infections or malignancies. No cases of tuberculosis were reported in either group [87].

Anti-TNF agents, therefore, provide rapid control of inflammation and have proven efficacy both in terms of clinical outcomes and regarding reduction of structural damage in early disease. They are, however, substantially more expensive than traditional DMARDs, limiting their widespread use in early disease. Selecting patients with poor prognostic factors may improve this cost–benefit balance [88]. These factors include a positive serum test for RF, the presence of anti-CCP antibodies, early radiographic evidence of erosive disease, impaired functional status and persistently active synovitis with high levels of disease activity [86].

INDUCTION WITH BIOLOGICALS AND MAINTENANCE WITH CONVENTIONAL DISEASE-MODIFYING ANTIRHEUMATIC DRUGS

Induction with biologicals and maintenance with conventional DMARDs is another therapeutic strategy. This concept was introduced in a placebo-controlled study by Quinn *et al.* [5]. The study demonstrated that patients with early RA and poor prognostic factors treated with infliximab and MTX showed a significant reduction in synovitis and developed fewer erosions on MRI at 12 months than patients treated with MTX alone. Furthermore, the functional and quality of life benefits obtained in patients treated with infliximab after 1 year was sustained at 2 years without further infliximab infusion (Figure 1.3).

Table 1.1 Trials comparing the efficacy of methotrexate, tumour necrosis factor inhibitors and combination tumour necrosis factor inhibitors and methotrexate in early rheumatoid arthritis

Trial	Treatment regimen	Number of patients	Disease duration	Follow-up (weeks)	Clinical outcomes at year 1				Radiographic outcome (mean change in total Sharp scores from baseline)	
					ACR20	ACR50	ACR70	Remission (DAS28 <2.6)	Year 1	Year 2
ERA [82, 95]	MTX+placebo	632	<3 years	54	65	45	22	–	0.47	1.3
	ETN 10 mg twice a week				60	35	15	–	1.03	3.2[a]
	ETN 25 mg twice a week				72	50	25	–		
ASPIRE [81]	MTX+placebo	1049	≥3 months and ≤3 years	54	54	32	21	15	3.7*	
	MTX+IFX 3 mg/kg				62	46[a]	33	21	0.5*[a]	
	MTX+IFX 6 mg/kg				66	50[a]	37[a]	31[a]	0.4*[a]	
PREMIER [65]	MTX	799	<3 years	104	63	46	28	21	5.7	10.4
	ADA 40 mg every other week				54	41	26	23	3.0[a]	5.5[a]
	MTX+ADA 40 mg every other week				73[b]	62[ab]	46[ab]	43[ab]	1.3[a]	1.9[ab]
COMET [87]	MTX	542	≥3 months and ≤2 years	52	67	49	28	28	2.44	
	MTX+ETN				86[a]	71[a]	48[a]	50[a]	0.27[a]	

ACR20, American College of Rheumatology 20% improvement criteria; ACR50, ACR 50% improvement criteria; ACR70, ACR 70% improvement criteria; ADA, adalimumab; ETN, etanercept; IFX, infliximab; MTX, methotrexate.

*van der Heijde modification.

[a] P <0.001 vs. MTX and placebo.

[b] P <0.001 vs. adalimumab alone.

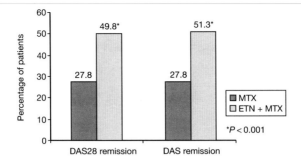

Figure 1.1 Percentage of patients achieving DAS28 remission (primary end-point) and DAS remission at week 52 in the groups receiving MTX versus MTX plus etanercept (ETN) [87]. Source: presentation at ACR, 2007, P. Emery.

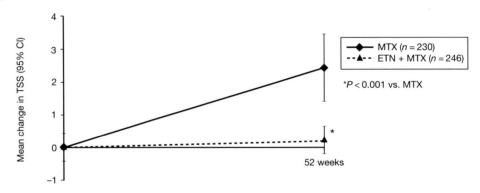

Figure 1.2 Comparison of the change in the modified total Sharp score (TSS) at 52 weeks between the group receiving MTX and the group receiving MTX plus etanercept (ETN) [87]. n, number of patients in each treatment group. Source: presentation at ACR, 2007, P. Emery.

COMPARISON OF TREATMENT OPTIONS

One study which compares the use of these various therapeutic options and addresses the optimal treatment paradigms for early RA is the BeSt trial. This multicentre single-blinded trial of 508 patients with RA and less than 2 years of symptoms compared four treatment strategies, including a sequential monotherapy (group 1), step-up combination therapy (group 2), a triple step-down strategy with MTX, SSZ and high-dose prednisolone (group 3) and infliximab plus MTX (group 4) [6]. Treatment was adjusted at 3-monthly intervals with a goal of achieving a DAS of 2.4 or less.

The two groups with initial intensive treatment (groups 3 and 4) showed a more rapid clinical response and a better radiographic outcome than groups 1 and 2. At 2 years, progression of joint damage was less in groups 3 and 4 (median Sharp–van der Heijde scores of 2.0, 2.0, 1.0 and 1.0 in groups 1, 2, 3 and 4, respectively; $P = 0.004$). In addition, fewer treatment adjustments were required in groups 3 and 4 to achieve suppression of disease activity and, after 2 years of treatment, approximately 50% of patients in group 4 were able to stop treatment with infliximab and maintain remission. By year 3, 15% of patients were in remission taking no DMARDs. No significant differences in toxicity were noted between the groups. At 4 years of follow-up, 455/508 patients were still in BeSt and 49% were in clinical

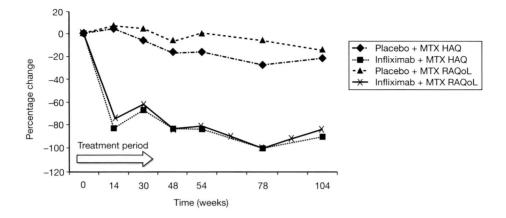

Figure 1.3 Percentage change in the median functional and quality-of-life scores over time in patients with poor-prognosis early RA [5]. HAQ, Health Assessment Questionnaire; MTX, methotrexate; RAQoL, rheumatoid arthritis quality of life. Source: Quinn MA *et al. Very early treatment with infliximab in addition to methotrexate in early, poor-prognosis rheumatoid arthritis reduces magnetic resonance imaging evidence of synovitis and damage, with sustained benefit after infliximab withdrawal: results from a twelve-month randomized, double-blind, placebo-controlled trial. Arthritis Rheum* 2005; 52:27–35.

remission (DAS < 1.6), with similar disease control across all groups. A small number (11%) of patients were able to successfully discontinue all therapies and were in treatment-free remission. In group 4, 51% of subjects were able to successfully discontinue infliximab with a mean infliximab period of 35 months. Overall, less radiographic progression was seen in those treated with infliximab than those in the other groups.

This study shows that good clinical outcomes were obtained in all patients irrespective of the initial treatment group, reinforcing the importance of early intervention and tight control in the treatment of RA. This strategy of frequent evaluation of disease activity and change of therapy to achieve low disease activity resulted in a sustained clinical and functional benefit for up to 4 years [89].

Further analysis from the BeSt trial comparing patients who received initial infliximab treatment (group 4) with patients receiving infliximab at a later stage (groups 1–3) showed that 56% of patients in group 4 were able to successfully stop infliximab compared with only 15% in the other groups at 2 years. This suggests that, by achieving remission within the 'therapeutic window of opportunity', patients may require less treatment later in the disease course [77].

A systematic review examined 23 head-to-head trials and compared the effectiveness and harms of the various disease-modifying agents for RA [90]. Similar clinical efficacy was found among synthetic DMARDs (limited to MTX, leflunomide and SSZ) and among anti-TNF agents (adalimumab, etanercept and infliximab). Monotherapy with anti-TNF agents resulted in better radiographic outcomes than did MTX alone, but no important differences in clinical outcomes (e.g. the ACR20, 50 and 70 response criteria) were found. Clinical response rates and functional outcomes were better with the various combinations of biological agents plus MTX compared with monotherapy with either MTX or biological agents alone. In patients whose monotherapy failed, combination therapy with synthetic DMARDs improved response rates. The comparative evidence, however, was not sufficient to firmly conclude which combination or therapeutic strategy was superior to the others for the early treatment of RA. In the trials that were reviewed, the numbers and types of short-term adverse events were similar for biological and synthetic DMARDs.

Newer biological therapies with different modes of action have been used in established RA. These include rituximab, a B-cell-depleting agent; abatacept, an inhibitor of T-cell co-stimulatory pathways; and tocilizumab, an interleukin 6 receptor antagonist. Clinical studies are ongoing to define their role in early disease.

PREVENTION OF RHEUMATOID ARTHRITIS

The goalpost for 'early' continues to move towards earlier diagnosis and treatment of patients with inflammatory arthritis. In randomized clinical trials, patients with early RA were included if they had a diagnosis of RA for less than 3 years. A survey from Europe and the USA, however, found that the majority of rheumatologists defined early RA as symptom duration less than 3 months [91]. Targeting early arthritis even before diagnosis of RA at the stage of undifferentiated inflammatory arthritis (UIA) is another area of research as a treatment strategy for obtaining better outcomes in RA. There is evidence which suggests treating undifferentiated arthritis (UA) with glucocorticosteroid, MTX or biological agents may delay or prevent development of RA.

An approach for patients who present with very early inflammatory arthritis (less than 12 weeks of symptoms) may be to give a single dose of glucocorticosteroid to provide rapid improvement symptoms and demonstrate the reversibility of disease. Green *et al.* [34] demonstrated the possible reversibility of early arthritis by treatment with glucocorticosteroid injections before diagnosis of RA. Results of an open study of 100 patients with UA suggest that a single dose of intramuscular or intra-articular steroids may induce remission [92].

In the PROMPT (Probable Rheumatoid Arthritis: Methotrexate versus Placebo Treatment) study, the first double-blind, randomized, controlled trial addressing early DMARD therapy in patients with UA before the stage of fulfilling ACR criteria for RA, 110 patients were randomized to treatment with MTX or placebo for 12 months. Outcomes at 30 months showed that MTX may delay the development of RA; this was mainly seen in the subgroup of patients who demonstrated the presence of anti-CCP antibodies [93].

In a recent study, Saleem *et al.* [94] evaluated the ability of TNF antagonist therapy to produce remission and prevent progression to RA in patients with poor prognosis UA. Seventeen patients with UA of less than 12 months' duration having relapsed after a single parenteral glucocorticosteroid injection were recruited into a double-blind, placebo-controlled trial of infliximab or placebo monotherapy administered at weeks 0, 2, 6 and 14. MTX was added at week 14 if no clinical response was achieved. The primary outcome was clinical remission at week 26. At week 14, the infliximab group had greater improvements in CRP and HAQ, but by week 26 there was just a trend favouring infliximab for early morning stiffness, tender joint count, swollen joint count and HAQ; there was no significant difference in DAS28 between the two groups. Furthermore, only three patients were in clinical remission (two infliximab, one placebo). By week 52, 100% (10/10) of patients in the infliximab group and 71% (5/7) of patients in the placebo group had developed RA. In this study, the use of a short course of TNF antagonist therapy in patients with poor-prognosis UA provided modest short-term relief but did not prevent the development of RA [94].

Managing patients in the earliest stages of inflammatory arthritis is an area of ongoing research. Further studies may enable one to assess the factors and therapeutic options that will influence the development and prevention of RA.

CONCLUSION

With effective therapies and advances in treatment strategies, the outcomes of patients with RA continue to improve. Studies have shown that early therapy with disease-modifying agents together with treatment escalation to achieve tight control results in significant clinical and radiographic benefits with a potential for (drug-free) remission or reduced biological or DMARD dependence. In determining optimum treatment strategies, issues such as drug safety and cost-efficacy will need to be taken into consideration. The biological agents, in particular TNF blockers, have been shown to be highly effective in the treatment of early RA but are more expensive than conventional DMARDs. With cost constraints, a pragmatic therapeutic option may be initial DMARD therapy, with steroids as adjunctive therapy, and early intervention with biological agents for those with poor prognostic features or inadequate disease control.

Treating patients with early inflammatory arthritis, or intervention in the preclinical stages for the prevention of RA, remains an area of interest and may be the way of the future.

TREATMENT STRATEGIES: PRACTICAL POINTS

- Early therapy with disease-modifying agents is the cornerstone of treatment for early RA.
- Disease activity should be monitored regularly, escalating treatment to achieve optimal disease control.
- Early use of TNF-blocking agents has been shown to improve clinical and radiographic outcomes in RA and may provide an opportunity for (drug-free) remission. Treatment with these agents should be considered early in the disease course, particularly if patients have an inadequate response to conventional DMARD therapy.

FURTHER RESEARCH

Areas for further research include:

- studies with an appropriate design to determine comparative effectiveness and cost-effectiveness of different therapeutic strategies;
- the effect of the temporary use of intensive treatments, such as biological agents in early arthritis, to assess whether prevention of erosions and cure (in terms of long-term, possibly drug-free, remission) of the disease is possible; and
- therapeutic strategies in early undifferentiated arthritis to prevent RA.

REFERENCES

1. Wolfe F, Mitchell DM, Sibley JT, Fries JF, Bloch DA, Williams CA *et al.* The mortality of rheumatoid arthritis. *Arthritis Rheum* 1994; 37:481–494.
2. Boers M, Verhoeven AC, Markusse HM, van de Laar MA, Westhovens R, van Denderen JC *et al.* Randomised comparison of combined step-down prednisolone, methotrexate and sulphasalazine with sulphasalazine alone in early rheumatoid arthritis. *Lancet* 1997; 350:309–318.
3. Korpela M, Laasonen L, Hannonen P, Kautiainen H, Leirisalo-Repo M, Hakala M *et al.* Retardation of joint damage in patients with early rheumatoid arthritis by initial aggressive treatment with disease-modifying antirheumatic drugs: five-year experience from the FIN-RACo study. *Arthritis Rheum* 2004; 50:2072–2081.
4. Klareskog L, van der Heijde D, de Jager JP, Gough A, Kalden J, Malaise M *et al.* Therapeutic effect of the combination of etanercept and methotrexate compared with each treatment alone in patients with rheumatoid arthritis: double-blind randomised controlled trial. *Lancet* 2004; 363:675–681.
5. Quinn MA, Conaghan PG, O'Connor PJ, Karim Z, Greenstein A, Brown A *et al.* Very early treatment with infliximab in addition to methotrexate in early, poor-prognosis rheumatoid arthritis reduces magnetic resonance imaging evidence of synovitis and damage, with sustained benefit after infliximab withdrawal: results from a twelve-month randomized, double-blind, placebo-controlled trial. *Arthritis Rheum* 2005; 52:27–35.

6. Goekoop-Ruiterman YP, de Vries-Bouwstra JK, Allaart CF, van Zeben D, Kerstens PJ, Hazes JM *et al*. Clinical and radiographic outcomes of four different treatment strategies in patients with early rheumatoid arthritis (the BeSt study): a randomized, controlled trial. *Arthritis Rheum* 2005; 52:3381–3390.

7. Emery P, Salmon M. Early rheumatoid arthritis: time to aim for remission? *Ann Rheum Dis* 1995; 54:944–947.

8. Majithia V, Geraci SA. Rheumatoid arthritis: diagnosis and management. *Am J Med* 2007; 120:936–939.

9. Quinn MA, Cox S. The evidence for early intervention. *Rheum Dis Clin North Am* 2005; 31:575–589.

10. Hannonen P, Mottonen T, Hakola M, Oka M. Sulfasalazine in early rheumatoid arthritis. A 48-week double-blind, prospective, placebo-controlled study. *Arthritis Rheum* 1993; 36:1501–1509.

11. Gough AK, Lilley J, Eyre S, Holder RL, Emery P. Generalised bone loss in patients with early rheumatoid arthritis. *Lancet* 1994; 344:23–27.

12. Deodhar AA, Brabyn J, Jones PW, Davis MJ, Woolf AD. Longitudinal study of hand bone densitometry in rheumatoid arthritis. *Arthritis Rheum* 1995; 38:1204–1210.

13. Devlin J, Lilley J, Gough A, Huissoon A, Holder R, Reece R *et al*. Clinical associations of dual-energy X-ray absorptiometry measurement of hand bone mass in rheumatoid arthritis. *Br J Rheumatol* 1996; 35:1256–1262.

14. Devlin J, Gough A, Huissoon A, Perkins P, Holder R, Reece R *et al*. The acute phase and function in early rheumatoid arthritis. C-reactive protein levels correlate with functional outcome. *J Rheumatol* 1997; 24:9–13.

15. van der Heijde DM, van Leeuwen MA, van Riel PL, van de Putte LB. Radiographic progression on radiographs of hands and feet during the first 3 years of rheumatoid arthritis measured according to Sharp's method (van der Heijde modification). *J Rheumatol* 1995; 22:1792–1796.

16. Nell VP, Machold KP, Eberl G, Stamm TA, Uffmann M, Smolen JS. Benefit of very early referral and very early therapy with disease-modifying anti-rheumatic drugs in patients with early rheumatoid arthritis. *Rheumatology* (Oxford) 2004; 43:906–914.

17. McGonagle D, Conaghan PG, O'Connor P, Gibbon W, Green M, Wakefield R *et al*. The relationship between synovitis and bone changes in early untreated rheumatoid arthritis: a controlled magnetic resonance imaging study. *Arthritis Rheum* 1999; 42:1706–1711.

18. Wakefield RJ, Gibbon WW, Conaghan PG, O'Connor P, McGonagle D, Pease C *et al*. The value of sonography in the detection of bone erosions in patients with rheumatoid arthritis: a comparison with conventional radiography. *Arthritis Rheum* 2000; 43:2762–2770.

19. McQueen FM, Benton N, Crabbe J, Robinson E, Yeoman S, McLean L *et al*. What is the fate of erosions in early rheumatoid arthritis? Tracking individual lesions using X rays and magnetic resonance imaging over the first two years of disease. *Ann Rheum Dis* 2001; 60:859–868.

20. Aho K, Heliovaara M, Maatela J, Tuomi T, Palosuo T. Rheumatoid factors antedating clinical rheumatoid arthritis. *J Rheumatol* 1991; 18:1282–1284.

21. Nielen MM, van Schaardenburg D, Reesink HW, van de Stadt RJ, van der Horst-Bruinsma IE, de Koning MH *et al*. Specific autoantibodies precede the symptoms of rheumatoid arthritis: a study of serial measurements in blood donors. *Arthritis Rheum* 2004; 50:380–386.

22. Rantapaa-Dahlqvist S, de Jong BA, Berglin E, Hallmans G, Wadell G, Stenlund H *et al*. Antibodies against cyclic citrullinated peptide and IgA rheumatoid factor predict the development of rheumatoid arthritis. *Arthritis Rheum* 2003; 48:2741–2749.

23. Nielen MM, van Schaardenburg D, Reesink HW, Twisk JW, van de Stadt RJ, van der Horst-Bruinsma IE *et al*. Increased levels of C-reactive protein in serum from blood donors before the onset of rheumatoid arthritis. *Arthritis Rheum* 2004; 50:2423–2427.

24. Conaghan PG, Ostergaard M, McGonagle D, O'Connor P, Emery P. The validity and predictive value of magnetic resonance imaging erosions in rheumatoid arthritis: comment on the article by Goldbach-Mansky *et al*. *Arthritis Rheum* 2004; 50:1009–1011.

25. Raza K, Falciani F, Curnow SJ, Ross EJ, Lee CY, Akbar AN *et al*. Early rheumatoid arthritis is characterized by a distinct and transient synovial fluid cytokine profile of T cell and stromal cell origin. *Arthritis Res Ther* 2005; 7:R784–795.

26. Singh JA, Pando JA, Tomaszewski J, Schumacher HR. Quantitative analysis of immunohistologic features of very early rheumatoid synovitis in disease modifying antirheumatic drug- and corticosteroid-naive patients. *J Rheumatol* 2004; 31:1281–1285.

27. Cush JJ. Early rheumatoid arthritis – is there a window of opportunity? *J Rheumatol* 2007; 80(Suppl.):1–7.

28. Lard LR, Visser H, Speyer I, vander Horst-Bruinsma IE, Zwinderman AH, Breedveld FC *et al*. Early versus delayed treatment in patients with recent-onset rheumatoid arthritis: comparison of two cohorts who received different treatment strategies. *Am J Med* 2001; 111:446–451.
29. Bukhari MA, Wiles NJ, Lunt M, Harrison BJ, Scott DG, Symmons DP *et al*. Influence of disease-modifying therapy on radiographic outcome in inflammatory polyarthritis at five years: results from a large observational inception study. *Arthritis Rheum* 2003; 48:46–53.
30. van Aken J, Lard LR, le Cessie S, Hazes JM, Breedveld FC, Huizinga TW. Radiological outcome after four years of early versus delayed treatment strategy in patients with recent onset rheumatoid arthritis. *Ann Rheum Dis* 2004; 63:274–279.
31. Mottonen T, Hannonen P, Korpela M, Nissila M, Kautiainen H, Ilonen J *et al*. Delay to institution of therapy and induction of remission using single-drug or combination-disease-modifying antirheumatic drug therapy in early rheumatoid arthritis. *Arthritis Rheum* 2002; 46:894–898.
32. Anderson JJ, Wells G, Verhoeven AC, Felson DT. Factors predicting response to treatment in rheumatoid arthritis: the importance of disease duration. *Arthritis Rheum* 2000; 43:22–29.
33. Finckh A, Choi HK, Wolfe F. Progression of radiographic joint damage in different eras: trends towards milder disease in rheumatoid arthritis are attributable to improved treatment. *Ann Rheum Dis* 2006; 65:1192–1197.
34. Green M, Marzo-Ortega H, McGonagle D, Wakefield R, Proudman S, Conaghan P *et al*. Persistence of mild, early inflammatory arthritis: the importance of disease duration, rheumatoid factor, and the shared epitope. *Arthritis Rheum* 1999; 42:2184–2188.
35. Grigor C, Capell H, Stirling A, McMahon AD, Lock P, Vallance R *et al*. Effect of a treatment strategy of tight control for rheumatoid arthritis (the TICORA study): a single-blind randomised controlled trial. *Lancet* 2004; 364:263–269.
36. Verstappen SM, Jacobs JW, van der Veen MJ, Heurkens AH, Schenk Y, ter Borg EJ *et al*. Intensive treatment with methotrexate in early rheumatoid arthritis: aiming for remission. Computer Assisted Management in Early Rheumatoid Arthritis (CAMERA, an open-label strategy trial). *Ann Rheum Dis* 2007; 66:1443–1449.
37. Fransen J, Moens HB, Speyer I, van Riel PL. Effectiveness of systematic monitoring of rheumatoid arthritis disease activity in daily practice: a multicentre, cluster randomised controlled trial. *Ann Rheum Dis* 2005; 64:1294–1298.
38. Combe B, Landewe R, Lukas C, Bolosiu HD, Breedveld F, Dougados M *et al*. EULAR recommendations for the management of early arthritis: report of a task force of the European Standing Committee for International Clinical Studies Including Therapeutics (ESCISIT). *Ann Rheum Dis* 2007; 66:34–45.
39. van der Heijde DM, van't Hof M, van Riel PL, van de Putte LB. Development of a disease activity score based on judgment in clinical practice by rheumatologists. *J Rheumatol* 1993; 20:579–581.
40. Prevoo ML, van't Hof MA, Kuper HH, van Leeuwen MA, van de Putte LB, van Riel PL. Modified disease activity scores that include twenty-eight joint counts. Development and validation in a prospective longitudinal study of patients with rheumatoid arthritis. *Arthritis Rheum* 1995; 38:44–48.
41. Aletaha D, Smolen J. The Simplified Disease Activity Index (SDAI) and the Clinical Disease Activity Index (CDAI): a review of their usefulness and validity in rheumatoid arthritis. *Clin Exp Rheumatol* 2005; 23(Suppl. 39):S100–108.
42. Felson DT, Anderson JJ, Boers M, Bombardier C, Furst D, Goldsmith C *et al*. American College of Rheumatology. Preliminary definition of improvement in rheumatoid arthritis. *Arthritis Rheum* 1995; 38:727–735.
43. Gotzsche PC, Johansen HK. Short-term low-dose corticosteroids vs placebo and nonsteroidal antiinflammatory drugs in rheumatoid arthritis. *Cochrane Database Syst Rev* 2004(3):CD000189.
44. Hansen TM, Kryger P, Elling H, Haar D, Kreutzfeldt M, Ingeman-Nielsen MW *et al*. Double blind placebo controlled trial of pulse treatment with methylprednisolone combined with disease modifying drugs in rheumatoid arthritis. *BMJ* 1990; 301(6746):268–270.
45. van Gestel AM, Laan RF, Haagsma CJ, van de Putte LB, van Riel PL. Oral steroids as bridge therapy in rheumatoid arthritis patients starting with parenteral gold. A randomized double-blind placebo-controlled trial. *Br J Rheumatol* 1995; 34:347–351.
46. Paulus HE, Di Primeo D, Sanda M, Lynch JM, Schwartz BA, Sharp JT *et al*. Progression of radiographic joint erosion during low dose corticosteroid treatment of rheumatoid arthritis. *J Rheumatol* 2000; 27:1632–1637.

47. Capell HA, Madhok R, Hunter JA, Porter D, Morrison E, Larkin J et al. Lack of radiological and clinical benefit over two years of low dose prednisolone for rheumatoid arthritis: results of a randomised controlled trial. *Ann Rheum Dis* 2004; 63:797–803.

48. Kirwan JR. The effect of glucocorticoids on joint destruction in rheumatoid arthritis. The Arthritis and Rheumatism Council Low-Dose Glucocorticoid Study Group. *New Engl J Med* 1995; 333:142–146.

49. van Everdingen AA, Jacobs JW, Siewertsz Van Reesema DR, Bijlsma JW. Low-dose prednisone therapy for patients with early active rheumatoid arthritis: clinical efficacy, disease-modifying properties, and side effects: a randomized, double-blind, placebo-controlled clinical trial. *Ann Intern Med* 2002; 136:1–12.

50. Rau R, Wassenberg S, Zeidler H. Low dose prednisolone therapy (LDPT) retards radiographically detectable destruction in early rheumatoid arthritis – preliminary results of a multicenter, randomized, parallel, double blind study. *Z Rheumatol* 2000; 59(Suppl 2):II/90–96.

51. Choy EH, Smith CM, Farewell V, Walker D, Hassell A, Chau L et al. Factorial randomised controlled trial of glucocorticoids and combination disease modifying drugs in early rheumatoid arthritis. *Ann Rheum Dis* 2008; 67:656–663.

52. Kirwan JR, Bijlsma JW, Boers M, Shea BJ. Effects of glucocorticoids on radiological progression in rheumatoid arthritis. *Cochrane Database Syst Rev* 2007; 2007(1):CD006356.

53. Durez P, Malghem J, Nzeusseu Toukap A, Depresseux G, Lauwerys BR, Westhovens R et al. Treatment of early rheumatoid arthritis: a randomized magnetic resonance imaging study comparing the effects of methotrexate alone, methotrexate in combination with infliximab, and methotrexate in combination with intravenous pulse methylprednisolone. *Arthritis Rheum* 2007; 56:3919–3927.

54. Hetland ML, Stengaard-Pedersen K, Junker P, Lottenburger T, Hansen I, Andersen LS et al. Aggressive combination therapy with intraarticular glucocorticoid injections and conventional disease modifying anti-rheumatic drugs in early rheumatoid arthritis. Two year clinical and radiographic results from the CIMESTRA study. *Ann Rheum Dis* 2008; 67:815–822.

55. Da Silva JA, Jacobs JW, Kirwan JR, Boers M, Saag KG, Ines LB et al. Safety of low dose glucocorticoid treatment in rheumatoid arthritis: published evidence and prospective trial data. *Ann Rheum Dis* 2006; 65:285–293.

56. Gonzalez-Gay MA. Glucocorticoid-related cardiovascular and cerebrovascular events in rheumatic diseases: myth or reality? *Arthritis Rheum* 2007; 57:191–192.

57. Davis JM, 3rd, Maradit Kremers H, Crowson CS, Nicola PJ, Ballman KV, Therneau TM et al. Glucocorticoids and cardiovascular events in rheumatoid arthritis: a population-based cohort study. *Arthritis Rheum* 2007; 56:820–830.

58. Georgiadis AN, Papavasiliou EC, Lourida ES, Alamanos Y, Kostara C, Tselepis AD et al. Atherogenic lipid profile is a feature characteristic of patients with early rheumatoid arthritis: effect of early treatment – a prospective, controlled study. *Arthritis Res Ther* 2006; 8:R82.

59. Haugeberg G, Strand A, Kvien TK, Kirwan JR. Reduced loss of hand bone density with prednisolone in early rheumatoid arthritis: results from a randomized placebo-controlled trial. *Arch Intern Med* 2005; 165:1293–1297.

60. Kirwan J, Power L. Glucocorticoids: action and new therapeutic insights in rheumatoid arthritis. *Curr Opin Rheumatol* 2007; 19:233–237.

61. Osiri M, Shea B, Robinson V, Suarez-Almazor M, Strand V, Tugwell P et al. Leflunomide for treating rheumatoid arthritis. Cochrane Database Syst Rev 2003(1):CD002047.

62. Maetzel A, Wong A, Strand V, Tugwell P, Wells G, Bombardier C. Meta-analysis of treatment termination rates among rheumatoid arthritis patients receiving disease-modifying anti-rheumatic drugs. *Rheumatology* (Oxford) 2000; 39:975–981.

63. Pincus T, Marcum SB, Callahan LF, Adams RF, Barber J, Barth WF et al. Long-term drug therapy for rheumatoid arthritis in seven rheumatology private practices: I. Nonsteroidal antiinflammatory drugs. *J Rheumatol* 1992; 19:1874–1884.

64. Weinblatt ME, Kaplan H, Germain BF, Block S, Solomon SD, Merriman RC et al. Methotrexate in rheumatoid arthritis. A five-year prospective multicenter study. *Arthritis Rheum* 1994; 37:1492–1498.

65. Breedveld FC, Weisman MH, Kavanaugh AF, Cohen SB, Pavelka K, van Vollenhoven R et al. The PREMIER study: a multicenter, randomized, double-blind clinical trial of combination therapy with adalimumab plus methotrexate versus methotrexate alone or adalimumab alone in patients with early, aggressive rheumatoid arthritis who had not had previous methotrexate treatment. *Arthritis Rheum* 2006; 54:26–37.

66. Machold KP, Stamm TA, Nell VP, Pflugbeil S, Aletaha D, Steiner G et al. Very recent onset rheumatoid arthritis: clinical and serological patient characteristics associated with radiographic progression over the first years of disease. *Rheumatology* (Oxford) 2007; 46:342–349.

67. Machold KP, Nell VP, Stamm TA, Smolen JS. Aspects of early arthritis. Traditional DMARD therapy: is it sufficient? *Arthritis Res Ther* 2006; 8:211.

68. Landewe RB, Boers M, Verhoeven AC, Westhovens R, van de Laar MA, Markusse HM et al. COBRA combination therapy in patients with early rheumatoid arthritis: long-term structural benefits of a brief intervention. *Arthritis Rheum* 2002; 46:347–356.

69. Mottonen T, Hannonen P, Leirisalo-Repo M, Nissila M, Kautiainen H, Korpela M et al. Comparison of combination therapy with single-drug therapy in early rheumatoid arthritis: a randomised trial. FIN-RACo trial group. *Lancet* 1999; 353:1568–1573.

70. Puolakka K, Kautiainen H, Mottonen T, Hannonen P, Korpela M, Julkunen H et al. Impact of initial aggressive drug treatment with a combination of disease-modifying antirheumatic drugs on the development of work disability in early rheumatoid arthritis: a five-year randomized follow-up trial. *Arthritis Rheum* 2004; 50:55–62.

71. Capell HA, Madhok R, Porter DR, Munro RA, McInnes IB, Hunter JA et al. Combination therapy with sulfasalazine and methotrexate is more effective than either drug alone in patients with rheumatoid arthritis with a suboptimal response to sulfasalazine: results from the double-blind placebo-controlled MASCOT study. *Ann Rheum Dis* 2007; 66:235–241.

72. Saunders SA, Capell HA, Stirling A, Vallance R, Kincaid W, McMahon AD et al. Triple therapy in early active rheumatoid arthritis: a randomized, single-blind, controlled trial comparing step-up and parallel treatment strategies. *Arthritis Rheum* 2008; 58:1310–1317.

73. Calguneri M, Pay S, Caliskaner Z, Apras S, Kiraz S, Ertenli I et al. Combination therapy versus mono-therapy for the treatment of patients with rheumatoid arthritis. *Clin Exp Rheumatol* 1999; 17:699–704.

74. Haagsma CJ, van Riel PL, de Jong AJ, van de Putte LB. Combination of sulphasalazine and methotrex-ate versus the single components in early rheumatoid arthritis: a randomized, controlled, double-blind, 52 week clinical trial. *Br J Rheumatol* 1997; 36:1082–1088.

75. Dougados M, Combe B, Cantagrel A, Goupille P, Olive P, Schattenkirchner M et al. Combination therapy in early rheumatoid arthritis: a randomised, controlled, double blind 52 week clinical trial of sulphasalazine and methotrexate compared with the single components. *Ann Rheum Dis* 1999; 58:220–225.

76. van der Kooij SM, de Vries-Bouwstra JK, Goekoop-Ruiterman YP, van Zeben D, Kerstens PJ, Gerards AH et al. Limited efficacy of conventional DMARDs after initial methotrexate failure in patients with recent onset rheumatoid arthritis treated according to the disease activity score. *Ann Rheum Dis* 2007; 66:1356–1362.

77. Castro-Rueda H, Kavanaugh A. Biologic therapy for early rheumatoid arthritis: the latest evidence. *Curr Opin Rheumatol* 2008; 20:314–319.

78. Feldmann M, Maini RN. Lasker Clinical Medical Research Award. TNF defined as a therapeutic target for rheumatoid arthritis and other autoimmune diseases. *Nat Med* 2003; 9:1245–1250.

79. Choo-Kang BS, Hutchison S, Nickdel MB, Bundick RV, Leishman AJ, Brewer JM et al. TNF-blocking therapies: an alternative mode of action? *Trends Immunol* 2005; 26:518–522.

80. Raza K, Buckley CE, Salmon M, Buckley CD. Treating very early rheumatoid arthritis. *Best Pract Res* 2006; 20:849–863.

81. St Clair EW, van der Heijde DM, Smolen JS, Maini RN, Bathon JM, Emery P et al. Combination of infliximab and methotrexate therapy for early rheumatoid arthritis: a randomized, controlled trial. *Arthritis Rheum* 2004; 50:3432–3443.

82. Genovese MC, Bathon JM, Martin RW, Fleischmann RM, Tesser JR, Schiff MH et al. Etanercept versus methotrexate in patients with early rheumatoid arthritis: two-year radiographic and clinical outcomes. *Arthritis Rheum* 2002; 46:1443–1450.

83. Lipsky PE, van der Heijde DM, St Clair EW, Furst DE, Breedveld FC, Kalden JR et al. Infliximab and methotrexate in the treatment of rheumatoid arthritis. Anti-Tumor Necrosis Factor Trial in Rheumatoid Arthritis with Concomitant Therapy Study Group. *New Engl J Med* 2000; 343:1594–1602.

84. Keystone EC, Kavanaugh AF, Sharp JT, Tannenbaum H, Hua Y, Teoh LS et al. Radiographic, clinical, and functional outcomes of treatment with adalimumab (a human anti-tumor necrosis factor monoclo-nal antibody) in patients with active rheumatoid arthritis receiving concomitant methotrexate therapy: a randomized, placebo-controlled, 52-week trial. *Arthritis Rheum* 2004; 50:1400–1411.

85. Smolen JS, Han C, Bala M, Maini RN, Kalden JR, van der Heijde D *et al.* Evidence of radiographic benefit of treatment with infliximab plus methotrexate in rheumatoid arthritis patients who had no clinical improvement: a detailed subanalysis of data from the anti-tumor necrosis factor trial in rheumatoid arthritis with concomitant therapy study. *Arthritis Rheum* 2005; 52:1020–1030.

86. Smolen JS, Van Der Heijde DM, St Clair EW, Emery P, Bathon JM, Keystone E *et al.* Predictors of joint damage in patients with early rheumatoid arthritis treated with high-dose methotrexate with or without concomitant infliximab: results from the ASPIRE trial. *Arthritis Rheum* 2006; 54:702–710.

87. Emery P, Breedeveld F, Hall S *et al.* Remission rate in subjects with active early rheumatoid arthritis –1 year results of the COMET trial: combination of methotrexate and etanercept in active early rheumatoid arthritis. ACR. Boston 2007.

88. Ikeda K, Cox S, Emery P. Aspects of early arthritis. Biological therapy in early arthritis – overtreatment or the way to go? *Arthritis Res Ther* 2007; 9:211.

89. Van Der Kooij S, Goekoop-Ruiterman YPM, de Vries-Bouwstra JK *et al.* Clinical and radiological efficacy of four different strategies in patients with recent onset rheumatoid arthritis: 4-year follow-up of the BeSt study. *Arthritis Rheum* 2007; 56(Suppl. 9):S299.

90. Donahue KE, Gartlehner G, Jonas DE, Lux LJ, Thieda P, Jonas BL *et al.* Systematic review: comparative effectiveness and harms of disease-modifying medications for rheumatoid arthritis. *Ann Intern Med* 2008; 148:124–134.

91. Aletaha D, Eberl G, Nell VP, Machold KP, Smolen JS. Practical progress in realisation of early diagnosis and treatment of patients with suspected rheumatoid arthritis: results from two matched questionnaires within three years. *Ann Rheum Dis* 2002; 61:630–634.

92. Quinn MA, Green MJ, Marzo-Ortega H, Proudman S, Karim Z, Wakefield RJ *et al.* Prognostic factors in a large cohort of patients with early undifferentiated inflammatory arthritis after application of a structured management protocol. *Arthritis Rheum* 2003; 48:3039–3045.

93. van Dongen H, van Aken J, Lard LR, Visser K, Ronday HK, Hulsmans HM *et al.* Efficacy of methotrexate treatment in patients with probable rheumatoid arthritis: a double-blind, randomized, placebo-controlled trial. *Arthritis Rheum* 2007; 56:1424–1432.

94. Saleem B, Mackie S, Quinn M, Nizam S, Hensor E, Jarrett S *et al.* Does the use of tumour necrosis factor antagonist therapy in poor prognosis, undifferentiated arthritis prevent progression to rheumatoid arthritis? *Ann Rheum Dis* 2008; 67:1178–1180.

95. Bathon JM, Martin RW, Fleischmann RM, Tesser JR, Schiff MH, Keystone EC *et al.* A comparison of etanercept and methotrexate in patients with early rheumatoid arthritis. *N Engl J Med* 2000; 343:1586–1593.

2

Established rheumatoid arthritis

Pieternella J. Barendregt, J. Mieke W. Hazes

INTRODUCTION AND DEFINITION OF ESTABLISHED RHEUMATOID ARTHRITIS

Chronic joint inflammation in rheumatoid arthritis (RA) often leads to destruction of bone and cartilage, joint dysfunction and disability. The ultimate goals in managing RA are to optimally control disease activity, prevent or control joint damage, and prevent loss of function. Treatment of RA has changed considerably in the past decades. New insights in the pathogenesis have led to new therapeutic strategies, such as powerful therapy with combinations of disease-modifying antirheumatic drugs (DMARDs) and the use of biologicals. Furthermore, early recognition and early treatment of RA has become more and more important, as has adequate treatment during all stages of the disease, constantly aiming at remission. These strategies are proven to be effective in preventing joint damage and lead to a better prognosis of the disease.

In recent years, research in RA has focused on early recognition and treatment. Nevertheless, treatment of long-standing, established RA must not be forgotten. This chapter will discuss the treatment of established RA, i.e. RA fulfilling the criteria of the American College of Rheumatology (ACR) [1] with a disease duration of more than 2 years.

NEW INSIGHTS IN THE TREATMENT OF RHEUMATOID ARTHRITIS: TIGHT CONTROL OF DISEASE ACTIVITY AND AIMING AT REMISSION

Rheumatoid arthritis is an aggressive disease that causes erosive joint damage even in its first 2 years [2, 3]. Therefore, it is important to start powerful treatment as soon as the diagnosis of RA is made. Several studies demonstrated the beneficial effect of starting early versus delayed treatment [4–6] on radiological progression. Approaches to early RA treatment vary from step-up treatment (in which, when the first DMARD shows an inadequate response, a second DMARD is added after 3 months) to aggressive treatment with a combination of DMARDs directly in the beginning of the disease (with subsequent discontinuation of individual agents when low disease activity is achieved). Studies on early combination therapy, such as the COBRA, FIN-RACo and BeSt studies, prove a better radiographic outcome from combination therapy, as compared with monotherapy [4, 7, 8].

Radiographic damage has been very well correlated with cumulative disease activity over the years [9, 10]. Also, there is a strong correlation between response to DMARDs and radiographic progression [11]. Furthermore, earlier data on disease activity and functional capacity in RA have taught us that even after 12 years of disease duration, disease activity is still a strong contributor to impaired function [12].

Considering the above, there is strong evidence for optimal treatment during all stages of the disease and for aiming at low disease activity/remission in all stages of RA. This is supported by the results of the TICORA study [13]. In this study, patients with RA were randomly allocated to either intensive management (frequent disease activity score [DAS] measurement and change in therapy if DAS score is > 2.4) or routine care. The strategy of intensive management of RA showed substantial improvement in disease activity, less radiographic disease progression and better physical function and quality of life.

DISEASE-MODIFYING ANTIRHEUMATIC DRUGS

Disease-modifying antirheumatic drugs are the mainstay of drug therapy in RA. Although chemically heterogeneous, the various DMARDs share several characteristics. They uniformly have a slow onset of action compared with non-steroidal anti-inflammatory drugs (NSAIDs) and glucocorticoids. Although their exact mechanism of action is not known, there is substantial *in vitro* evidence suggesting that these agents modulate distinct facets of immune and inflammatory responses. An overview of the various DMARDs and their mechanism of action is given in Table 2.1.

With respect to efficacy, traditional DMARDs are known to have several benefits. They improve the clinical signs and symptoms of RA by reducing inflammation. Also, they improve functional status in comparison with NSAIDs, and slow down radiographic progression. Most DMARDs have well-known toxicity and drug interaction profiles. However, they also have several important limitations. In addition to the delayed onset of action, some have less proven effectiveness on radiographic disease progression and health-related quality of life, and they seldom yield treatment-free remissions. They also require close monitoring because of multiple toxicities and sometimes difficult and complex dosing regimens are necessary [14].

The DMARDs commonly used in RA include methotrexate (MTX), hydroxychloroquine (HCQ), sulfasalazine (SSZ), leflunomide and gold salts.

METHOTREXATE

Initially developed as a chemotherapeutic agent, MTX is the most commonly used DMARD and has been the gold standard for the treatment of RA since the 1990s. MTX has also been used as the 'anchor' agent for regimens of combination therapy. MTX acts as a dihydrofolate reductase inhibitor which induces adenosine release, leading to anti-inflammatory effects. Subsequent placebo-controlled trials confirmed the efficacy of MTX in the treatment of RA, especially in doses routinely used nowadays (15–25 mg/week).

Methotrexate is usually given orally once weekly (if necessary divided over several doses on one day [15]), which has proved to be efficient and well tolerated in doses up to 30 mg/week. Parenteral administration may sometimes be desirable because it results in higher serum levels compared with oral regimes [16, 17]. In clinical practice, folic acid is generally used to minimize the occurrence of some adverse events, such as stomatitis, nausea, bone marrow suppression, liver function abnormalities and diarrhoea [18, 19].

As the most frequent adverse reaction to MTX is elevation of liver enzyme levels and leucopenia, liver function and blood cell counts must be monitored. MTX is teratogenic, thus appropriate contraceptive measures during MTX treatment are essential.

HYDROXYCHLOROQUINE

Hydroxychloroquine (HCQ), an antimalarial drug, is not as effective as other DMARDs in improving clinical measures such as disease activity. Furthermore, HCQ has not been shown to alter radiographic progression significantly [20]. Nevertheless, HCQ is still used, particularly in cases of mild or very early RA. Early treatment with HCQ has a significant

Table 2.1 Overview of the disease-modifying antirheumatic drugs used in rheumatoid arthritis

Therapeutic agent	Mechanism of action	Contraindications	Side-effects	Dosage
Disease-modifying antirheumatic drugs				
Sulfasalazine	Modulates B-cell responses and angiogenesis	Allergy to sulphate, severe renal failure, liver insufficiency	GI intolerance, hepatotoxicity, rash, headache, BM suppression	1000–1500 mg twice daily
Methotrexate	Inhibits dihydrofolate reductase; induces adenosine release → anti-inflammatory effects	Severe renal failure, bone marrow suppression, liver insufficiency	GI intolerance, alopecia, oral ulcers, liver function abnormality, BM suppression, pulmonary fibrosis	15–30 mg once weekly, p.o., s.c. or i.m. Add folic acid 5–10 mg once weekly or 1 mg daily (not on MTX day)
Leflunomide	Inhibits pyrimidine synthesis; inhibits DNA synthesis and cellular proliferation	Severe renal failure, liver insufficiency, bone marrow suppression	Hypertension, liver function abnormality, diarrhoea/nausea, alopecia, rash, BM suppression	20 mg once daily p.o.
Hydroxychloroquine	Modulates cytokine secretion and macrophage function	Retinopathy	Retinopathy, rash, hyperpigmentation, GI intolerance	200–400 mg once daily p.o.
Gold	Not clear	Severe renal failure, liver insufficiency, bone marrow suppression	Dermatitis, BM suppression, proteinuria	Test dose of 10 mg i.m., followed by weekly injections of 50 mg. After +/– 20 weeks: 50 mg i.m. monthly
Immunosuppressive drugs				
Glucocorticosteroids	Suppresses leucocyte cell migration and phagocytosis, less production of antibodies in high dose, suppresses granulation tissue and inflammation	Active infections	Skin atrophy, hyperglycaemia, weight gain/moonface, osteoporosis, hypertension, increased risk of infection	Depends on indication
Azathioprine	Inhibits purine metabolism; inhibits DNA synthesis and cellular proliferation	Severe renal failure, liver insufficiency, bone marrow suppression	Liver function abnormalities, BM suppression, GI intolerance	1.5–2.5 mg/kg/day
Ciclosporin	Inhibits IL-2 and other cytokine production	Renal failure, hypertension	Hypertension, nephropathy, GI intolerance, hirsutism	2.5 mg/kg/day

BM, bone marrow; GI, gastrointestinal; IL, interleukin; i.m., intramuscular.

impact on long-term outcome. Also, HCQ is known to be effective in combination with MTX and SSZ [21, 22]. Because of the generally favourable safety profile, HCQ treatment can be considered in patients with co-morbidity. No routine laboratory monitoring is required. Rash, diarrhoea and abdominal cramps are infrequent adverse effects. Before starting HCQ, a baseline ophthalmological examination is recommended for patients over the age of 40 or patients with previous eye disease [23]. Annual ophthalmological examination is recommended in high-risk patients, defined as patients over 60 years of age having more than 5 years' HCQ use in doses greater than 6.5 mg/kg/day [23, 24].

SULFASALAZINE

Sulfasalazine, a combination of sulphapyridine and 5-salicylic acid, alters folate metabolism, suppresses various leucocyte functions and lymphocyte subtypes and, like methotrexate, leads to extracellular adenosine release. SSZ is effective for the treatment of mild to moderate RA. Multiple open-label and placebo-controlled studies have validated its efficacy [25, 26]. Also, SSZ has been shown to reduce radiographic progression compared with placebo or antimalarials [26, 27]. In a meta-analysis, SSZ was similar to gold and a modest dose of MTX [28].

Sulfasalazine has been a frequent compound in combination therapies, although the benefit of some combinations is controversial. SSZ is usually well tolerated, with most side-effects, which include nausea and abdominal discomfort, occurring in the first few months of therapy. Leucopenia and liver function abnormalities are occasional, more serious, side-effects that may occur at any time, and periodic laboratory monitoring is therefore necessary.

LEFLUNOMIDE

Leflunomide, developed in the early 1980s, is the latest addition to the current list of DMARDs. It modulates the immune response through inhibiting cell activation by altering the enzymes important for the activation of T cells (pyrimidine synthesis inhibitor). In multicentre, head-to-head comparative studies comparing leflunomide with SSZ and a modest-dosage MTX, leflunomide proved to be equally efficacious. These trials have established leflunomide as an alternative to MTX monotherapy, especially for patients who cannot tolerate MTX or have an inadequate response. Also, leflunomide has been shown to improve functional status and delay the progression of joint damage, although to a lesser extent than MTX [29–31]. Common side-effects of leflunomide include diarrhoea, abdominal pain, elevation of liver transaminases, hypertension, rash, alopecia and headaches. Haematological reactions have also been observed [29, 30].

It is recommended that liver enzyme levels and blood counts are monitored every 2 weeks for the first 6 months of treatment and every 8 weeks thereafter. Leflunomide has a very long half-life; elimination of the drug would take as long as 2 years. Also, leflunomide is a potent teratogen. In cases of side-effects or a wish to conceive, wash-out procedures with cholestyramine or activated charcoal are necessary.

GOLD THERAPY

Parenteral organic gold compounds have been used since the 1920s for the treatment of RA. The clinical efficacy of gold therapy has been shown in several older double-blind studies [32, 33]. Furthermore, these studies showed radiographic efficacy, as measured by the total Sharp score [33, 34].

After a test dose of 10 mg intramuscular (i.m.), followed by 25 mg i.m. after 1 week, weekly injections of 50 mg gold are required until a response is achieved, approximately after 20 weeks. At that point, injections of 50 mg are given monthly. Injections have to be stopped earlier if toxicity develops. Adverse effects include mucocutaneous reactions, proteinuria and (serious) cytopenias. In patients treated with gold, careful monitoring of renal function (including urine tests) is necessary, and blood counts need to be measured at monthly intervals for the duration of the therapy.

In the past few years, use of i.m. gold in the treatment of RA has become less important, mostly due to the availibility of several new drugs such as the biologicals, but also because of the high incidence of side-effects and toxicity of gold. Nevertheless, if treatment with i.m. gold is tolerated, it can be very effective and sustained remission for long periods is described in some patients (J.M.W. Hazes, personal communication).

Oral gold compounds were developed in order to prevent the serious adverse events, but have been shown to be not very efficacious and are virtually unused now [28].

COMBINATION THERAPY

Conventional treatment with monotherapy DMARDs often fails to control the disease activity adequately. Therefore, in practice, an increasing number of rheumatologists are prescribing a combination of DMARDs [35]. The goal of combination therapy is to control inflammation as completely and quickly as possible before permanent joint damage occurs. Theoretically, by combining agents with complementary mechanisms of action, greater efficacy might be achieved. Combination therapy can be used in different ways: first, one can choose a continuous approach, with two or more DMARDs, with the intention of continuing them all; second, a step-up approach can be chosen, in which the rheumatologist begins with conventional monotherapy and adds subsequent DMARDs if adequate efficacy is not achieved; and third, the most aggressive of the three, the so-called step-down approach, in which the rheumatologist starts a combination of DMARDs at the beginning of the disease, with the intention of stopping the most toxic or the most expensive DMARD once disease activity is low. Research results are controversial. However, many of the data suggest that combination therapy is more efficacious than monotherapy, and not necessarily more toxic [4, 8, 21, 36].

Although results suggest benefits of combination therapy among patients with established RA, they have not been as substantial as those in early RA, as most combination studies were performed in early RA.

Ciclosporin and methotrexate
Ciclosporin added to MTX was proven to be more effective than MTX alone in the treatment of RA, resulting in a greater ACR20 response. However, long-term follow-up data showed development of hypertension and elevated creatinine levels in the combination group, similar to those observed in prior studies with ciclosporin alone [37, 38].

Methotrexate, sulfasalazine and hydroxychloroquine
In a randomized controlled clinical trial in patients with RA, the combination of MTX, HCQ and SSZ demonstrated a substantially increased efficacy compared with MTX alone or the combination of HCQ and SSZ. Furthermore, in this study no evidence was found for increased toxicity in the combination group [21].

The increased efficacy without additional toxicity of this three-DMARD combination was confirmed in another randomized trial in patients with early RA (FIN-RACo trial), but in this study the treatment regimen included low-dose prednisolone in a subset of patients [22].

More recent studies confirmed the superiority of the combination of MTX, SSZ and HCQ as compared with MTX and SSZ or MTX and HCQ, in early as well as in more advanced RA [39, 40].

Methotrexate and leflunomide
Several studies showed an increased efficacy on disease activity when adding leflunomide to MTX in the treatment of RA.

First, in two open-label studies leflunomide was administered to patients with active RA who had been receiving long-term MTX therapy. No significant pharmacokinetic interactions between leflunomide and MTX were noted. This combination therapy was generally well tolerated clinically, with the exception of elevations of liver enzyme levels. Both studies suggested improved clinical response with combination therapy [41, 42].

In a 24-week multicentre randomized double-blind placebo-controlled trial, leflunomide or placebo was added in patients with persistent RA despite receiving MTX for at least 6 months. In this study, the combination therapy of leflunomide and MTX provided statistically significant clinical benefits for the ACR20 response and Health Assessment Questionnaire (HAQ). Leflunomide plus MTX was generally well tolerated. Results of these studies suggest that the combination of MTX and leflunomide can be used relatively safely with appropriate liver enzyme and haematological monitoring [43]. However, in daily practice, one has to be careful when prescribing the combination MTX and leflunomide because of several post-marketing reports about serious elevation of liver enzymes when these agents are combined.

Methotrexate, sulfasalazine and prednisolone (COBRA study)
In a double-blind randomized, step-down design trial the combination of SSZ (2000 mg/day), MTX 7.5 mg/week and high-dose prednisolone (tapering dosage) was compared with SSZ alone in 155 patients with early RA. Prednisolone was stopped after 28 weeks and MTX after 40 weeks. In this study, the combination group reached the ACR response quicker than the SSZ group and, more importantly, the combination group demonstrated a greater and sustained radiographic protection [7, 36].

Biologicals and methotrexate
Combinations with the current tumour necrosis factor (TNF)-α inhibitors (infliximab, etanercept and adalimimab) with MTX will be discussed elsewhere in this chapter. In all studies in patients with partial response to MTX monotherapy, combinations with TNF-α inhibitors were found to be beneficial [44, 45].

IMMUNOSUPPRESSIVE DRUGS AND GLUCOCORTICOIDS

GLUCOCORTICOIDS

Glucocorticoids are important, but also controversial, in the treatment of RA [46]. They have very good short-term anti-inflammatory properties, but at high doses or during long-term treatment they may cause serious side-effects, such as osteoporosis, hypertension, weight gain, hyperglycaemia, fluid retention, skin fragility and increased risk of infection.

Low-dose oral glucocorticoids ($\leq$ 10 mg of prednisolone daily) are highly effective in slowing disease activity and reducing pain and functional disability, especially in the very early stage of the disease when other DMARDs have not yet reached their effect on disease activity [47].

Also, recent evidence suggests that low-dose glucocorticoids slow the rate of joint damage [47–49]. Most studies show that glucocorticoids are inadequate as sole treatment for RA, but, on the other hand, many patients with RA are functionally dependent on glucocorticoids and continue them for a long time [46]. For long-term disease control, it is important to keep the glucocorticoid dose as low as possible to prevent adverse events. Moreover, patients with chronic steroid use should receive 1500 mg of calcium per day (including dietary intake) and

400–800 IU of vitamin D per day to prevent osteoporosis. Antiresorptive agents, especially bisphosphonates, prevent bone loss and should also be considered at the time glucocorticoid therapy is started. Glucocorticoid injections of joints and peri-articular structures are very effective, especially when a patient has a disease flare in only one or a few joints. The need for repeated or multiple injections indicates the need to reassess the current DMARD regime.

Finally, use of high-dose glucocorticoids is indicated in cases of life-threatening organ involvement in RA. This subject will be discussed elsewhere in this chapter.

AZATHIOPRINE

Azathioprine (AZA), a purine analogue myelosuppressive drug, has been extensively used in the treatment of systemic lupus erythematosus. AZA has demonstrated moderate benefits in controlling RA, but a number of patients cannot tolerate AZA therapy due to toxicity (bone marrow suppression). Because of its modest clinical effect, its toxicity and the availability of new biological agents and other therapeutic options, AZA is typically reserved for patients with refractory RA who have failed other agents and for severe extra-articular disease in combination with steroids [50]. Therefore, AZA is rarely used nowadays for the treatment of uncomplicated RA.

CICLOSPORIN A

Ciclosporin A (CSA), an immunosuppressive drug used for prevention of rejection after organ transplantation, was initially assessed for the treatment of RA because of its effect on T-cell function. Several studies demonstrated dose-dependent clinical superiority of CSA over placebo, but also many types of dose-dependent toxicity. Studies on radiographic outcome during CSA therapy show conflicting results. Adverse events such as hypertension and nephrotoxicity make long-term use of CSA in the treatment of RA difficult [51–53]. Currently, CSA is mainly reserved for refractory cases of RA (in combination with MTX) and for treatment of RA with refractory leucopenia.

CYCLOPHOSPHAMIDE

Cyclophosphamide, an alkylating agent, is of limited benefit for the treatment of RA synovitis and has high toxicity, including bone marrow toxicity, infertility, bladder toxicity and oncogenicity. Its use in RA is restricted to treatment of glucocorticoid-refractory systemic vasculitis or other life-threatening organ involvement.

TUMOUR NECROSIS FACTOR ALPHA INHIBITORS

The treatment of RA has changed dramatically over the past decade with the introduction of biological agents that selectively block cytokines. The most clinically effective anticytokine agents are antagonists to TNF-α, an essential mediator of the cytokine inflammatory cascade in RA (see also Table 2.2). Three anti-TNF-α agents are available for the treatment of RA: infliximab (a chimeric mouse–human anti-TNF monoclonal antibody), etanercept (a recombinant soluble TNF-Fc fusion protein) and adalimumab (a fully human monoclonal antibody to TNF-α).

Many randomized, double-blind, placebo-controlled trials have demonstrated the efficacy of etanercept, adalimumab and infliximab in early as well as in patients with established RA in whom previous DMARD therapy had failed. Those studies were performed with or without MTX as concomitant therapy. All TNF blockers show good clinical improvement, in both monotherapy and in combination therapy studies. However, clinical responses, according to the ACR improvement criteria, were found to be higher when a TNF blocker was given in combination with MTX. Also, all three TNF blockers showed significant decrease in radiographic progression and increase in physical function, especially in combination with MTX [44, 45, 54–63].

Despite some differences in their structure, all TNF inhibitors have a relatively quick onset of action, with most patients experiencing significant improvement within a few weeks. However, although there is a good effect of TNF blockers on disease activity, drug-free remission is rarely achieved and most patients experience increased disease activity after discontinuation of therapy. Data from the STURE registry in Sweden about the continuation of TNF-α blockers showed that after 5 years 74.8% of patients were still on treatment. These data are better than the overall survival of treatment with one specific TNF blocker (after 5 years, 43.9%) [64]. If treatment with any of the TNF blockers fails, there is no evidence for increasing the dose above the recommended dosage [65], but switching to another TNF blocker after primary or secondary failure has shown to be useful [66–68].

Nowadays, TNF blockers have a prominent place in the treatment of RA. However, rheumatologists have to be aware of some practical problems when prescribing these agents. First, due to the immunosuppressive effects of TNF inhibitors, one should be aware of higher rates of infections. The increased risk of (opportunistic) infections, in particular granulomatous infections such as tuberculosis, has been confirmed in most of the recent cohort studies and is now generally accepted [69–72].

The risk of serious infections during TNF-α blocker treatment observed in daily practice was much higher than in phase III trials evaluating TNF-α blockers [73]. Some cohort studies show conflicting results about infections (no increased risk for pneumonia, only increased risk for skin and soft-tissue infections) during TNF-α blockers [72, 74].

However, in a recent meta-analysis in which nine anti-TNF trials were included, a pooled odds ratio of 2.0 (95% confidence interval [CI] 1.3–3.1) for serious infections was found [75]. Therefore, routine screening (and treatment) for tuberculosis before starting anti-TNF therapy is necessary, and is included in the treatment guidelines, as is close monitoring for (opportunistic) infections during treatment [69, 73]. The notion of the possible increased risk of malignancy with anti-TNF therapy is much less appreciated, mainly because of the relative rare occurrence of malignancies.

Earlier publications did show a potentially increased risk of lymphoma with anti-TNF treatment [76], although other studies did not confirm these results [77, 78]. This finding could have been explained by the possibility of confounding by indication, in that patients with the most severe and active disease are more likely to receive anti-TNF therapy [79] and severe, active disease is associated with a substantially increased risk of lymphoma [80].

In a recent meta-analysis of nine anti-TNF trials, a threefold increased risk (pooled odds ratio 3.3, 95% CI 1.2–9.1) for malignancies was found; confounding by indication was ruled out as all patients in the studies included in this meta-analysis started with the same indication for treatment. Also, the authors found a dose-dependent relationship between antibodies to TNF and the risk of malignancy [75]. On the other hand, rather reassuring results were seen in large cohort studies which did not show an increased incidence of malignancies in patients with RA treated with anti-TNF [76, 81]. In practice, clinicians have to balance the risks of anti-TNF therapy against the risk of lymphoma in active RA.

In both clinical trials and clinical practice, cases of severe demyelinating disease have been reported in patients on TNF inhibitors. Development of autoimmune diseases, such as systemic lupus erythematosus (SLE)-like disease, are also described during anti-TNF therapy. Autoantibodies, especially antinuclear antibodies (ANAs) and antibodies against dsDNA, are described in up to 60% and 15% of treated patients (especially during infliximab therapy). TNF inhibitors should be avoided in patients with congestive heart failure, as studies showed worsening of heart failure during anti-TNF treatment [82].

INTERLEUKIN-I RECEPTOR ANTAGONIST (IL-I RA)

ANAKINRA

Anakinra is a recombinant human interleukin 1 (IL-1) receptor antagonist which prevents the binding of IL-1 to its receptor, thereby preventing target cell signalling (see also Table 2.2). The efficacy of anakinra has been studied as monotherapy as well as in combination with other drugs. It was shown that anakinra monotherapy gives a clinically significant improvement in ACR response and in patient function, and also slows the rate of radiographic progression [83, 84]. The combination of anakinra with MTX has been demonstrated to be superior to MTX alone for ACR responses and patient function. Also, the rate of radiographic progression was lower in the combination group [85]. However, compared with the results seen with TNF inhibitors, responses were more modest with anakinra.

ANTI-B-LYMPHOCYTE THERAPY

RITUXIMAB (ANTI-CD20 ANTIBODY)

Until recently, most treatments for RA were targeted at T cells. Since data suggest that B-cell depletion in RA can cause sustained improvement of disease activity [86], there has been renewed interest in the role of B cells in RA. B cells not only produce the potentially pathological rheumatoid factor and other autoantibodies, but also present antigens and provide co-stimulatory signals to T cells. B-cell depletion can be achieved using rituximab, a genetically engineered chimeric anti-CD20 monoclonal antibody.

CD20, a B-cell surface antigen, is expressed on pre-B and mature B cells. Rituximab, first designed for lymphoma treatment, causes a selective transient depletion of the CD20-positive B-cell population (see also Table 2.2). Several controlled studies demonstrate rituximab to be efficacious in refractory RA [87–89].

In 2006 the results of two important studies were published. First, in the DANCER study, the efficacy and safety of different rituximab doses were studied in patients with active RA resistant to DMARDs including biological agents. A total of 465 patients were randomized in nine treatment groups to either placebo or rituximab (500 mg or 1000 mg on days 1 and 15), each also taking either placebo, glucocorticosteroids, intravenous (i.v.) methylprednisolone premedication or i.v. methylprednisolone premedication plus oral prednisolone for 2 weeks. All patients received concomitant MTX 10–25 mg weekly.

Significantly more patients who received either 500 mg or 1000 mg of rituximab met the ACR20 criteria at week 24 (55% and 54%, respectively) compared with placebo (28%). ACR50 response was achieved by 33%, 34% and 13% respectively, and ACR70 response was achieved by 13%, 20% and 5% of the patients. Glucocorticoids did not contribute significantly to the primary efficacy end-point, but i.v. glucocorticoid premedication reduced the frequency and intensity of infusion-associated events. In this study rituximab was well tolerated with both the type and the severity of infections being similar to those for placebo [90].

In the REFLEX study, the efficacy and safety of treatment with rituximab plus MTX was studied in patients with active RA who had an inadequate response to anti-TNFα. In this 2-year, multicentre, randomized, double-blind, placebo-controlled phase III study, 520 patients were randomized to receive one course of i.v. rituximab (i.e. two infusions of 1000 mg each) or placebo, both with background MTX. At week 24, significantly more rituximab-treated patients than placebo-treated patients demonstrated ACR20 (51 vs. 18%), ACR50 (27 vs. 5%) and ACR70 (12% vs. 1%) responses. Also, the rituximab-treated patients had clinically meaningful improvements in fatigue, disability and health-related quality of life and showed a trend towards less radiographic progression. In this study, the rate of serious infections was a little higher in the rituximab group (5.2 vs. 3 per 100 patient-years) compared with placebo and the infusion reactions were mild to moderate [91].

Table 2.2 Overview of the biological agents used in rheumatoid arthritis

Biological agent	Mechanism of action	Contraindications	Side-effects	Dosage
TNF-alpha blockers				
Infliximab	Chimeric monoclonal antibody, binds soluble TNF-a. Inhibits the binding of TNF-a to TNF receptors	Active infection, untreated TB, multiple sclerosis, congestive heart failure, malignancies	Risk of TB reactivation, increased infection risk, drug-induced SLE, autoantibody formation, infusion reactions, serum sickness-like reactions	3–10 mg/kg i.v. every 8 weeks
Etanercept	Recombinant TNF-Fc fusein protein. Competitive inhibitor of TNF receptor	Similar to infliximab	Risk of TB reactivation, increased infection risk, injection site reactions	50 mg s.c. once a week or 25 mg s.c. twice a week
Adalimumab	Human monoclonal antibody, binds soluble TNF-α. Inhibits the binding of TNF-α to TNF receptors	Similar to infliximab	Risk of TB reactivation, increased infection risk, injection site reactions	40 mg s.c. once every 2 weeks
IL-1 blockers				
Anakinra	Recombinant IL-1 receptor antagonist. Prevents binding of IL-1 to its receptor	Serious infections, impaired renal function	Risk of infection, injection site reactions, headache, neutropenia	100 mg s.c. daily
Anti-B-lymphocyte				
Rituximab	Anti-CD20 monoclonal antibody. Depletion of CD20-positive B-lymphocytes	Serious infections	Increased risk of infection, infusion reactions	Two infusions of 1000 mg i.v. on day 1 and day 15. Premedication of 100 mg methylprednisolone i.v. is recommended
T-cell co-stimulation blocker				
Abatacept	CTLA-4-Ig, a selective co-stimulation modulator. Inhibits T-cell activation	Serious infections	Increased risk of infections, headache	Once-monthly 500, 750 or 1000 mg i.v. (depending on body weight)
IL-6 blockers				
Tocilizumab	Humanized monoclonal antibody against IL-6	Serious infections	Increased risk of infection, infusion reactions, neutropenia, headache	8 mg/kg i.v. every 4 weeks

IL, interleukin; i.v., intravenous; s.c., subcutaneous; SLE, systemic lupus erythematosus; TB, tuberculosis; TNF, tumour necrosis factor.

Results of these two studies suggest that a single course of rituximab with concomitant MTX therapy provides meaningful improvements in patients with active, longstanding RA who have an inadequate response to anti-TNF therapy.

T-CELL CO-STIMULATION BLOCKERS

Abatacept, also known as CTLA-4-Ig, is the first selective co-stimulation modulator inhibiting T-cell activation that is approved for the management of RA. Abatacept is a fusion protein developed to modulate the T-cell co-stimulatory signal that is mediated through the CD28–CD80/86 pathway (see also Table 2.2).

Early clinical studies demonstrated efficacy in the treatment of RA [92]. More recently, in 2006, the results were published of a study in which patients with active RA (despite MTX treatment) were treated with abatacept. In this 1-year, multicentre, randomized, double-blind, placebo-controlled trial, 652 patients with active RA, despite MTX treatment, received a once-monthly infusion of a fixed dose of abatacept (approximately 10 mg/kg of body weight) or placebo.

After 1 year, ACR responses were 73.1% for abatacept versus 39.7% for placebo (ACR20), 48.3% versus 18.2% (ACR50) and 28.8% versus 6.1% (ACR70). Also, physical function significantly improved in 63.7% versus 39.3% of patients ($P < 0.001$). After 1 year, abatacept statistically significantly slowed the progression of structural joint damage compared with placebo. Abatacept-treated patients had a similar incidence of adverse events [93].

Another randomized, placebo-controlled study in 2006 demonstrated safety data for abatacept. In this study, patients were randomized 2:1 to receive abatacept at a fixed dose approximating 10 mg/kg, or placebo. The abatacept and placebo groups exhibited similar frequencies of adverse events and serious adverse events. Serious infections were more frequent in the abatacept group than in the placebo group (2.9% vs. 1.9%). The incidence of neoplasms was 3.5% in both groups. When evaluated according to background therapy, serious adverse events occurred more frequently in the subgroup receiving abatacept plus a biological agent (22.3%) than in the other subgroups. Therefore, abatacept is not recommended for use in combination with other biological therapy. Also, this study showed that abatacept in combination with DMARDs improved physical function and physician- and patient-reported disease outcomes [94].

Finally, in clinical studies abatacept was demonstrated to improve physical health in patients with RA who have inadequate response on MTX [95] and to improve health-related quality of life in patients with an inadequate response on anti-TNF therapy [96].

ANTIBODIES AGAINST INTERLEUKIN 6

TOCILIZUMAB

One of the newest IL blockers is tocilizumab, a humanized monoclonal antibody against the interleukin 6 receptor. Several studies have shown beneficial results of this agent in patients with active RA. One of the earliest studies, the CHARISMA (Chugai Humanized Anti-human Recombinant Interleukin-Six Monoclonal Antibody) study (in patients with active RA despite MTX use), showed statistically higher ACR20, ACR50 and ACR70 responses in the tocilizumab group, compared with the placebo group. In this study, tocilizumab was mostly well tolerated, with a safety profile similar to that of other biologic therapies [97]. These results were confirmed in the AMBITION study [98], in which the efficacy and safety of tocilizumab monotherapy in patients with active RA (who had not previously failed methotrexate and/or biologics treatment) was evaluated. This 24-week, double-blind study, randomized 673 patients with RA to either tocilizumab 8 mg/kg every 4 weeks, methotrexate (start 7.5 mg/week, increasing dosage to 20 mg/week), or placebo for 8 weeks followed by tocilizumab 8 mg/kg. The results of this study showed that tocilizumab was superior to methotrexate treatment, with a higher ACR20 response (69.9% vs. 52.5%; $P<0.0001$) and DAS28 <2.6 rate (33.6% vs. 12.1%) at week 24.

The incidence of serious adverse events (AEs) with tocilizumab was 3.8% and 2.8% with methotrexate ($P=0.50$). Serious infections were reported in 1.4% and 0.7%, respectively, of the patients. In another double-blind, randomized, placebo-controlled, study (OPTION study), 623 patients with moderate to severe active RA were randomly assigned to receive tocilizumab 8 mg/kg, tocilizumab 4 mg/kg, or placebo intravenously every 4 weeks, with methotrexate at stable pre-study doses (10–25 mg/week). At 24 weeks, ACR20 responses were seen in more patients receiving tocilizumab than in those receiving placebo; however, more people receiving tocilizumab had at least one adverse event. The most common serious adverse events were infections, reported by six patients in the 8 mg/kg group, three in the 4 mg/kg group and two in the placebo group [99].

Tocilizumab combined with conventional DMARDs was studied in 1220 patients with active RA in the TOWARD study [100]. Patients remained on stable doses of DMARDs and received tocilizumab 8 mg/kg or placebo every 4 weeks for 24 weeks. At week 24, the proportion of patients achieving an ACR20 improvement was significantly greater in the tocilizumab plus DMARD group than in the control group (61% vs. 25%; $P<0.0001$). Secondary end-points including ACR50/70 improvement, DAS28 score, DAS28 remission responses (DAS28<2.6), EULAR (European League Against Rheumatism) responses and systemic markers, such as the C-reactive protein and haemoglobin levels, also demonstrated superiority of tocilizumab plus DMARDs over DMARDs alone.

Finally, the RADIATE study [101], examined the efficacy and safety of tocilizumab, in 499 patients with rheumatoid arthritis (RA) refractory to tumour necrosis factor (TNF) antagonist therapy. The patients were randomly assigned to receive 8 mg/kg or 4 mg/kg tocilizumab or placebo intravenously every 4 weeks with stable methotrexate dosage for 24 weeks. At 24 weeks, ACR20 was achieved by 50.0%, 30.4% and 10.1% of patients in the 8 mg/kg, 4 mg/kg and control groups, respectively ($P<0.001$ for both tocilizumab groups vs. control).

Furthermore, patients responded regardless of most recently failed anti-TNF or the number of failed treatments. DAS28 remission (DAS28 <2.6) rates at week 24 were clearly dose related, being achieved by 30.1%, 7.6% and 1.6% of in the 8 mg/kg, 4 mg/kg and control groups, respectively. Most adverse events were mild or moderate, the most common adverse events with higher incidence in tocilizumab groups were infections, gastrointestinal symptoms, rash and headache. The incidence of serious adverse events was higher in controls (11.3%) than in the 8 mg/kg (6.3%) and 4 mg/kg (7.4%) groups.

The studies mentioned above, indicate that tocilizumab plus methotrexate is an effective treatment for patients with RA, even after an inadequate response to TNF antagonists, and also that tocilizumab has a manageable safety profile.

TREATMENT OF EXTRA-ARTICULAR DISEASE MANIFESTATIONS

Being a systemic disease, RA not only affects the joints and tendons, but may also cause a variety of extra-articular disease manifestations, such as vasculitis, Felty's syndrome, pulmonary disease, secondary Sjogren's syndrome and other eye problems. The advances in treating RA, particularly the use of MTX and powerful biological agents, have led to less extra-articular disease. However, because of the life-threatening properties of some extra-articular complications, one has to be aware of these possible complications and the necessary treatment.

Most non-life-threatening complications of RA, such as skin vasculitis, can be treated with adequate DMARD therapy including MTX or AZA and low-dose prednisolone [50]. In cases of severe organ involvement, such as systemic vasculitis or interstitial lung disease, prompt treatment with a combination of high-dose glucocorticoids (1 mg/kg) and cyclophosphamide pulse i.v. or oral daily is necessary [102, 103].

A short review of extra-articular complications and treatment is presented in Table 2.3.

CONCLUSION

In the last decade, the outcome of patients with early and established RA has dramatically improved. Early recognition and early (intensive) treatment of the disease, as well as tight disease control, has led to less cumulative disease activity and eventually to less radiographic damage.

Moreover, new insights in therapeutic strategies, such as higher dosages and combination of DMARDs, are very helpful in reaching the ultimate treatment goal of disease remission.

Table 2.3 Extra-articular complications of RA and treatment

Extra-articular complication	Pharmacological management
Vasculitis	
Severe vasculitis with organ involvement	High-dose glucocorticosteroids and cyclophosphamide (i.v. pulse) [102, 103]
Only skin involvement	Adequate DMARD therapy (MTX or azathioprine); if necessary, low-dose prednisolone [50]
Leucopenia	
Felty's syndrome/LGL syndrome	Methotrexate, cyclosporin A. If necessary, high-dose steroids or rG-CSF [104–106]
Pulmonary disease	
Interstitial lung disease	High-dose glucocorticosteroids combined with azathioprine (if not effective, cyclophosphamide) [107]
Pleural effusions	Adequate antirheumatic treatment, including DMARDs
Cardiac complications	
Acute rheumatic pericarditis (with congestive heart failure)	Diuretics, high-dose steroids with or without cyclophosphamide
Eye complications	
Secondary Sjogren's syndrome/sicca syndrome	Artificial tears, eye salves, tear conservation suffices
Episcleritis (simple or nodular)	Oral NSAIDs, ice compresses
Anterior scleritis (diffuse or nodular)	Oral NSAIDs
Scleritis and diffuse stromal keratitis	Local steroids or short course of systemic steroids
Necrotizing scleritis	High-dose steroids with adequate antirheumatic treatment. If granulomatizing scleritis, high-dose glucocorticosteroids i.v. and cyclophosphamide [108, 109]
Osteoporosis	Avoid steroids. If doses higher than 7.5 mg daily are necessary, add bisphosphonates. Advise sufficient daily intake of calcium and vitamin D, and if necessary prescribe calcium/vitamin D. In selected cases consider hormone replacement therapy to prevent postmenopausal loss of bone
Amyloidosis	Adequate disease control. Renal amyloidosis: consider cyclophosphamide [110]

DMARD, disease-modifying antirheumatic drug; LGL, large granular lymphocyte; MTX, methotrexate; NSAID, non-steroidal anti-inflammatory drug; RA, rheumatoid arthritis; rG-CSF, recombinant granulocyte colony-stimulating factor.

A great advance in the treatment of RA is the introduction of biological agents that selectively block cytokines. The three TNF-α blockers – infliximab, etanercept and adalimumab – have proven to be effective and relatively safe. New agents for the treatment of RA, such as rituximab, abatacept and tocilizumab, also show promising results on disease activity and radiographic progression.

REFERENCES

1. Arnett FC, Edworthy SM, Bloch DA et al. The American Rheumatism Association 1987 revised criteria for the classification of rheumatoid arthritis. *Arthritis Rheum* 1988; 31:315–324.
2. Fuchs HA, Kaye JJ, Callahan LF et al. Evidence of significant radiographic damage in rheumatoid arthritis within the first two years. *J Rheumatol* 1989; 16:585–591.
3. Van der Heijde DM, van Leeuwen MA, van Riel PL et al. Radiographic progression on radiographs of hands and feet during the first 3 years of rheumatoid arthritis measured according to Sharp's method (van de Heijde modification). *J Rheumatol* 1995; 22:1792–1796.
4. Makinen H, Kautiainen H, Hannonen P et al. Sustained remission and reduced radiographic progression with combination disease modifying antirheumatic drugs in early rheumatoid arthritis. *J Rheumatol* 2007; 34:316–321.
5. Van Aken J, Lard LR, le Cessie S et al. Radiological outcome after four years of early versus delayed treatment strategy in patients with recent onset rheumatoid arthritis. *Ann Rheum Dis* 2004; 63:274–279.
6. Lard LR, Visser H, Speyer I et al. Early versus delayed treatment in patients with recent-onset rheumatoid arthritis: comparison of two cohorts who received different treatment strategies. *Am J Med* 2001; 111:446–451.
7. Landewe RB, Boers M, Verhoeven AC et al. COBRA combination therapy in patients with early rheumatoid arthritis: long-term structural benefits of a brief intervention. *Arthritis Rheum* 2002; 46:347–356.
8. Goekoop-Ruiterman YP, de Vries-Bouwstra JK, Allaart CF et al. Clinical and radiographic outcomes of four different treatment strategies in patients with early rheumatoid arthritis (the BeSt study): a randomized, controlled trial. *Arthritis Rheum* 2005; 52:3381–3390.
9. Van Leeuwen MA, van der Heijde DM, Van Rijswijk MH et al. Interrelationship of outcome measures and process variables in early rheumatoid arthritis. A comparison of radiologic damage, physical disability, joint counts, and acute phase reactants. *J Rheumatol* 1994; 21:425–429.
10. Boers M, Kostense PJ, Verhoeven AC et al. Inflammation and damage in an individual joint predict further damage in that joint in patients with early rheumatoid arthritis. *Arthritis Rheum* 2001; 44:2242–2246.
11. Van der Heijde D. Radiographic progression in rheumatoid arthritis: does it reflect outcome? Does it reflect treatment? *Ann Rheum Dis* 2001; 60(Suppl. 3):iii47–50.
12. Drossaers- Bakker KW, de Buck M, van Zeben D et al. Long-term course and outcome of functional capacity in rheumatoid arthritis: the effect of disease activity and radiologic damage over time. *Arthritis Rheum* 1999; 42:1854–1860.
13. Grigor C, Capell H, Stirling A et al. Effect of a treatment strategy of tight control for rheumatoid arthritis (the TICORA study): a single-blind randomised controlled trial. *Lancet* 2004; 364:263–269.
14. Breedveld FC, Kalden JR. Appropriate and effective management of rheumatoid arthritis. *Ann Rheum Dis* 2004; 63:627–633.
15. Hoekstra M, Haagsma C, Neef C et al. Splitting high-dose oral methotrexate improves bioavailibility: a pharmacokinetic study in patients with rheumatoid arthritis. *J Rheumatol* 2006; 33:481–485.
16. Wegrzyn J, Adeleine P, Miossec P. Better efficacy of methotrexate given by intramuscular injection than orally in patients with rheumatoid arthritis. *Ann Rheum Dis* 2004; 63:1232–1234.
17. Freeman-Narrod M, Gerstley BJ, Engstrom PF. Comaprison of serum concentrations of MTX after various routes of administration. *Cancer* 1975; 36:1619–1624.
18. Van Ede AE, Laan RF, Rood MJ et al. Effect of folic or folinic acid supplementation on the toxicity and efficacy of methotrexate in rheumatoid arthritis: a forty-eight week, multicenter, randomized, double-blind, placebo-controlled study. *Arthritis Rheum* 2001; 44:1515–1524.
19. Morgan SL, Bagott JE, Vaughn WH et al. The effect of folic acid supplementation on the toxicity of low-dose methotrexate in patients with rheumatoid arthritis. *Arthritis Rheum* 1990; 33:9–18.
20. Van der Heijde DM, van Riel PL, Nuver-Zwart IH et al. Effects of hydroxychloroquine and sulfasalazine on progression of joint damage in rheumatoid arthritis. *Lancet* 1989; 1:1036–1038.

21. O'Dell JR, Haire CE, Erikson N. Treatment of rheumatoid arthritis with methotrexate alone, sulfasalazine and hydroxychloroquine, or a combination of all three medications. *N Engl J Med* 1996; 334:1287–1291.
22. Mottonen T, Hannonen P, Leirisalo-Lepo M *et al.* Comparison of combination therapy with single drug therapy in early rheumatoid arthritis: a randomised trial. *Lancet* 1999; 353:1568–1573.
23. American College of Rheumatology Subcommittee on Rheumatoid Arthritis Guidelines. Guidelines for the management of rheumatoid arthritis. 2002 update. *Arthritis Rheum* 2002; 46:328–346.
24. Marmor MF, Carr RE, Easterbrook M *et al.* Recommendations on screening for chloroquine and hydroxychloroquine retinopathy. *Ophthalmology* 2002; 109:1377–1382.
25. Pinals RS, Kaplan SB, Lawson JG *et al.* Sulfasalazine in rheumatoid arthritis. *Arthritis Rheum* 1986; 29:1427–1434.
26. Box SA, Pullar T. Sulfasalazine in the treatment of rheumatoid arthritis. *Br J Rheumatol* 1997; 36:382–386.
27. Mottonen T, Hannonen P, Hakola M *et al.* Sulfasalazine in early RA. *Arthritis Rheum* 1993; 36:1501–1509.
28. Felson DT, Andersson JJ, Meenan RF. The comparative efficacy and toxicity of second-line drugs in rheumatoid arthritis: results of two meta-analyses. *Arthritis Rheum* 1990; 33:1449–1461.
29. Strand V, Cohen S, Schiff M *et al.* Treatment of active rheumatoid arthritis with leflunomide compared with placebo and methotrexate. *Arch Int Med* 1999; 159:2542–2550.
30. Emery P, Breedveld FC, Lemmel EM *et al.* A comparison of the efficacy and safety of leflunomide and methotrexate for the treatment of rheumatoid arthritis. *Rheumatology* 2000; 39:655–665.
31. European Leflunomide Study Group. Smolen JS, Kalden JR, Scott DL *et al.* Efficacy and safety of leflunomide compared with placebo and sulphasalazine in active rheumatoid arthritis: a double-blind randomized multicenter trial. *Lancet* 1999; 353:259–266.
32. Sigler JW, Bluhm GB, Duncan H. Gold salts in the treatment of rheumatoid arthritis. A double blind study. *Ann Int Med* 1974; 80:21–26.
33. Luukkainen R. Chrysotherapy in rheumatoid arthritis with particular amphasis on radiographic changes and on the optimal time of initiation of therapy. *Scand J Rheum* 1980; 34(Suppl.):1–56.
34. Gordan DA, Klinkhoff AV. Gold and penicillamine. In: Ruddy S, ed. *Kelley's Textbook of Rheumatology*, 6th edn. St Louis, MO: WB Saunders Company, 2001.
35. Pincus T, O'Dell JR, Kremer JM. Combination therapy with multiple disease-modifying antirheumatic drugs in rheumatoid arthritis: a preventive strategy. *Ann Int Med* 1999; 131:768–774.
36. Boers M, Verhoeven AC, Markusse HM *et al.* Randomised comparison of combined step-down prednisolone, methotrexate and sulphasalazine with sulphasalazine alone in early rheumatoid arthritis. *Lancet* 1997; 350:309–318.
37. Salaffi F, Carotti M, Cervini C. Combination therapy of cyclosporine A with methotrexate or hydroxychloroquine in refractory rheumatoid arthritis. *Scand J Rheumatol* 1996; 25:16–23.
38. Tugwell P, Pincus T, Yocum D *et al.* Combination therapy with cyclosporine and methotrexate in severe rheumatoid arthritis. *N Engl J Med* 1996; 333:137–141.
39. Calguneri M, Pay S, Caliskaner Z *et al.* Combination therapy versus monotherapy for the treatment of patients with rheumatoid arthritis. *Clin Exp Rheumatol* 1999; 17:699–704.
40. O'Dell J, Leff R, Paulsen G *et al.* Treatment of rheumatoid arthritis with methotrexate and hydroxychloroquine, methotrexate and sulfasalazine, or a combination of the three medications: results of a two-year, randomized, double-blind placebo-controlled trial. *Arthritis Rheum* 2002; 46:1164–1170.
41. Weinblatt ME, Kremer JM, Coblyn JS *et al.* Pharmacokinetics, safety, and efficacy of combination treatment with leflunomide and methotrexate in patients with active rheumatoid arthritis. *Arthritis Rheum* 1999; 42:1322–1328.
42. Mroczkowski PJ, Weinblatt ME. Methotrexate and leflunomide combination therapy for patients with active rheumatoid arthritis. *Clin Exp Rheumatol* 1999; 17(Suppl. 18):S66–68.
43. Kremer JM, Genovese MC, Cannon GW *et al.* Concomitant leflunomide therapy in patients with active rheumatoid arthritis despite stable doses of methotrexate. A randomized, double-blind, placebo-controlled trial. *Ann Intern Med* 2002; 137:726–733.
44. Lipsky PE, van de Heijde DM, St. Clair EW *et al.* Infliximab and methotrexate in the treatment of rheumatoid arthritis. Anti-Tumor Necrosis Factor Trial in Rheumatoid Arthritis with Concomitant Therapy Study Group. *N Engl J Med* 2000; 343:1594–1602.
45. Weinblatt ME, Kremer JM, Bankhurst AD *et al.* A trial of etanercept, a recombinant tumor necrosis factor receptor:Fc fusion protein, in patients with rheumatoid arthritis receiving methotrexate. *N Engl J Med* 1999; 340:253–259.
46. Wilder RL. Corticosteroids. In: Klippel JH, Crofford LJ, Stone JH, Weyand CM, eds. *Primer on the Rheumatic Diseases*, 12th edn. Atlanta, GA: The Arthritis Foundation, 2001, pp. 593–598.

47. Van Everdingen AA, Jacobs JW, Siewertsz Van Reesema DR *et al.* Low-dose prednisone therapy for patients with early active rheumatoid arthritis: clinical efficacy, disease-modifying properties, and side-effects: a randomized, double-blind, placebo-controlled clinical trial. *Ann Intern Med* 2002; 136:1–12.

48. Kirwan JR. The effect of glucocorticoids on joint destruction in rheumatoid arthritis. The Arthritis and Rheumatism Council Low-Dose Glucocorticoid Study Group. *N Engl J Med* 1995; 333:142–146.

49. Jacobs JW, van Everdingen AA, Verstappen SM *et al.* Followup radiographic data on patients with rheumatoid arthritis who participated in a two-year trial of prednisone therapy or placebo. *Arthritis Rheum* 2006; 54:1422–1428.

50. Heurkens AHM, Westedt ML, Breedveld FC. Prednisone plus azathioprine treatment in patients with rheumatoid arthritis complicated by vasculitis. *Arch Int Med* 1991; 51:224–254.

51. Dougados M, Awada H, Amor B. Cyclosporin in rheumatoid arthritis: a double blind, placebo controlled study in 52 patients. *Ann Rheum Dis* 1988; 47:127–133.

52. Tugwell P, Bombardier C, Gent M *et al.* Low-dose cyclosporin versus placebo in patients with rheumatoid arthritis. *Lancet* 1990; 335:1051–1055.

53. Drosos AA, Voulgari PV, Papadopoulos IA *et al.* Cyclosporine A in the treatment of early rheumatoid arthritis. A prospective, randomized 24-month study. *Clin Exp Rheumatol* 1998; 16:695–701.

54. Moreland LW, Schiff MH, Baumgartner SW *et al.* Etanercept therapy in rheumatoid arthritis: a randomized controlled trial. *Ann Int Med* 1999; 130:478–486.

55. Maini RN, Breedveld FC, Kalden JR *et al.* Therapeutic efficacy of multiple intravenous infusions of anti-tumor necrosis factor alpha monoclonal antibody combined with low-dose weekly methotrexate in rheumatoid arthritis. *Arthritis Rheum* 1998; 41:1552–1563.

56. Maini R, St. Clair EW, Breedveld F *et al.* Infliximab (chimeric anti-tumour necrosis factor alpha monoclonal antibody) versus placebo in rheumatoid arthritis patients receiving concomitant methotrexate: a randomised phase III trial. ATTRACT Study Group. *Lancet* 1999; 354:1932–1939.

57. Kavanaugh A, St. Clair EW, McCune WJ *et al.* Chimeric anti-tumor necrosis factor-alpha monoclonal antibody treatment of patients with rheumatoid arthritis receiving methotrexate therapy. *J Rheumatol* 2000; 27:841–850.

58. Bathon JM, Martin RW, Fleishmann RM *et al.* A comparison of etanercept and methotrexate in patients with early rheumatoid arthritis. *N Engl J Med* 2000; 343:1586–1593.

59. Weinblatt ME, Keystone EC, Furst DE. Adalimumab, a fully human anti-tumor necrosis factor α monoclonal antibody for the treatment of rheumatoid arthritis patients taking concomitant methotrexate. *Arthritis Rheum* 2003; 48:35–45.

60. Burmeister GR, van der Putte LB, Rau *et al.* Long-term efficacy and safety of adalimumab monotherapy in patients with DMARD refractory rheumatoid arthritis – results from a 2-year study (Abstract). *Arthritis Rheum* 2002; 46:1436.

61. Keystone EC, Kavanaugh AF, Sharp JT *et al.* Radiographic, clinical, and functional outcomes of treatment with adalimumab (a human anti-tumor necrosis factor monoclonal antibody) in patients with active rheumatoid arthritis receiving concomitant methotrexate therapy: a randomized, placebo-controlled, 52-week trial. *Arthritis Rheum* 2004; 50:1400–1411.

62. Van der Heijde D, Klareskog L, Rodriguez-Valverde V *et al.* Comparison of etanercept and methotrexate, alone and combined, in the treatment of rheumatoid arthritis: two-year clinical and radiographic results from the TEMPO study, a double-blind, randomized trial. *Arthritis Rheum* 2006; 54:1063–1074.

63. Weinblatt M, Keystone E, Furst D *et al.* Adalimumab, a fully human anti-tumor necrosis factor alpha monoclonal antibody, for the treatment of rheumatoid arthritis in patients taking concomitant methotrexate: the ARMADA trial. *Arthritis Rheum* 2003; 48:35–45.

64. Van Vollenhoven RF. Six-year report of the STURE Registry for Biologicals in Rheumatology: satisfactory overall results, but plenty of room for improvement. *Arthritis Rheum* 2005; 52(Suppl.): Abstract 273.

65. Van Vollenhoven RF, Breedveld FC, Kavanauagh AF *et al.* The clinical and radiographic efficacy of every-other-week vs. weekly dosing frequency of adalimumab in the treatment of early rheumatoid arthritis (RA). *Arthritis Rheum* 2005; 52(Suppl.):Abstract 271.

66. Wick MC, Ernestam S, Lindblad S *et al.* Adalimumab (Humira) restores clinical response in patients with secondary loss of efficacy from infliximab (Remicade) or etanercept (Enbrel): results from the STURE registry at Karolinska University Hospital. *Scand J Rheumatol* 2005; 34:353–358.

67. Bombardieri S, Ruiz AA, Fardelione P *et al.* Effectiveness of adalimumab for rheumatoid arthritis in patients with a history of TNF-antagonist therapy in clinical practice. *Rheumatology* 2007; 46:1191–1199.

68. Van Vollenhoven R, Harju A, Brannemark S *et al.* Treatment with infliximab (Remicade) when etanercept (Enbrel) has failed or vice versa: data from the STURE registry showing that switching tumour necrosis factor alpha blockers can make sense. *Ann Rheum Dis* 2003; 62:1195–1198.
69. Keane J, Gershon S, Wise RP *et al.* Tuberculosis associated with infliximab, a tumor necrosis factor alpha-neutralizing agent. *N Engl J Med* 2001; 345:1098–1104.
70. Askling J, Fored CM, Brandt L *et al.* Risk and case characteristics of tuberculosis in rheumatoid arthritis associated with tumor necrosis factor antagonists in Sweden. *Arthritis Rheum* 2005; 52:1986–1992.
71. Askling J, Fored CM, Brandt L *et al.* Time-dependent increase in risk of hospitalisation with infection among swedish ra-patients treated with TNF- antagonists. *Ann Rheum Dis* 2007; Jan 29 [Epub ahead of print].
72. Dixon WG, Watson K, Lunt M *et al.* Rates of serious infection, including site-specific and bacterial intracellular infection, in rheumatoid arthritis patients receiving anti-tumor necrosis factor therapy: results from the British Society for Rheumatology Biologics Register. *Arthritis Rheum* 2006; 54:2368–2376.
73. Salliot C, Gossec L, Ruyssen-Witrand A *et al.* Infections during tumour necrosis factor-alpha blocker therapy for rheumatic diseases in daily practice: a systematic retrospective study of 709 patients. *Rheumatology* 2007; 46:327–334.
74. Wolfe F, Caplan L, Michaud K. Treatment for rheumatoid arthritis and the risk of hospitalization for pneumonia: associations with prednisone, disease-modifying antirheumatic drugs, and anti-tumor necrosis factor therapy. *Arthritis Rheum* 2006; 54:628–634.
75. Bongartz T, Sutton AJ, Sweeting MJ *et al.* Anti-TNF antibody therapy in rheumatoid arthritis and the risk of serious infections and malignancies: systematic review and meta-analysis of rare harmful effects in randomized controlled trials. *JAMA* 2006; 295:2275–2285.
76. Geborek P, Bladstrom A, Turesson C *et al.* Tumour necrosis factor blockers do not increase overall tumour risk in patients with rheumatoid arthritis, but may be associated with an increased risk of lymphomas. *Ann Rheum Dis* 2005; 64:699–703.
77. Wolfe F, Michaud K. The effect of methotrexate and anti-tumor necrosis factor therapy on the risk of lymphoma in rheumatoid arthritis in 19,562 patients during 89,710 person-years of observation. *Arthritis Rheum* 2007; 56:1433–1439.
78. Askling J, Fored CM, Baecklund E *et al.* Haematopoietic malignancies in rheumatoid arthritis: lymphoma risk and characteristics after exposure to tumour necrosis factor antagonists. *Ann Rheum Dis* 2005; 64:1414–1420.
79. Franklin JP, Symmons DP, Silman AJ. Risk of lymphoma in patients with RA treated with anti-TNFalpha agents. *Ann Rheum Dis* 2005; 64:657–658.
80. Baecklund E, Iliadou A, Askling J *et al.* Association of chronic inflammation, not its treatment, with increased lymphoma risk in rheumatoid arthritis. *Arthritis Rheum* 2006; 54:692–701.
81. Askling J, Fored CM, Brandt L *et al.* Risks of solid cancers in patients with rheumatoid arthritis and after treatment with tumour necrosis factor antagonists. *Ann Rheum Dis* 2005; 64:1421–1426.
82. Sarzi- Puttini P, Atzeni F, Shoenfeld Y *et al.* TNF-alpha, rheumatoid arthritis, and heart failure: a rheumatological dilemma. *Autoimmun Rev* 2005; 4:153–161.
83. Bresnihan B, Alvaro-Garcia JM, Cobby M *et al.* Treatment of rheumatoid arthritis with recombinant human interleukine-1 receptor antagonist. *Arthritis Rheum* 1998; 41:2196–2204.
84. Jiang Y, Genant HK, Watt I *et al.* A multicenter, double-blind, dose-ranging, randomized, and placebo-controlled study of recombinant human interleukin-1 receptor antagonist in patients with rheumatoid arthritis: radiological progression and correlation of Genant and Larsen scores. *Arthritis Rheum* 2000; 43:1001–1009.
85. Cohen SB, Hurd E, Cush JJ *et al.* Treatment of rheumatoid arthritis with anakinra, a recombinant human interleukin-1 receptor antagonist, in combination with methotrexate. *Arthritis Rheum* 2002; 46:614–624.
86. Edwards JC, Cambridge G. Sustained improvement in RA following a protocol designed to deplete B lymphocytes. *Rheumatology* 2001; 40:205–211.
87. Edwards JC, Szczepanski L, Szechinsky J *et al.* Efficacy of B-cell-targeted therapy with rituximab in patients with rheumatoid arthritis. *N Engl J Med* 2004; 350:2572–2581.
88. De Vita S, Zaja F, Sacco S *et al.* Efficacy of selective B cell blockade in the treatment of rheumatoid arthritis. *Arthritis Rheum* 2002; 46:2029–2933.
89. Leandro MJ, Edwards JC, Cambridge G. Clinical outcome in 22 patients with rheumatoid arthritis treated with B-lymphocyte depletion. *Ann Rheum Dis* 2002; 61:883–888.

90. Emery P, Fleischmann R, Filipowicz-Sosnowska A *et al.* The efficacy and safety of rituximab in patients with active rheumatoid arthritis despite methotrexate treatment: results of a phase IIB randomized, double-blind, placebo-controlled, dose-ranging trial. *Arthritis Rheum* 2006; 54:1390–1400.

91. Cohen SB, Emery P, Greenwald MW *et al.* Rituximab for rheumatoid arthritis refractory to anti-tumor necrosis factor therapy: results of a multicenter, randomized, double-blind, placebo-controlled, phase III trial evaluating primary efficacy and safety at twenty-four weeks. *Arthritis Rheum* 2006; 54:2793–2806.

92. Kremer JM, Dougados M, Emery P *et al.* Treatment of rheumatoid arthritis with the selective costimulation modulator abatacept: twelve-month results of a phase IIb, double-blind, randomized, placebo-controlled trial. *Arthritis Rheum* 2005; 52:2263–2271.

93. Kremer JM, Genant HK, Moreland LW *et al.* Effects of abatacept in patients with methotrexate-resistant active rheumatoid arthritis: a randomized trial. *Ann Int Med* 2006; 144:865–876.

94. Weinblatt M, Combe B, Covucci A *et al.* Safety of the selective costimulation modulator abatacept in rheumatoid arthritis patients receiving backgroud biologic and non-biologic disease-modifying anti-rheumatic drugs: a one-year randomized, placebo-controlled study. *Arthritis Rheum* 2006; 54:2807–2816.

95. Russell AS, Wallenstein GV, Li T *et al.* Abatacept improves both the physical and mental health of patients with rheumatoid arthritis who have inadequate response to methotrexate treatment. *Ann Rheum Dis* 2007; 66:189–194.

96. Westhovens R, Cole JC, Li T *et al.* Improved health-related quality of life for rheumatoid arthritis patients treated with abatacept who have inadequate response to anti-TNF therapy in a double-blind, placebo-controlled, multicentre randomized clinical trial. *Rheumatology* 2006; 45:1238–1246.

97. Maini RN, Taylor PC, Szechinsky J *et al.* Double-blind randomized controlled trail of the interleukin-6 receptor antagonist, tocilizumab, in European patients with rheumatoid arthritis who had an incomplete response to methotrexate. *Arthritis Rheum* 2006; 54:2817–2829.

98. Jones G, Sebba A, Gu J *et al.* Comparison of tocilizumab monotherapy versus methotrexate monotherapy in patients with moderate to severe rheumatoid arthritis: the AMBITION study. *Ann Rheum Dis* 2010; 69:88–96.

99 Smolen JS, Beaulieu A, Rubbert-Roth A *et al.* Effect of interleukin-6 receptor inhibition with tocilizumab in patients with rheumatoid arthritis (OPTION study): a double-blind, placebo-controlled, randomised trial. *Lancet* 2008; 371:987–997.

100. Genovese MC, McKay JD, Nasonov EL *et al.* Interleukin-6 receptor inhibition with tocilizumab reduces disease activity in rheumatoid arthritis with inadequate response to disease-modifying antirheumatic drugs: the tocilizumab in combination with traditional disease-modifying antirheumatic drug therapy study. *Arthritis Rheum* 2008; 58:2968–2980.

101. Emery P, Keystone E, Tony HP *et al.* IL-6 receptor inhibition with tocilizumab improves treatment outcomes in patients with rheumatoid arthritis refractory to anti-tumour necrosis factor biologicals: results from a 24-week multicentre randomised placebo-controlled trial. *Ann Rheum Dis* 2008; 67:1516–1523.

102. Turesson C, Matteson EL. Management of extra-articular disease manifestations in rheumatoid arthritis. *Curr Opin Rheumatol* 2004; 16:206–211.

103. Guillivin L, Cohen P, Howie AJ *et al.* Treatment of polyarteritis nodosa and microscopic polyangiitis with poor prognosis factors: a prospective trial comparing glucocorticoids and six or twelve cyclophosphamide pulses in sixty five patients. *Arthritis Rheum* 2003; 49:93–100.

104. Burks EJ, Loughran TP Jr. Pathogenesis of neutropenia in large granular lymphocyte leukemia and Felty's syndrome. *Blood Rev* 2006; 20:245–266.

105. Rosenstein ED, Kramer N. Felty's and pseudo-Felty's syndromes. *Semin Arthritis Rheum* 1991; 21:129–142.

106. Hellmich B, Scnabel A, Gross WL. Treatment of severe neutropenia due to Felty's syndrome or systemic lupus erythematosus with granulocyte colony-stimulating factor. *Semin Arthritis Rheum* 1999; 29:82–89.

107. Jindal SK, Agarwal R. Autoimmunity and interstitial lungdisease. *Curr Opin Pulm Med* 2005; 11:438–446.

108. Watson PG, Hazleman BL, Pavesio CE *et al.* *The Sclera and Systemic Disorders*, 2nd edn. Oxford: Butterworth-Heinemann, 2004.

109. Jabs DA, Rosenbaum JT, Foster CS *et al.* Guidelines for the use of immunosuppressive drugs in patients with ocular inflammatory disorders: recommendations of an expert panel. *Am J Ophthal* 2000; 130:492–513.

110. Chevrel G, Jenvrin C, McGregor B, Miossec P. Renal type AA amyloidosis associated with rheumatoid arthritis: a cohort study showing improved survival on treatment with pulse cyclophosphamide. *Rheumatology* 2001; 40:821–825.

3

Beyond anti-TNF: other biological drugs in inflammatory arthritis

Peter C. Taylor

INTRODUCTION

The armamentarium of potential therapeutics for rheumatoid arthritis (RA) has grown with the identification of relevant disease molecules. Of these, biological therapeutics targeting tumour necrosis factor (TNF)-α, particularly when used in combination with oral methotrexate (MTX), have enjoyed notable success in suppressing inflammation and markedly inhibiting the progression of structural damage previously thought to be an unavoidable characteristic of RA [1, 2]. However, despite the unprecedented clinical and commercial successes of TNF inhibitors, their availability is restricted by high costs, and a substantial proportion of patients with RA fail to demonstrate significant clinical responses. The apparent failure of some patients to achieve clinically meaningful responses to TNF blockade may imply that other cytokines drive a syndrome with the same phenotypic manifestations. Various proinflammatory cytokines other than TNF-α have also been targeted in RA. These include interleukin 1 (IL-1), IL-6 and IL-15. Of these, the only one to reach the clinic so far is interleukin 1 receptor antagonist (IL-1ra; anakinra), an approach to IL-1 inhibition that has been met with only limited success.

An alternative approach is to target cells implicated in the persistence of RA. The main focus of this chapter is on biologicals with specificity for cellular targets, in particular rituximab, an antibody that selectively depletes a B-cell subset, and abatacept, a fusion protein that selectively modulates a co-stimulatory signal necessary for T-cell activation. Rituximab is approved in the USA and Europe for use in combination with MTX to treat RA by reducing the signs and symptoms in adult patients who have moderately to severely active disease and have failed one or more anti-TNF drugs. Abatacept is the first selective co-stimulation modulator to be approved in the USA for the treatment of patients with RA who show an inadequate response to other non-biological or biological disease-modifying antirheumatic drugs (DMARDs).

TARGETING B CELLS

INTRODUCTION

The role of B cells in the pathogenesis of RA is not fully understood. Nonetheless, B-cell functions of likely relevance include their role in antigen presentation, secretion of proinflammatory cytokines, production of rheumatoid factor and thus their role in immune complex formation, and co-stimulation of T cells. Of note, immune complexes are one trigger to production of TNF and other pro-inflammatory cytokines.

In the late 1990s, Edwards and colleagues suggested that the (assumed) underlying autoreactive response in RA might be driven by self-perpetuating B cells and that initiation of inflammation results from ligation of the low-affinity immunoglobulin G (IgG) receptor, FcRγIIIa, by immune complexes [3, 4]. They also proposed that such rheumatoid factor-producing B cells might become self-perpetuating by an amplification signal arising from co-ligation of the B-cell receptor and small immune complexes formed by IgG rheumatoid factor bound to the complement component C3d, providing a survival signal [5]. In contrast, co-ligation of certain other B-cell surface receptors with the B-cell receptor may provide a negative survival signal. In the rare event that self-perpetuating, autoreactive B cells arise having escaped normal regulatory mechanisms, this theory predicts that a B-cell depletion strategy would remove the autoreactive B-cell clones and their antibody products. Because CD20 is not internalized and is highly expressed on a range of B lineage cells including pre-B cells, immature B cells, activated cells and memory cells, but is not found on stem, dendritic or plasma cells, it is an ideal target for B-cell depletion by monoclonal antibodies.

INTRODUCTION TO RITUXIMAB

Rituximab is a chimaeric mouse–human monoclonal antibody, directed against the extracellular domain of the CD20 antigen located in the B-cell membrane with 44 amino acids exposed to the extracellular space. Its function is unknown, although it may have a role in cell signalling or in calcium mobilization [6]. CD20-positive B cells represent a prominent population in the rheumatoid synovial tissue in the majority of patients. CD20 initiates complement-mediated B-cell lysis and may permit antibody-dependent, cell-mediated cytotoxicity when the Fc portion of the antibody is recognized by corresponding receptors on cytotoxic cells. Rituximab may also initiate apoptosis [7] and influence the ability of B cells to respond to antigen or other stimuli [8]. Rituximab initially found a role in the clinic as a single-agent treatment for relapsed or refractory low-grade or follicular CD20-positive B-cell non-Hodgkin's lymphoma, for which it was approved. For this reason, there was a wide experience of rituximab in haematological oncology prior to clinical trials of this drug in RA, and it has recently gained approval in the USA and Europe for treatment of patients with active TNF inhibitor-refractory RA.

CLINICAL STUDIES OF RITUXIMAB IN RHEUMATOID ARTHRITIS

The clinical effects of B-cell depletion therapy in RA were initially tested using rituximab in several small studies using treatment regimes based on those derived from the rituximab–CHOP (cyclophosphamide, doxorubicin, vincristine and prednisone) regime used in non-Hodgkin's lymphoma patients [9–11]. The encouraging early efficacy findings pointed to a possible therapeutic potential for rituximab in RA.

In a phase IIa study, the efficacy of rituximab in active RA was tested in 161 patients who had failed to respond adequately to treatment with methotrexate [12]. Patients were assigned to one of four groups: a 1-g infusion of intravenous (i.v.) rituximab alone on days 1 and 15; MTX alone as a comparator arm; i.v. rituximab with cyclophosphamide infusions at a dose of 750 mg on days 3 and 17; or rituximab and MTX. All patients received 100 mg methylprednisolone just before each treatment, in addition to prednisolone 60 mg daily on day 2 and days 4–7 and 30 mg daily on days 8–14. At week 24, a significantly greater proportion of patients achieved the designated ACR50 primary end-point in the rituximab and MTX combination group (43%; $P = 0.005$), and the rituximab and cyclophosphamide combination group (41%; $P = 0.005$) than in the group receiving MTX as monotherapy (13%)

Table 3.1 The table illustrates the percentage of patients achieving ACR20, 50 and 70 responses at 24 weeks following treatment with either methotrexate plus placebo infusions or methotrexate plus two infusions of 1 g rituximab, 2 weeks apart in the phase IIa, phase IIb DANCER and phase III REFLEX studies

Study	Treatment	ACR20	ACR50	ACR70
Phase IIa study [19]	1 g Rituximab×2, plus methotrexate	65	35	15
	Methotrexate	20	5	0
Phase IIb study DANCER [20]	1 g Rituximab×2, plus methotrexate	54	34	20
	Methotrexate	28	13	5
Phase III study REFLEX [21]	1 g Rituximab×2, plus methotrexate	51	27	12
	Methotrexate	18	5	1

(Table 3.1). Thirty-three per cent of the patients receiving rituximab alone achieved an ACR50 response, but this failed to reach statistical significance compared with MTX alone ($P = 0.059$). In all the rituximab groups, the mean change from baseline in disease activity score was significant compared with MTX alone, and patients were noted to have a substantial and rapid reduction in the concentration of serum rheumatoid factor [12].

The phase IIb 'DANCER' study (Dose-ranging Assessment: International Clinical Evaluation of Rituximab in RA) was designed to examine the efficacy and safety of rituximab at different doses, with or without glucocorticosteroids, in patients with active RA resistant to DMARDs, including biologicals [13]. A total of 465 patients with active disease were recruited. They had to have failed at least one DMARD other than MTX and/or biological response modifiers, and to have been treated with 4 weeks of stable MTX monotherapy at a dose of at least 10 mg weekly. All other DMARDs were withdrawn several weeks prior to randomization. Patients received either placebo infusions or rituximab at a dose of 500 mg or 1 g on days 1 and 15, together with one of three glucocorticosteroid options, comprising glucocorticosteroid placebo, 100 mg i.v. methylprednisolone prior to each rituximab infusion, or 100 mg of methylprednisolone prior to each infusion, in addition to oral glucocorticosteroid. The results at 24 weeks confirmed the significant efficacy of a single course of rituximab in active RA when combined with continuing MTX. This benefit was independent of glucocorticosteroids, although methylprednisolone on day 1 reduced the incidence and severity of first rituximab infusion reactions by about one-third. Both rituximab doses were efficacious. At the most stringent ACR70 response level, the difference between the percentages of responders in the placebo, lower and higher rituximab groups was most marked at the higher rituximab dose of 1 g 2 weeks apart (5%, 13% and 20% respectively, $P < 0.05$).

Primary efficacy and safety data at 24 weeks into the phase III 'REFLEX' (A Randomised Evaluation of Long-term Efficacy of Rituximab in RA) trial have recently been published [14], and preliminary results of supplementary data at 12 months of follow-up are available [15]. This trial was designed to determine the efficacy and safety of rituximab when used in combination with MTX in patients with active RA who have an inadequate response to one or more anti-TNF therapies. The recruited cohort comprised 520 patients, with a mean disease duration of 12 years, on a background regime of 10–25 mg of once-weekly MTX. All patients recruited had radiographic evidence of at least one joint with definite erosion attributable to RA. After a wash-out period during which other DMARDs and anti-TNFs were withdrawn, patients were randomized to receive a single course of 1 g rituximab, or placebo, infusions on days 1 and 15. All patients were given 100 mg i.v. methylprednisolone prior to each infusion and a brief course of oral prednisolone between the two doses; 60 mg daily from days 2 to 7 and 30 mg daily from days 8 to 14 [14].

Of the patients assigned to rituximab, 82% completed 6 months compared with only 54% assigned to placebo. The major reason for study withdrawal was lack of response reported in 40% of placebo and 12% of rituximab-treated patients. At 6 months, significantly more patients receiving rituximab achieved ACR20, 50 and 70 responses, at 51%, 27% and 12%, respectively, than patients receiving placebo infusions, at 18%, 5% and 1%, respectively (Table 3.1). Intention-to-treat analyses showed that patients who received rituximab infusions achieved a reduction in disease activity score (DAS28) of 1.83 from baseline compared with a reduction of 0.34 in the placebo group [14]. Maximal clinical responses to rituximab were observed at 24 weeks. Thereafter, patients were eligible to exit the study and receive further rituximab treatment based on clinical need. Of the patients in the rituximab plus MTX group, 37% (114/308) remained in the study over 48 weeks, indicating continued clinical benefit following a single initial treatment course. The majority of patients who withdrew did so to receive further courses of rituximab between weeks 24 and 48 of the study [15].

Disease modification with rituximab

Preliminary analyses of REFLEX radiographic data set at 1 year showed a mean change of 2.31 in Genant–modified Sharp score in the placebo plus MTX arm compared with 1.0 in the rituximab plus MTX group ($P = 0.0043$). Significant differences were also reported for joint space narrowing and bone erosions, comprising both components of the score. The proportion of patients with no progression in erosion score was 61% in the rituximab arm, significantly higher than the 52% in the placebo arm [16]. These represent the first data to indicate that B-cell depletion therapy can inhibit progressive destruction to joints in a population refractory to anti-TNF treatment.

SAFETY ISSUES

A common concern regarding all therapies directed at B cells is the potential for toxicities related to modulation of humoral immunity, although rituximab has the advantage of an oncology safety database based on more than 350 000 non-Hodgkin's lymphoma patient treatments since 1997 [17]. The overall conclusions are that serious adverse events are infrequent and often associated with well-defined risk factors such as cardiopulmonary disease or high numbers of circulating cancer cells. Of note, in this lymphoma population, prolonged peripheral B-cell depletion has not been associated with cumulative toxicity or increased occurrence of opportunist infections [18–20]. However, it cannot be assumed that the toxicity profile will be identical in distinct disease phenotypes with differing pathogenic processes.

In the phase II study, the overall incidence of infection reported was similar in the control and rituximab groups at 24 and 48 weeks. By week 24, four patients in the rituximab groups had suffered a serious infection, and one in the control group. Infusion reactions of any type were reported in 36% of patients receiving rituximab and 30% of patients receiving placebo, although most were characterized as mild or moderate. The reactions included hypotension, hypertension, flushing, pruritus and rash.

In RA open-label [21] phase II [12, 13] and III [14] studies, although decreases in serum total immunoglobulin levels were observed in patients receiving rituximab, concentrations remained within normal limits. Of note, existing antibody titres against tetanus toxoid appear to be unaffected by a single course of rituximab treatment [22]. However, there is some emerging evidence that total serum immunoglobulin concentrations fall below the normal range in those patients receiving multiple cycles of rituximab treatment over a number of years in open-label studies [5]. It is unclear at this stage whether this results in increased risk of infection. In the phase II studies, the majority of adverse events were mild to moderate and associated with infusions including headache, nausea and rigors.

DURATION OF BENEFIT FOLLOWING RITUXIMAB

Among patients with RA who are achieving clinical responses to rituximab treatment, the time to clinical relapse is heterogeneous. In some patients, relapse is closely correlated to the reappearance of peripheral blood B cells, but, in others, it may be delayed by years [23]. Restoration of peripheral B-cell numbers takes about 8 months after depletion treatment, although re-treatment may need to be earlier. Clinical relapse is more closely associated with increases in autoantibody levels but there remains a need for better biomarkers reliably informing optimal management strategies on an individual patient basis.

CURRENT POSITIONING OF RITUXIMAB IN THE MANAGEMENT OF RHEUMATOID ARTHRITIS

Rituximab is a promising addition to the therapeutic armamentarium for the treatment of RA. It is not clear at this point in time to what extent there are differences in efficacy of rituximab in rheumatoid factor-positive and -negative patients, although available data from the REFLEX study indicate that the effect of treatment on ACR responses was not dependent on baseline rheumatoid factor status [14]. However, new data were recently presented from a study exploring the relationship between baseline autoantibodies (rheumatoid factor and anti-cyclic citrullinated peptide [anti-CCP] antibodies) and clinical response after the first cycle of rituximab treatment in patients with RA who show an inadequate response to one or more anti-TNF agents [24]. Patients seronegative for both types of autoantibodies achieved some clinical benefit (28% ACR20 responses at week 24 after rituximab vs. 6% after placebo), but the ACR responses were lower than in patients seropositive for one or both antibodies (50% ACR20 responses at week 24 after rituximab versus 18% after placebo). Higher-level ACR responses were not seen in the group seronegative for rheumatoid factor and anti-CCP.

Based on the DANCER study findings, it is recommended that rituximab is given in combination with once-weekly MTX, usually at doses of at least 15 mg/week, to optimize efficacy. Furthermore, administration of 100 mg i.v. methylprednisolone is recommended prior to each rituximab infusion as standard care to reduce frequency and severity of infusion reactions.

At present, the major use for rituximab in the treatment of RA is confined to the TNF inhibitor-refractory population. It may also have a role in those patients for whom TNF blockade is relatively contraindicated, such as those with connective tissue disease overlap syndromes. There are uncertainties regarding the implications of long-term peripheral B-cell depletion and the timing and need for re-dosing with rituximab in patients who respond. In a series of 155 patients with prior exposure to TNF inhibitors, a first course of rituximab gave rise to ACR20, 50 and 70 responses of 65%, 33% and 12%, respectively and 72%, 42% and 21%, respectively for a second treatment course, relative to original baseline. In 82 of these patients going on to receive a third rituximab course, the median interval between first and second courses was very similar to that between second and third courses, at between 30 and 31 weeks [25]. Further studies are needed to identify the optimum regimes that can be used for maintenance therapy that will provide efficacy and limit toxicity.

OTHER B-CELL-TARGETED THERAPIES

Other therapies targeting CD20 in clinical trails include ocrelizumab, a humanized version of rituximab, and HuMax-CD 20/ofatumumab, a fully human anti-CD20. Many other approaches to B-cell targeted therapy are in clinical testing, including the use of antibodies to

CD22 and BLyS. Belimumab, or LymphoStat-B, is a human anti-BLyS monoclonal antibody currently in clinical development for the treatment of RA and other rheumatic indications. An alternative approach to BLyS inhibition in early stages of clinical development is to block signalling through BLyS receptors using a soluble receptor such as a transmembrane activator and calcium modulator and cyclophilin ligand interactor immunoglobulin (TACI-Ig). Preliminary results of a phase II double-trial of belimumab in 283 patients with active RA have been presented [26]. Patients were randomized to receive i.v. belimumab at a dose of 1, 4 or 10 mg/kg or placebo infusions on days 0, 14 and 28, then every 28 days through 24 weeks. The ACR20 response at week 24 in the combined belimumab groups was 29%, compared with 16% in the placebo group, with no dose–response effect observed. The antibody was well tolerated. Further results are awaited with interest.

TARGETING CO-STIMULATORY MOLECULES

INTRODUCTION

Co-stimulation is an essential step in the induction of adaptive immune responses. Although the role of T cells in the perpetuation of RA has been debated and remains poorly understood, it has long been believed that T-cell activation is a key event in the pathogenesis. Successful T-cell activation requires multiple signals. One signal is provided by presentation of an antigen bound to cell surface major histocompatibility complex (MHC) molecules on antigen-presenting cells to a specific T-cell receptor. In the absence of further signals, T cells become unresponsive and may ultimately be eliminated through apoptosis. An important co-stimulatory signal is provided by an interaction between members of the B-7 family (either CD80 or 86) on antigen-presenting cells, and CD28 on T cells. After activation, T cells express CTLA-4, which interferes with the B-7–CD-28 interaction and helps to return the cells to the quiescent state.

INTRODUCTION TO ABATACEPT

Abatacept is a novel, fully human, fusion protein comprising the extracellular portion of CTLA-4 and the Fc fragment of a human IgG-1 (CTLA4Ig). In December 2005, abatacept became the first co-stimulatory blocker to be approved by the Food and Drug Administration (FDA) in the USA for the treatment of patients with RA who have had an inadequate response to other drugs. Abatacept binds to CD80 and CD86 on antigen-presenting cells, thus preventing these molecules from binding their ligand, CD28, on T cells, with consequent inhibition of optimal T-cell activation. *In vitro*, abatacept decreases T-cell proliferation and inhibits production of TNF-α, interferon-γ and interleukin 2. CTLA4Ig showed promising activity in rodent collagen-induced arthritis models, prompting its evaluation in several clinical trials in patients with RA [27, 28].

CLINICAL STUDIES OF ABATACEPT IN RHEUMATOID ARTHRITIS

In an initial 3-month phase IIa double-blind pilot study, patients with DMARD-refractory active RA were randomized to receive one of two different biological inhibitors of co-stimulation (abatacept or belatacept) or placebo infusions [29]. Active drug was given at doses of 0.5, 2 or 10 mg/kg i.v. to 214 patients, for a total of four infusions on days 1, 15, 29 and 57. The proportion of patients achieving ACR20 responses on day 85 were dose dependent and suggested clinical efficacy for both co-stimulatory blocking molecules, particularly at the higher doses.

The findings were confirmed in a multicentre phase IIb study of abatacept plus MTX in 339 patients with active RA despite MTX treatment [30]. In this study, patients were

Table 3.2 The percentage of patients achieving ACR20, 50 and 70 responses at 24 weeks following treatment with either methotrexate plus placebo infusions or methotrexate plus abatacept at day 0, 15 and 29 then once monthly at a dose approximating 10 mg/kg in the phase IIb and phase III AIM and ATTAIN studies

Study		*ACR20*	*ACR50*	*ACR70*
Phase IIb study [42]	Abatacept 10 mg/kg plus methotrexate	60	37	17
	Methotrexate	35	12	2
Phase III study AIM [45]	Abatacept 10 mg/kg plus methotrexate	68	40	20
	Methotrexate	40	17	7
Phase III study ATTAIN [46]	Abatacept 10 mg/kg plus methotrexate	50	20	10
	Methotrexate	20	4	1

randomized to receive infusions of either placebo or abatacept at a dose of 2 mg/kg or 10 mg/kg at baseline, 2 weeks, 4 weeks, and then monthly through to 6 months. ACR20 responses were achieved in 60%, 41.9% and 35.3% of patients receiving abatacept at 10 mg/kg, 2 mg/kg, or placebo infusions, respectively. At the more stringent ACR50 response level, the figures were 36.5%, 22.9% and 11.8%, respectively (Table 3.2). Patients continued on blinded therapy for an additional 6 months, during which time response to therapy was maintained [31]. From day 90 onwards, there were statistically significant and progressively rising differences in remission rates between the group receiving MTX plus abatacept at 10 mg/kg and the group assigned to MTX and placebo infusions. By 1 year of treatment, 34.8% of patients on abatacept plus MTX achieved a DAS28 remission (< 2.6), in contrast to 10.1% of the MTX plus placebo-treated patients ($P < 0.001$) [31]. Patients completing the double-blind phase over 12 months became eligible to enter a long-term extension phase in which all participants received abatacept at 10 mg/kg. At year 3, abatacept-treated patients experienced > 70% improvements in swollen and tender joint counts, and approximately 50% improvement in pain and physical function [32]. Patients who received placebo infusions during the double-blinded phase and then switched to abatacept during the long-term extension rapidly achieved equivalent efficacy to those treated with abatacept throughout.

The findings of two large phase III studies of abatacept in different RA populations have recently been reported. One population, the AIM (Abatacept in Inadequate Responders to Methotrexate) trial, comprised MTX-refractory patients [33]. The other phase III study comprised a population of patients with RA with an inadequate response to TNF antagonist therapy, the Abatacept Trial in Treatment of Anti-TNF Inadequate Responders (ATTAIN) trial [34].

In the AIM study, in a population of 652 patients with RA who show an inadequate response to MTX, 219 were randomly assigned to receive placebo and 433 to a fixed dose of abatacept approximating 10 mg/kg on days 1, 15 and 29, and every 4 weeks thereafter for a year, all patients remaining on background MTX therapy [33]. Both patient groups exhibited high disease activity at baseline with DAS28 of 6.4. Patients receiving abatacept showed greater improvement in all ACR response criteria at 6 and 12 months than placebo-treated patients (Table 3.2). Abatacept plus MTX induced DAS28 remission (< 2.6) in 14.8% at 6 months and 23.8% at 12 months compared with 2.8% and 1.9% of MTX plus placebo-treated patients at the corresponding time points ($P < 0.001$). Furthermore, patients on the abatacept and MTX combination also showed slowing of the progression of mean structural damage at 1.2 total Sharp score points over 1 year compared with MTX alone, for which the rate of progression was 2.3 Sharp score points [33]. When assessed by conventional clinical outcome measures such as European League Against Rheumatism (EULAR) response, the data suggest that a plateau of clinical efficacy is achieved with abatacept between 4 and 6 months of treatment. However, using more stringent measures for analyses, such as the time to low disease activity score (defined by DAS28 ≤ 3.2) or time to sustained low disease activity score, a plateau of efficacy was not observed over the first 12 months, suggesting an ongoing recruitment of clinical benefit with abatacept plus MTX [35].

Patients completing the double-blind phase of the AIM study over 12 months became eligible to enter a long-term extension phase in which all participants received methotrexate plus abatacept at a fixed dose approximating 10 mg/kg every 4 weeks. Clinically meaningful reductions in disease activity were maintained through 2 years [36]. Furthermore, inhibition of structural damage to joints was sustained as evaluated by plain radiography, and the effect determined after 2 years of abatacept was significantly greater than that at year 1, with minimal radiographic progression observed over the second year of treatment [37].

In the ATTAIN phase III study, abatacept therapy was evaluated in 391 patients with active disease, receiving conventional DMARDs or anakinra, who failed to respond adequately to at least 3 months of therapy with etanercept, infliximab or both agents at the approved dose regimes [34]. Anti-TNF therapy was discontinued at the time of enrolment if it had not been done previously. Following a wash-out period, patients were randomly assigned in a 2:1 ratio to receive either the same fixed dose of abatacept (10 mg/kg) or placebo. Patients receiving abatacept showed significantly greater improvement in all ACR response criteria through 6 months (Table 3.2) than placebo-treated patients (ACR20 response 50.4% vs. 19.5%, $P < 0.001$; ACR50 response 20.3% vs. 3.8%, $P < 0.001$; and ACR70 response 10.2% vs. 1.5%, $P = 0.003$). Furthermore, a DAS28 remission was achieved in 10% of patients receiving abatacept versus only 1% of patients receiving placebo infusions plus DMARDs. ACR20 responses were seen irrespective of whether the patients had been exposed to prior etanercept or infliximab treatment or both anti-TNF therapies without adequate response.

All patients who completed the 6-month double-blind phase of the ATTAIN study were eligible to enter a 1-year, long-term extension phase during which all patients received a once-monthly fixed dose of abatacept in addition to at least one conventional DMARD [38]. Of 258 patients randomized to abatacept during the double-blind phase, 223 completed 6 months of treatment and 218 entered the long-term extension. Of these, 168 completed 18 months' treatment. The ACR20 responses observed at the end of the double-blind phase were sustained throughout the 1-year extension phase, with the proportion of patients achieving the more stringent ACR50 and ACR70 responses rising to 35% and 18%, respectively, at 18 months. The proportion of patients meeting DAS28 remission criteria doubled to 22.5% by the end of the 1-year extension. Similarly, of all patients initially treated with abatacept and DMARDs who entered the long-term extension phase, the mean reduction in DAS28 from baseline to the end of the double-blind phase was –1.99, falling further to a mean reduction of –2.81 from baseline at the end of 18 months. In the double-blind phase, patients assigned to placebo infusions together with DMARDs had a mean reduction from baseline in DAS28 of –0.93 and at the end of the long-term extension after crossing over to abatacept infusions, the reduction from baseline was –2.72 [39]. These data again emphasize the sustained, but relatively slow and incremental, clinical responses observed following abatacept therapy.

SAFETY ISSUES

In clinical practice, it is commonplace to use conventional DMARDs in combination regimes in the belief that there are additive benefits in terms of efficacy without the penalty of unacceptable toxicity. It is important to know whether these same principles apply to the use of abatacept in clinical practice, and this question was addressed in the ASSURE trial (Abatacept Study of Safety in Use with other RA Therapies) [40]. In this multicentre, randomized, double-blind study, safety was compared for the addition of abatacept or placebo infusions with a background treatment regime of at least one of the traditional non-biological or biological DMARDs currently approved for RA treatment for at least 3 months.

A total of 1456 patients were randomized 2:1 to receive abatacept or placebo. In the study as a whole, the proportion of serious adverse events occurring in each treatment arm was similar at 13% for abatacept and 12% for placebo, with 5% discontinuations due to adverse events in the abatacept group and 4% in the placebo group. Serious infections occurred more frequently in the abatacept group (2.9%) than in the placebo group (1.9%). There were five deaths in the abatacept group and four in the placebo group, all but one of which in each group was thought unlikely to be related to the study drug. All of the deaths occurred in patients without concomitant biological background therapy. However, when a subanalysis of the data was performed according to whether patients were receiving biological or non-biological background therapy, it became clear that serious adverse events occurred almost twice as frequently in the subgroup receiving abatacept plus another biological agent (22.3%) than in the other subgroups (12.5%). A particularly important observation in this study was the increased number of serious infections observed when abatacept was combined with other biological therapies (5.8% vs. 1.6% for the subgroup on background biological therapy plus placebo infusions). Furthermore, the clinical benefits of abatacept tended to be less in the patients receiving background biological therapy than in those with a background of non-biological DMARDs. There were no reported cases of lymphoma, demyelinating disorders or tuberculosis.

The ASSURE trial findings regarding safety of abatacept in patients on background biological therapy mirrored those in a smaller, recently reported randomized, placebo-controlled, double-blind phase pilot study. This phase IIb trial investigated the efficacy and safety of the addition of abatacept infusions at 2 mg/kg over 1 year in patients with at least 8/66 swollen and 10/68 tender joints, despite at least 3 months' treatment with twice-weekly 25 mg subcutaneous etanercept [41]. The biological combination had limited clinical benefit over etanercept and placebo infusions but was associated with an increase in the proportion of patients experiencing serious adverse events (16.5% vs. 2.8%) and serious infections (3.5% vs. 0%). On the basis of these observations, the use of abatacept is not advised in combination with other biological therapies.

In ATTAIN, the incidence of infection was slightly higher in the abatacept group than in the placebo group, although no specific infection was clearly more frequent, and the intensity of infections appeared similar in the two groups. There were no significant differences in the numbers of patients discontinuing treatment as a result of infection or in the incidence of serious infections.

CURRENT POSITIONING OF ABATACEPT IN THE MANAGEMENT OF RHEUMATOID ARTHRITIS

Abatacept may be used as monotherapy or concomitantly with DMARDs other than TNF antagonists. It is not recommended for use concomitantly with IL-1 or TNF antagonists. The encouraging clinical trial data indicate that abatacept, like rituximab, represents a new addition to the therapeutic armentarium for patients with RA who have not responded adequately to TNF blockade.

There are emerging data concerning the comparative efficacy, safety and kinetics of response for the anti-TNF-α antibody infliximab and abatacept [42]. In a 1-year double-blind study, patients with RA who show an inadequate response to MTX (mean baseline DAS28 6.8) and no previous anti-TNF therapy were randomized to receive abatacept at 10 mg/kg every 4 weeks (156 patients), infliximab at 3 mg/kg every 8 weeks (165 patients) or placebo every 4 weeks (110 patients). Patients randomized to placebo were switched to abatacept after 6 months but were not included in the 1-year analyses. At the end of the first 6 months, the frequency of serious adverse events was 5.1%, 11.5% and 11.8% for abatacept, infliximab and placebo, respectively. In the same group order, the frequency of acute infusion-related adverse events was 5.1%, 18.2% and 10%. Over the 1-year period, infections reported as serious adverse events were more frequent with infliximab at 8.5% than abatacept at 1.9%. These included two cases of tuberculosis, both in infliximab-treated patients. Over 6 months, ACR response rates, changes in DAS28, HAQ and SF-36 were similar following treatment with either abatacept or infliximab. However, abatacept was observed to have increasing efficacy beyond 6 months, in contrast to the infliximab group in which measures had apparently reached a plateau or diminished over time. For example, the mean change from baseline in DAS28 for abatacept was –2.3 at 6 months and –2.9 at 1 year in comparison to –2.3 at 6 and 12 months for infliximab.

T-CELL-TARGETED THERAPIES

Data from several different preclinical animal models of inflammatory arthritis suggest a pathogenic role for CD4+ T cells in response to various arthritogenic antigens presented in the context of MHC class II molecules [43]. These observations led to a number of experimental protocols designed to investigate the effect of depleting and non-depleting antibodies directed at CD4 as well as other T-cell-associated molecules. Early randomized, placebo-controlled clinical studies exploring the potential of biological therapies targeting T cells in the treatment of RA have had generally disappointing results. Some anti-T-cell agents were non-efficacious, whereas other preliminary trials demonstrating some clinical efficacy were terminated owing to adverse events, particularly profound and prolonged T-cell depletion [44]. However, the primatized monoclonal anti-CD4 antibody keliximab results in dose-dependent clinical responses when administered once weekly over four consecutive weeks and the clinical response correlates with CD4+ T-cell coating with keliximab [45] rather than T-cell depletion.

Examples of biological therapies targeting other T-cell-associated molecules include Campath-1H, a monoclonal antibody directed against CD52 (a polypeptide expressed on all lymphocytes). Campath-1H was tested as a treatment for refractory RA in two small trials, and, although a single i.v. dose of between 1 and 100 mg resulted in significant CD4+ T-cell depletion and clinical improvements in over half of patients, there was poor correlation between biological action and clinical response [46, 47]. Furthermore, therapy was associated with significant acute toxicity, presumed to reflect a cytokine release syndrome, including headache, nausea and hypotension. Arthritis activity returned over time, despite prolonged suppression of peripheral blood CD4+ T-cell numbers.

IL-1 BLOCKADE

Another proinflammatory cytokine abundantly expressed in RA synovium is interleukin 1 (IL-1). It stimulates resorption of cartilage and bone through activation of osteoclasts and inhibits synthesis of proteoglycan and articular collagen [48–50]. Proof of principle for IL-1 blockade has been established, not with antibodies but by means of once-daily, subcutaneously administered IL-1 receptor antagonist (IL-1ra; anakinra), a naturally occurring inhibitor of IL-1 [51]. The combination of anakinra and MTX is well tolerated and provides significantly greater clinical benefit than MTX alone [52]. Analysis of hand radiographs, by two different methodologies, after 24 weeks of treatment in the phase II rHuIL-1ra study, have led to claims of retardation of the rate of development of structural damage to joints in patients receiving active drugs [51, 53].

However, the overall magnitude of clinical responses and changes in acute phase reactants were relatively modest, at 20–35% from baseline, compared with those reported for TNF-α blockade. These observations do not necessarily imply that IL-1 is not a good target for therapy in RA, but may reflect pharmacokinetic challenges for IL-1ra as a means to achieve IL-1 blockade. For example, the kidneys excrete IL-1ra rapidly, and therapeutic levels persist for a few hours only. Furthermore, IL-1 receptors are ubiquitously expressed and have a rapid turnover. Alternative strategies for IL-1 inhibition are in clinical trials. These include the use of monoclonal antibodies with specificity for IL-1β, and the IL-1 trap, an engineered protein comprising the two high-affinity signalling chains of the cell surface IL-1 receptor, linked by the Fc portion of IgG1.

IL-6 BLOCKADE

IL-6 regulates the production of acute-phase proteins by hepatocytes and activates osteoclasts to absorb bone. The therapeutic potential of a humanized anti-IL-6 receptor mAb without agonist activity has been assessed in randomized trials in Europe and Japan [54, 55]. In a European multicentre randomized clinical trial, tocilizumab was used, either as monotherapy (by discontinuation of MTX) or concomitantly with MTX therapy, and compared with placebo infusions in patients maintained on a fixed dose of MTX over 20 weeks (CHARISMA; Chugai Humanized Anti-human Recombinant Interleukin-Six Monoclonal Antibody). A total of 359 patients with established RA and an inadequate response to MTX were recruited [56]. In this study, the percentage of patients receiving MTX alone achieving ACR20, 50 and 70 responses was 41%, 29% and 16%, respectively. Tocilizumab was given at one of three dose regimes, 2 mg/kg, 4 mg/kg or 8 mg/kg, either as a monotherapy or in combination with MTX. A dose–response effect was seen, with the best responses at the highest doses of tocilizumab. As a monotherapy, 8 mg/kg of tocilizumab gave rise to ACR20, 50 and 70 responses in 63%, 41% and 16%, respectively. In combination with MTX, the corresponding figures were 74%, 53% and 37%, significantly higher than the MTX and placebo infusion group. In general, tocilizumab was well tolerated in the CHARISMA study. Antitocilizumab antibodies were observed in the monotherapy groups receiving the two lowest doses of antibody, but none occurred in the 8 mg/kg group, whether given as monotherapy or in combination. A small proportion of patients who started the study with a normal neutrophil count experienced neutropenia when treated with the higher dose of tocilizumab at 8 mg/kg. Three new cases of serious infection were noted in the combination therapy group receiving 8 mg/kg of tocilizumab but four serious infections were noted in the 2 mg/kg monotherapy group, with none noted in the MTX monotherapy group. Four cases of anaphylactic reaction were reported out of 107 patients treated with the two lower doses of tocilizumab as a monotherapy. As in the Japanese study, moderate but reversible increases in mean non-fasting total cholesterol and triglycerides were observed over the study period. However, there was also a rise in HDL cholesterol and the mean atherogenic index was unchanged.

These studies validate IL-6 as a target for therapy in RA and a potentially promising means of controlling disease activity. Tocilizumab treatment, either as monotherapy or combination therapy with MTX, is well tolerated in the majority of cases, with a safety pattern that is consistent with other biological and immunosuppressive therapies. Further phase III studies are under way to further investigate IL-6 blockade.

IL-15 BLOCKADE

IL-15 is another potential therapeutic target of interest across a range of inflammatory pathologies. In RA it is detectable in inflamed joints and serves as a powerful T-cell chemoattractant. T cells from rheumatoid synovial membranes have the capability to induce TNF-α synthesis by blood- or synovial-derived macrophages through cell membrane contact, and there is evidence that IL-15 is one factor capable of sustaining this activity [57]. Blockade of IL-15 ameliorates animal models of RA, and IL-15 levels in the rheumatoid synovium correlate with TNF-α activity.

In a phase I/II 12-week, dose-ascending, placebo-controlled, double-blind, proof-of-concept study, a fully human IgG-1 anti-IL-15 antibody, AMG 714, was tested in 30 patients with RA. The antibody was administered in dose-ascending order to six cohorts of five patients by single subcutaneous infusion. The patients were followed up for 28 days and, in the absence of dose-limiting toxicity by day 28, all patients received four additional doses of AMG 714 at weekly intervals by open-label extension. The antibody was well tolerated clinically, with no significant effects on T-lymphocyte subsets and natural killer cell numbers. Substantial improvements in disease activity were observed, with 63% achieving an ACR20 response, 38% achieving ACR50, and 25% achieving ACR70 [58].

AMG 714 is being tested in ongoing clinical trials, and interim analyses have been presented for a phase II study [59]. Rheumatoid patients with active disease, despite treatment with at least one conventional DMARD but naive to biological therapy, were randomized to receive placebo or one of four doses of AMG 714 injected subcutaneously once every 2 weeks over 12 weeks. All patients received two loading doses of AMG 714 or placebo, according to treatment allocation. Stable background MTX, non-steroidal anti-inflammatory drugs and low-dose glucocorticosteroids were continued. Preliminary data analysis showed that 62% of patients receiving the highest 280-mg dose achieved an ACR20 response compared with 26% of placebo-treated patients. There were no differences in adverse events, infections or serious adverse events between the groups in this interim analysis.

These preliminary data are promising, but must be interpreted with some caution because of the small numbers studied to this point. However, IL-15 represents a potentially interesting target because of its multifaceted proinflammatory role in RA. In particular, in addition to its involvement in the proinflammatory cascade, IL-15 is required for the maintenance of CD8+ memory T cells. Theoretically, therefore, IL-15 blockade might diminish the inflammatory component of disease and the self-directed T-cell immunological memory that characterizes the autoimmune response [60, 61]. The full data set is therefore awaited with great interest.

CONCLUSION

Advances in the understanding of disease pathogenesis in RA with the identification of a number of molecular and cellular targets for therapy together with advances in molecular biotechnology permitting the production of large quantities of clinical grade protein inhibitors has led to a range of new therapies for RA. Several have already been approved for use in the clinic and many more are in development.

As yet, however, the comparative effects of abatacept, rituximab and TNF blockade on structural damage are unknown. It is clear that where clinical responses are unsatisfactory, combination therapy with MTX and an anti-TNF agent may still confer significant joint protection compared with MTX alone. Thus, the merits of switching a patient from an anti-TNF inhibitor to abatacept or rituximab on the basis of an inadequate clinical response are not yet clearcut with respect to disease modification. Other factors likely to determine the future uptake and relative positioning of new biologicals in the clinic include further long-term safety data, comparative cost-effectiveness analyses and the perceived convenience of i.v. administration.

REFERENCES

1. Klareskog L, van der Heijde D, de Jager JP *et al.* Therapeutic effect of the combination of etanercept and methotrexate compared with each treatment alone in patients with rheumatoid arthritis: double-blind randomised controlled trial. *Lancet* 2004; 363:675–681.
2. Lipsky PE, van der Heijde DM, St Clair EW *et al.* Anti-tumor necrosis factor trial in rheumatoid arthritis with concomitant therapy study group: infliximab and methotrexate in the treatment of rheumatoid arthritis. *N Engl J Med* 2000; 343:1594–1602.
3. Bhatia A, Blades S, Cambridge G *et al.* Differential distribution of FcγRIIIa in normal human tissues and co-localisation with DAF and fibrillin-1: implications for immunological microenvironments. *Immunology* 1998; 94:56–63.

4. Abrahams VM, Cambridge G, Edwards JC. Induction of tumour necrosis factor α by human monocytes: a key role for FcγRIIIa in rheumatoid arthritis. *Arthritis Rheum* 2002; 43:608–616.
5. Edwards JCW, Cambridge G. B cell targeting in rheumatoid arthritis and other diseases. *Nat Rev Immunol* 2006; 6:394–405.
6. Riley JK, Sliwkoski MX. CD20: a gene in search of a function. *Semin Oncol* 2000; 27(Suppl. 12):17–24.
7. Szodoray P, Alex P, Dandapani V *et al.* Apoptotic effect of rituximab on peripheral B cells in RA. *Scand J Immunol* 2004; 60:209–218.
8. Tsokos GC. B cells, be gone – B-cell depletion in the treatment of rheumatoid arthritis. *N Engl J Med* 2004; 350:2546–2548.
9. Edwards JC, Cambridge G. Sustained improvement in rheumatoid arthritis following a protocol designed to deplete B lymphocytes. *Rheumatology* (Oxford) 2001; 40:205–211.
10. De Vita S, Zaja F, Sacco S *et al.* Efficacy of selective B cell blockade in the treatment of rheumatoid arthritis: evidence for a pathogenetic role of B cells. *Arthritis Rheum* 2002; 46:2029–2033.
11. Leandro MJ, Edwards JC, Cambridge G. Clinical outcome in 22 patients with rheumatoid arthritis treated with B lymphocyte depletion. *Ann Rheum Dis* 2002; 61:883–888.
12. Edwards JC, Szczepanski L, Szechinski J *et al.* Efficacy of B-cell-targeted therapy with rituximab in patients with rheumatoid arthritis. *N Engl J Med* 2004; 350:2572–2581.
13. Emery P, Fleischmann R, Filipowicz-Sosnowska A *et al.*; for the DANCER study group. The efficacy and safety of rituximab in patients with active rheumatoid arthritis despite methotrexate treatment: results of a phase IIB randomized, double-blind, placebo-controlled, dose-ranging study. *Arthritis Rheum* 2006; 54:1390–1400.
14. Cohen SB, Emery P, Greenwald MW *et al.* Rituximab for rheumatoid arthritis refractory to anti-tumor necrosis factor therapy: results of a multicenter, randomized, double-blind, placebo-controlled, phase III trial evaluating primary efficacy and safety at twenty-four weeks. *Arthritis Rheum* 2006; 54:2793–2806.
15. Cohen S, Emery P, Greenwald M *et al.* Prolonged efficacy of rituximab in rheumatoid arthritis patients with inadequate response to one or more TNF inhibitors: 1-year follow-up of a subset of patients receiving a single course in a controlled trial (reflex study). *Ann Rheum Dis* 2006; 65(Suppl. II):183.
16. Keystone E, Emery P, Peterfy CG *et al.* Prevention of joint structural damage at 1 year in rheumatoid arthritis patients with an inadequate response to one or more TNF inhibitors (REFLEX). *Ann Rheum Dis* 2006; 65(Suppl II):58.
17. Morbacher A. B cell non-Hodgkin's lymphoma: rituximab safety experience. *Arthritis Res Ther* 2005; 7(Suppl. 3): S19–S25.
18. McLaughlin P, Grillo-Lopez AJ, Link BK *et al.* Rituximab anti-CD20 monoclonal antibody therapy for relapsed indolent lymphoma: half of patients respond to a four dose treatment program. *J Clin Oncol* 1998;16:2825–2833.
19. McLaughlin P, Hagemeister FB, Grillo-Lopez AJ. Rituximab in indolent lymphoma: the single agent pivotal trial. *Semin Oncol* 1999; 26(Suppl. 14):79–87.
20. Coffier B, Lepage E, Brier J *et al.* CHOP chemotherapy plus rituximab compared with CHOP alone in elderly patients with diffuse large B cell lymphoma. *N Engl J Med* 2002; 346:235–242.
21. Higashida J, Wun T, Schmidt S *et al.* Safety and efficacy of rituximab in patients with rheumatoid arthritis refractory to disease modifying anti-rheumatic drugs and anti-TNFα treatment. *J Rheumatol* 2005; 32:2109–2115.
22. Emery P, Fleischman RM, Filipowicz-Sosnowska A *et al.* Rituximab in rheumatoid arthritis: a double-blind, placebo-controlled, dose ranging study. *Arthritis Rheum* 2005; 52(Suppl.):S709.
23. Cambridge G, Leandro MJ, Edwards JC *et al.* Serologic changes following B lymphocyte depletion therapy for rheumatoid arthritis. *Arthritis Rheum* 2003; 48:2146–2154.
24. Tak PP, Cohen S, Emery P *et al.* Baseline autoantibody status (RF, anti-CCP) and clinical response following the first treatment course with rituximab. *Arthritis Rheum* 2006; 54(Suppl.):833.
25. van Vollenhoven RF, Cohen S, Pavelka K *et al.* Response to rituximab in patients with rheumatoid arthritis is maintained by repeat therapy: results of an open-label trial. *Ann Rheum Dis* 2006; 65(Suppl. II):510.
26. McKay J, Chwalinska-Sadowska H, Boling E *et al.* Efficacy and safety of belimumab (BMAB), a fully human monoclonal antibody to B lymphocyte stimulator (BLyS) for the treatment of rheumatoid arthritis. *Arthritis Rheum* 2005; 52(Suppl.):S710.
27. Knoerzer DB, Karr RW, Schwartz BD *et al.* Collagen-induced arthritis in the BB rat. Prevention of disease by treatment with CTLA-4-Ig. *J Clin Invest* 1995; 96:987–993.

28. Webb LM, Walmsley MJ, Feldmann M. Prevention and amelioration of collagen-induced arthritis by blockade of the CD28 co-stimulatory pathway: requirement for both B7–1 and B7–2. *Eur J Immunol* 1996; 26:2320–2328.

29. Moreland LW, Alten R, Van den Bosch F *et al*. Co-stimulatory blockade in patients with rheumatoid arthritis: a pilot, dose-finding, double-blind, placebo-controlled clinical trial evaluating CTLA-4Ig and LEA29Y eighty-five days after the first infusion. *Arthritis Rheum* 2002; 46:1470–1479.

30. Kremer JM, Westhovens R, Leon M *et al*. Treatment of rheumatoid arthritis by selective inhibition of T-cell activation with fusion protein CTLA4Ig. *N Engl J Med* 2003; 349:1907–1915.

31. Kremer JM, Dougados M, Emery P *et al*. Treatment of rheumatoid arthritis with the selective costimulation modulator abatacept: twelve-month results of a phase IIb, double-blind, randomized, placebo-controlled trial. *Arthritis Rheum* 2005; 52:2263–2271.

32. Westhovens R, Emery P, Aranda R *et al*. Abatacept provides sustained clinical benefit through 3 years in rheumatoid arthritis patients with inadequate responses to methotrexate. *Ann Rheum Dis* 2006; 65(Suppl. II):512.

33. Kremer JM, Genant HK, Moreland LW *et al*. Effects of abatacept in patients with methotrexate-resistant active rheumatoid arthritis: a randomized trial. *Ann Intern Med* 2006; 144:865–876.

34. Genovese MC, Becker JC, Schiff M *et al*. Abatacept for rheumatoid arthritis refractory to tumor necrosis factor alpha inhibition. *N Engl J Med* 2005; 353:1114–1123.

35. Dougados M, LeBars MA, Schmidely N. Low disease activity in rheumatoid arthritis treated with abatacept in the AIM (Abatacept in Inadequate response to Methotrexate) trial. *Ann Rheum Dis* 2006; 65(Suppl. II):188.

36. Kremer JM, Emery P, Becker JC *et al*. Abatacept provides significant and sustained benefits in clinical and patient-reported outcomes through 2 years in rheumatoid arthritis and an inadequate response to methotrexate: the long-term extension (LTE) of the AIM trial. *Ann Rheum Dis* 2006; 65(Suppl. II):327.

37. Genant HK, Peterfy C, Westhovens R *et al*. Abatacept sustains inhibition of radiographic progression over 2 years in rheumatoid arthritis patients with an inadequate response to methotrexate: results form the long-term extension (LTE) of the AIM trial. *Ann Rheum Dis* 2006; 65(Suppl. II):57.

38. Genovese MC, Luggen M, Schiff M *et al*. Sustained improvements through 18 months with abatacept in rheumatoid arthritis patients with an inadequate response to anti-TNF therapy. ACR 2005 late breaking abstract (not included in abstract supplement).

39. Siblia J, Schiff M, Genovese MC *et al*. Sustained improvement in disease activity score 28 (DAS28) and patient reported outcomes (PRO) with abatacept in rheumatoid arthritis patients with an inadequate response to anti-TNF therapy: the long-term extension of the ATTAIN trial. *Ann Rheum Dis* 2006; 65(Suppl. II):501.

40. Weinblatt M, Combe B, Covucci A *et al*. Safety of the selective co-stimulation modulator abatacept in rheumatoid arthritis patients receiving background biologic and nonbiologic disease-modifying antirheumatic drugs: a one-year randomized, placebo-controlled study. *Arthritis Rheum* 2006; 54:2807–2816.

41. Weinblatt ME, Schiff MH, Goldman A *et al*. Selective co-stimulation modulation using abatacept in patients with active rheumatoid arthritis while receiving etanercept: a randomized clinical trial. *Ann Rheum Dis* 2007; 66:228–234.

42. Schiff M, Keiserman M, Codding C *et al*. The efficacy and safety of abatacept or infliximab in RA patients with an inadequate response to MTX: results from a 1 year double-blind, randomised, placebo controlled trial. ACR 2006 late breaking abstract (not included in abstract supplement).

43. Weyand CM, Goronzy JJ. T-cell-targeted therapies in rheumatoid arthritis. *Nat Clin Pract Rheumatol* 2006; 2:201–210.

44. Taylor PC. Antibody therapy for rheumatoid arthritis. *Curr Opin Pharmacol* 2003; 3:323–328.

45. Mason U, Aldrich J, Breedveld F *et al*. CD4 coating, but not CD4 depletion, is a predictor of efficacy with primatized monoclonal anti-CD4 treatment of active rheumatoid arthritis. *J Rheumatol* 2002; 29:220–229.

46. Weinblatt ME, Maddison PJ, Bulpitt KJ *et al*. CAMPATH-1H, a humanized monoclonal antibody, in refractory rheumatoid arthritis: an intravenous dose-escalation study. *Arthritis Rheum* 1995; 38:1589–1594.

47. Schnitzer TJ, Yocum DE, Michalska M *et al*. Subcutaneous administration of CAMPATH-1H: clinical and biological outcomes. *J Rheumatol* 1997; 24:1031–1036.

48. van de Loo AA, Arntz OJ, Bakker AC, van Lent PL, Jacobs MJ, van den Berg WB. Role of interleukin-1 in antigen-induced exacerbations of murine arthritis. *Am J Pathol* 1995; 146:239–249.

49. Fantuzzi G, Dinarello CA. The inflammatory response in IL-1β deficient mice. Comparison with other cytokine-related knock-out mice. *J Leukocyte Biol* 1996; 59:489–493.
50. van de Loo FAJ, Joosten LAB, van Lent PL, Arntz OJ, van den Berg WB. Role of interleukin-1 tumor necrosis factor α, and interleukin-6 in cartilage proteoglycan metabolism and destruction: effect of in situ blocking in murine antigen- and zymosan-induced arthritis. *Arthritis Rheum* 1995; 38:164–172.
51. Bresnihan B, Alvaro-Gracia JM, Cobby M *et al.* Treatment of rheumatoid arthritis with recombinant human interleukin-1 receptor antagonist. *Arthritis Rheum* 1998; 41:2196–2204.
52. Cohen S, Hurd E, Cush J *et al.* Treatment of rheumatoid arthritis with Anakinra, a recombinant human interleukin-1 receptor antagonist, in combination with methotrexate. *Arthritis Rheum* 2002; 46:614–624.
53. Jiang Y, Genant HK, Watt I *et al.* A multicenter, double-blind, dose-ranging, randomised, placebo-controlled study of recombinant human interleukin-1 receptor antagonist in patients with rheumatoid arthritis. Radiologic progression and correlation of Genant and Larsen Scores. *Arthritis Rheum* 2000; 43:1001–1009.
54. Choy E, Isenberg D, Garrood T *et al.* The effect of anti-interleukin 6 (IL-6) receptor monoclonal antibody, MRA, in rheumatoid arthritis. *Ann Rheum Dis* 2002; 61(Suppl. 1): 54.
55. Nishimoto N, Yoshizaki K, Miyasaka N *et al.* A multi-centre, randomised, double-blind, placebo-controlled trial of humanised anti-interleukin-6 receptor monoclonal antibody (MRA) in rheumatoid arthritis (RA). *Arthritis Rheum* 2002; 46(Suppl.):S559.
56. Maini RN, Taylor PC, Szechinski J *et al.* for the CHARISMA Study Group. Randomised clinical trial of the IL-6 receptor antagonist, Tocilizumab (MRA), in rheumatoid arthritis patients with an incomplete response to methotrexate in Europe (CHARISMA). *Arthritis Rheum* 2006; 54:2817–2829.
57. Liew FY, McInnes IB. Role of interleukin 15 and interleukin 18 in inflammatory response. *Ann Rheum Dis* 2002; 61(Suppl. 2):ii100–102.
58. Baslund B, Tvede N, Danneskiold-Samsoe B *et al.* Targeting interleukin-15 in patients with rheumatoid arthritis: a proof-of-concept study. *Arthritis Rheum* 2005; 52:2686–2692.
59. McInnes I, Martin R, Zimmerman-Gorska I *et al.* Safety and efficacy of a human monoclonal antibody to IL-15 (AMG 714) in patients with rheumatoid arthritis (RA): results from a multi-center, randomized, double-blind, placebo-controlled trial. *Arthritis Rheum* 2004; 50:S241, 527.
60. Zhang X, Sun S, Hwang I, Tough DF, Sprent J. Potent and selective stimulation of memory-phenotype CD8+ T cells in vivo by IL-15. *Immunity* 1998; 8:591–599.
61. Ku CC, Murakami M, Sakamoto A, Kappler J, Marrack P. Control of homeostasis of CD8+ memory T cells by opposing cytokines. *Science* 2000; 288:675–678.

4

Pharmacogenetics of inflammatory arthritis

Judith A. M. Wessels, Tom W. J. Huizinga, Henk-Jan Guchelaar

Rheumatoid arthritis (RA) is the most common form of chronic inflammatory joint disease, affecting approximately 1% of the population [1]. No treatment cures RA. Therefore, reducing disease activity with early therapeutic intervention is key to minimizing the joint damage and functional decline [2, 3]. Initiation of therapy with disease-modifying antirheumatic drugs (DMARDs) within a few months after the diagnosis of RA is essential. A delay of 3 months in the introduction of medication has been shown to result in substantially more radiographic damage at 5 years [4].

Treatment of RA usually follows a stepwise approach (Figure 4.1) [5]. First, patients are treated with monotherapy DMARDs, with methotrexate (MTX), administered weekly in low doses, being the most commonly used drug [6–8]. If there is insufficient response and/or adverse drug events, the DMARD may be switched to another DMARD, a second DMARD may be added to the monotherapy, or therapy may be changed to a newer subgroup of DMARDs, so-called biological agents, either alone or in combination with other DMARDs [9–12]. Currently available biological agents inhibit the actions of tumour necrosis factor (TNF)-α and interleukin 1 (IL-1), two proinflammatory cytokines thought to play a pivotal role in the pathogenesis of RA [13]. More recently, drugs targeting other cytokines or altering the activation of T cells or eliminating pre-B cells have gained interest for treating patients with RA. Examples of these new agents are anti-CTLA4Ig (abatacept) and anti-CD20 (rituximab) [14–16].

Despite the fact that the understanding of the pathophysiology of RA has led to different treatment options and strategies for patients with RA, the response to treatment with DMARDs is often suboptimal. For example, only 46% of patients show a good clinical response with MTX monotherapy and 30% discontinue treatment because of toxicity, whereas for anti-TNF (adalimumab) therapy approximately 60% show good response and 22% discontinue treatment [11, 17, 18]. Remarkably, studies in the field of identifying determinants for effective and safe drug treatment for individual patients with RA are still scarce. To date, the choice of drug for therapeutic intervention is made empirically.

A key challenge is to improve drug therapy by targeting DMARDs in RA to those patients who are most likely to respond, thereby predicting the individual response with maximum efficacy and avoiding toxicity [13, 19–21]. The interindividual variability in toxicity and drug response has become the basis of current pharmacogenetic research. This chapter will discuss the principles of pharmacogenetics, address genetic variability in genes contributing to outcome in DMARD treatment and, finally, will consider future research perspectives and implications of pharmacogenetic testing in improving RA therapy.

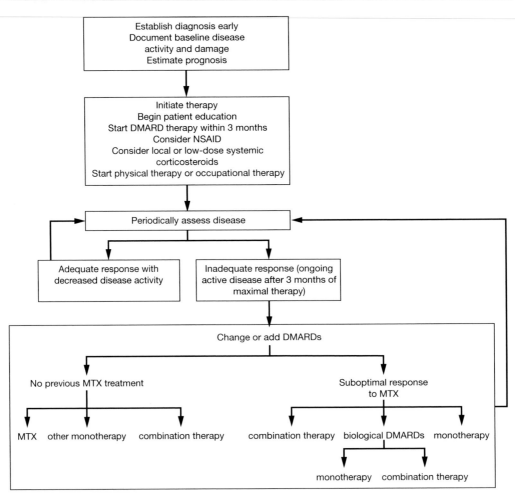

Figure 4.1 Stepwise approach of treating patients with rheumatoid arthritis. DMARD, disease-modifying antirheumatic drug; MTX, methotrexate; NSAID, non-steroidal anti-inflammatory drug.

PHARMACOGENETICS

Pharmacogenetics is the field that studies the influence of variations of DNA sequence on drug response [22]. Single nucleotide polymorphisms (SNPs) represent the most abundant source of genetic variation in humans. An SNP is a genetic variation characterized by a single nucleotide base change due to alteration, deletion or insertion of the base. Genetic variants are designated as polymorphic when the minor allele frequency of the SNP is at least 1% and the allele leads to small phenotypic changes.

Single nucleotide polymorphisms occur every few hundred bases in promoter regions, coding and non-coding sequences. Functional SNPs can alter promoter activity (regulatory SNPs), DNA, pre-mRNA conformation or mature RNA (alternative splicing), and they can influence the function or expression of the gene product – the protein [13]. In addition, copy number variants (CNVs) – defined as DNA segments that are 1 kb or larger in size present at variable copy number in comparison with reference genome – have also been shown to lead to phenotypic changes as a result of altering gene dosage, disrupting coding sequences or perturbing long-range gene regulation [23]. Moreover, variable numbers of tandem repeats (VNTR), especially in the promoter region of a gene, have shown to influence gene expression and are another source of genetic variation.

The current strategies used in pharmacogenetic studies include association studies of drug response with SNPs in 'candidate genes', which are genes selected on the basis of the pharmacokinetic and pharmacodynamic properties of the drug under study. Another strategy is the genome-wide analysis of SNPs, for example between responders and non-responders. This latter approach intends to associate independently evenly distributed SNPs across the human genome in (or in linkage with) candidate genes with response, without using any *a priori* knowledge about the pharmacology of a drug.

Although the candidate gene approach is appealing, it may fail for several reasons. This method does not take into account the potential role of other genes, including those genes whose function is not yet understood. It also does not account for gene duplications and other mechanisms that alter protein function, for example post-translational modifications. On the other hand, genome-wide analysis has the advantage of considering genes whose function in relation to the studied phenotype is not yet understood or recognized, but has limitations with regard to generating relatively high costs and requiring more sophisticated statistical approaches. For instance, testing thousands of SNPs for their association with clinical outcome increases the number of false-positive results, whereas a stringent adjustment for multiple testing with Bonferroni correction reduces study power and may lead to false-negative associations [24–26]. Even though the term 'genome-wide' indicates that allelic variants across the human genome are covered, currently available scans with 100000–500000 SNP arrays cover, at most, 5% of the estimated allelic variations in our genome. Therefore, associations in genome-wide studies do not only depend on association between genotype and clinical phenotype, power and sample size of the study to detect a significant difference, but also on allele frequencies at the marker and the candidate gene locus and the amount of linkage disequilibrium between genetic variants [27].

An interesting step between the candidate gene and the whole-genome pharmacogenetic analysis is the study of drug response in the downstream and interacting signalling pathways [20, 28]. Pathways of genes with allelic variants may be more important than individual genes, with the effects of polymorphisms in networks of genes acting together to create one phenotype. Thus, variability in drug response may reflect genetically determined changes in the biological environment in which drugs interact.

Nevertheless, it has to be realized that genetic factors are estimated to account for 15–30% of the interindividual variation in drug response. Only for certain drugs has an exceptionally high degree of interindividual variation in response been attributed to genetic variants [29]. Drug efficacy and safety are more likely to be a complex result of the influence of many genes interacting with environmental and behavioural factors [29, 30]. For that reason, the current examples of clinically applied pharmacogenetics represent genetic variations with relatively high penetrance in a monogenic trait; an allelic variant has a profound effect on the pharmacokinetic and pharmacodynamic factors of a drug, and that individual difference in one gene accounts for clearly recognizable phenotypes [28, 29]. An approach to increase the explained variation in drug response and to improve the usefulness of clinical pharmacogenetic testing is to develop models in which genetic and non-genetic factors important for the phenotype are combined.

Pharmacogenetic studies in complex traits such as RA are, as yet, developing. To date, the extent to which genetic factors influence drug response in RA is largely unknown. The unidentified nature of the disease makes the precise mechanisms of action of DMARDs uncertain and the candidate gene approach of limited use. In addition, disease activity fluctuations and disease progression may affect treatment response. However, recent reports do indicate that genetic variants affect DMARD response in patients with RA.

PHARMACOGENETICS IN RHEUMATOID ARTHRITIS

Disease-modifying antirheumatic drugs exhibit a variety of pharmacological actions, and the clinical effects can probably be attributed to multiple targets, such as reducing cell proliferation, increasing the rate of apoptosis of T and B cells, altering the expression of cellular adhesion molecules responsible for cell migration to the synovium and altering proinflammatory cytokine production or blocking their function [6, 12, 14–16]. Accordingly, it is expected that many genes influence DMARD treatment.

Current pharmacogenetic studies in RA concentrate mainly on two kinds of polymorphisms: those that could modulate the response to the drug (pharmacokinetic and pharmacodynamic effects) and those that could modulate the (inflammatory) pathway itself. For example, TNF-α and IL-1 genes are plausible subjects of investigation because of their pivotal role in the initiation and maintenance of inflammation in RA, whereas the 5-aminoimidazole-4-carboxamide-ribo-nucleotide transformylase (*ATIC*) gene is a subject because it encodes an enzyme that is inhibited by polyglutamated MTX.

Polymorphic genes likely to, or reported to, influence DMARD treatment outcome are listed in Table 4.1. However, it is beyond the scope of this chapter to discuss completely the DMARD pharmacogenetic data. For this reason, only the pharmacogenetics of MTX and

Table 4.1 Disease-modifying antirheumatic drugs (DMARDs) of interest for pharmacogenetic studies

DMARD	Polymorphic genes reported or likely to influence DMARD response and/or safety
Sulfasalazine	Metabolizing enzyme *N*-acetyltransferase 2 (NAT2) Drug transporter reduced folate carrier (RFC)
Hydroxychloroquine	Drug transporter of the ATP-binding cassette type A (ABCA4)
Azathioprine	Metabolizing enzyme thiopurine methyltransferase (TPMT) Drug targets such as enzymes in the purine synthesis
Ciclosporin	Metabolizing cytochrome P450 enzymes Drug transporter multidrug resistance protein (MRP)
Leflunomide	Metabolizing cytochrome P450 enzymes Drug targets dihydroorotate dehydrogenase (DHODH) and enzymes in the pyrimidine syntheses
Methotrexate	Drug transporters reduced folate carrier, P-glycoprotein and multiresistant proteins (RFC, ABCB1, MRP) Drug targets such as enzymes in the pyrimidine and purine syntheses Biological milieu genes such as genes in the major histocompatibility complex region
Anakinra	Drug target interleukin 1 gene Biological milieu genes such as genes in the major histocompatibility complex region
Etanercept Infliximab Adalimumab	Drug target TNF gene and promoter region, TNF-α receptor gene Drug target immunoglobulin G fragment C receptor type IIa, type IIIa and b Biological milieu genes such as genes in the major histocompatibility complex region
Abatacept	Drug target CTLA4 Biological milieu genes such as genes in the major histocompatibility complex region
Rituximab	Drug target immunoglobulin G fragment C receptor type IIa and type IIIa Biological milieu genes such as genes in the major histocompatibility complex region

anti-TNF-α blockers (anti-TNF-α agents) will be discussed in detail, as their drug responses have been mainly studied in relation to genetic variants.

PHARMACOGENETICS OF METHOTREXATE

Methotrexate is thought to act mainly via the direct or indirect inhibition of purine and pyrimidine pathway enzymes, although it has probably more targets which are likely to account for its immunosuppressive and antiproliferative effects in RA [6, 31]. Yet, genetic variants in genes coding for enzymes responsible for purine and pyrimidine synthesis have been extensively studied in relation to treatment outcome. Studies linking responses of MTX monotherapy in patients with RA who have SNPs in these pathway genes have yielded mixed results [32–41]. Table 4.2 presents the pharmacogenetic data of patients with RA treated with MTX monotherapy.

The best-studied association is the SNP in the gene methylene tetrahydrofolate reductase (*MTHFR*), an enzyme that catalyses the formation of 5-methyltetrahydrofolate (methyl-THF), a methyl donor for a variety of metabolic reactions. Two common polymorphisms in *MTHFR* enzyme at position 677, wild-type C-allele replaced by a variant T-allele (C>T) and 1298A>C, are associated with diminished enzyme activity, leading to homocysteinaemia. Increased homocysteine plasma levels have been associated with MTX toxicity [42–44]. As a consequence, several reports studied the association between the 1298 and 677 polymorphisms with MTX toxicity, especially gastrointestinal (GI) and liver toxicity (Table 4.2) [32, 35, 37–40, 42, 45, 46]. In addition, the effects of these *MTHFR* polymorphisms on MTX efficacy were assessed [32, 35, 39, 40, 45, 46].

Seven studies found no association of *MTHFR* 677C>T with overall MTX-induced toxicity [32, 35, 37, 38, 40, 42, 45], whereas three studies found associations with GI toxicity for the CT genotype [42], increased MTX discontinuation because of increased liver enzyme levels for 677 T-allele carriers [39], and overall toxicity [39, 46]. The *MTHFR* 677C>T was found not to be associated with the decrease of disease activity score (DAS), C-reactive protein (CRP) levels and erythrocyte sedimentation rate (ESR) levels in four reports [39, 40, 45, 46], whereas two studies found that patients with the 677CC genotype were more likely to achieve clinical improvement as defined by the decrease of DAS [32, 35].

The results for the *MTHFR* 1298A>C polymorphism are even more conflicting. Two reports found associations with efficacy, but with 1298AA genotypes and a decrease in DAS, which is in contrast to the association of C-allele carriers with decreased CRP and ESR levels (Table 4.2) [32, 46]; yet three reports did not find association of *MTHFR* 1298A>C with efficacy [35, 40, 45].

Regarding toxicity, *MTHFR* 1298 A-allele carriers were related to side-effects in two reports [38, 45]; one group found no association [40], and two groups detected an association between 1298 C-allele carriers with overall toxicity and GI toxicity [32, 35].

Unfortunately, it is difficult to summarize the results of clinical studies when different clinical outcome measures are used (CRP levels, number of swollen joints, DAS). Lack of uniform validated methodology makes meta-analysis impossible. Only two groups performed data analysis from controlled trials with clear end-points and calculated haplotypes (linkage of SNPs) for the *MTHFR* gene [32, 45]. However, different cut-off levels for treatment outcome evaluation and different number of SNPs to design the haplotypes were used. Moreover, the ethnicities differed between these two groups. Since allele frequencies differ among different ethnic groups, any comparison is weak [47].

Based on current data, it is tempting to speculate that *MTHFR* 1298–677 A–C haplotype is favourable for MTX reducing RA disease activity, given the fact that we found an increased likelihood of a decreased DAS with increased number of copies of the haplotype [32]. However, a prospective longitudinal study testing this association of number of copies of the alleles and outcome is needed to strengthen these findings regarding efficacy.

Table 4.2 Pharmacogenetic association studies of methotrexate with treatment outcome in rheumatoid arthritis

Gene	Role in pathways, relation with MTX	SNP	Postulated effect SNP	Clinical effects
MTHFR	Catalyses methylene THF to methyl-THF; indirect target MTX	677C>T	Thermolabile MTHFR with decreased activity and increased homocysteine levels	Increases homocysteine level [42]; no increased homocysteine level [44]; effect on GI toxicity [42]; T-allele associated with increased liver enzyme levels [39]; T-allele associated with toxicity [46]; no association with toxicity [32, 35, 37, 38, 40, 42, 45]; no association with efficacy [39, 40, 45]; association with efficacy [32, 35]
		1298A>C	May further decrease MTHFR activity and increase homocysteine levels	A-allele associated with toxicity [38, 45]; C-allele associated with toxicity and GI toxicity [32, 35]; no association with toxicity [40]; no association with efficacy [35, 40, 45]; association with efficacy [32, 46]
ATIC	Conversion of AICAR to 10-formyl-AICAR; target of polyglutamated MTX	347C>G	May decrease ATIC activity, affect AICAR accumulation and adenosine release	Association with efficacy [33, 37, 51]; no association with efficacy [35]; GG associated with toxicity and GI toxicity [33, 35, 37]; no effect on toxicity [49]
DHFR	Reduction of DHF to THF; target of MTX	−473G>A 35389G>A	Possibly affecting mRNA transcription, affinity of MTX	No effect on efficacy or toxicity [32]
MTHFD1	Catalyses interconversion of 1-carbon derivatives of THF; indirect target MTX	1958G>A	May decrease enzyme activity	AA associated with inefficacy [51]
SHMT1	Catalyses conversion of serine and THF to glycine and methylene-THF; indirect target MTX	1420C>T	May decrease enzyme activity	No association with efficacy [35]; CC associated with efficacy [51]; no association with toxicity [35, 37]; CC associated with alopecia and CNS side-effects [37]
TSER	Enhancer region of TYMS; indirect target of MTX	5′ UTR 28-bp repeat	May increase enzyme activity	No association with efficacy [35, 40, 51]; no association with toxicity [35, 40]; association with toxicity and alopecia [37]
TYMS	Conversion of dUMP to dTMP; target of MTX	3′ UTR 6-bp deletion	May decrease TYMS mRNA stability and expression	May affect MTX efficacy [40]; no effect on efficacy as defined by MTX dose [49]; no effect on toxicity [49]
AMPD1	Conversion of AMP to ADP and ATP; indirect target MTX	34C>T	Decreased enzyme activity, may enhance conversion to adenosine	T-allele associated with efficacy [33, 51]; no association with toxicity [33]

Gene	Function	SNP	Effect	Association
MTR	Methylation of homocysteine to methionine; indirect target MTX	2756A>G	May decrease enzyme activity; increase homocysteine levels	No association with efficacy [33, 35]; AA associated with toxicity [35]; no association with toxicity [33]
MTRR	Methylation of cofactors required for MTR action; indirect target MTX	66A>G	May decrease MTRR activity; increase homocysteine levels	No effect on efficacy [33, 35]; no association with toxicity [33]; association with toxicity [35]
ITPA	Conversion IMP to ITP; indirect target MTX	94C>A	Decreased enzyme activity; may enhance conversion to AMP and adenosine	CC associated with efficacy [33, 51]; association with toxicity [33]
FPGS	Adding polyglutamates to MTX; prolonging cellular retention MTX	1994A>G 114G>A	May affect MTX polyglutamation	No association with efficacy [41]; no association with toxicity [41]
GGH	Conversion of long-chain polyglutamated MTX into short chain by removing polyglutamates	452C>T 16C>T −401C>T	Decreased binding affinity for polyglutamated MTX May affect polyglutamated MTX levels	May affect efficacy [41]; no association with efficacy [51]; no association with toxicity [41] No association with efficacy [35]; May affect efficacy [36]; CC associated with toxicity [35]
ABCB1	Efflux transporter on cells; efflux of MTX	3435C>T	May decrease enzyme expression or mRNA stability; may increase intracellular MTX levels	TT associated with increased MTX dose [49]; T-allele associated with inefficacy [50]
RFC	Folate entry in the cell	80G>A	May affect transcriptional activity and increased MTX entry in the cell	No effect efficacy as defined by MTX dose [49]; no association with efficacy [32, 35]; no association with toxicity [32, 35, 49]

In addition, only a number of MTX-induced side-effects are supposed to be folate pathway enzyme dependent, for example GI effects [6]. Thus, it may be that the current associations between *MTHFR* and toxicity are flawed findings: increased efficacy through the inhibition of folate pathway enzymes may only lead to increased side-effects which are related to the inhibition of these enzymes. Moreover, folic acid reduces MTX-induced side-effects [48], whereas concomitant non-steroidal anti-inflammatory drug (NSAID) use is likely to increase toxicity. Additionally, the lack of objective measures to evaluate toxicity may lead to further confounding. These differences may be the explanation for the conflicting associations of *MTHFR* with toxicity.

Only one group tested *MTHFR* haplotypes with toxicity, but in a population not 100% supplemented with folic acid [45]. Then again, if efficacy and toxicity are positively associated to some extent, our group would have found increased toxicity in responders to MTX, which was not detected [32]. Therefore, future association analysis of *MTHFR* haplotypes and side-effects, which are most likely to be related to folate pathway enzymes, should preferably be carried out in patients receiving folic acid supplementation.

Interestingly, an additional number of SNPs in the purine and pyrimidine synthesis pathway, in addition to one drug efflux transporter, have been associated with MTX efficacy (Table 4.2) [33, 35, 40, 41, 49–51]. However, nearly all results were single reports concerning MTX response. Only ATIC and P-glycoprotein (*ABCB1* gene) have been positively associated with efficacy in two independent studies [33, 37, 49, 50]. In contrast, Dervieux *et al.* [35] found no association of ATIC with efficacy. Furthermore, the positive association of *ABCB1* gene and MTX inefficacy has only been established in cross-sectional study designs [49, 50]. Therefore, current results should be regarded as preliminary data.

The relation of serine hydroxymethyltransferase (*SHMT1*) polymorphism with MTX efficacy is conflicting in two studies; Dervieux *et al.* [35] found an association with response, whereas we did not [51]. Additionally, so far there is no evidence from single or multiple studies that purine and pyrimidine enzymes dihydrofolate reductase (*DHFR*), reduced folate carrier (*RFC1*), thymidylate synthetase enhancer region (*TSER*), 5-methyltetrahydrofolate–homocysteine methyltransferase (*MTR*), 5-methyltetrahydrofolate–homocysteine methyltransferase reductase (*MTRR*) or folylpoly-glutamate synthetase (*FPGS*) polymorphisms are related to MTX efficacy in patients with RA [32, 33, 35, 40, 41, 49, 51].

Our group identified the association of ATIC polymorphism in combination with adenosine monophosphate deaminase (*AMPD1*), inosine triphosphatase (*ITPA*) and methylenetetrahydrofolate dehydrogenase (*MTHFD1*) polymorphisms with MTX response. Next, we developed a pharmacogenetic model in combination with clinical factors to predict MTX efficacy in recent-onset RA [51]. This concept is appealing because this model predicts MTX efficacy before starting treatment with baseline variables only. In this study it was found that the clinical factors gender, rheumatoid factor combined with smoking status and disease activity at baseline were predictive for MTX response. The prediction resulted in the classification of 60% of the patients with RA into MTX responders and non-responders, with 95% and 86% as true positive and negative response rates, respectively. Evaluation of this predictive model in a second group of 38 patients with RA supported our results. Although this is an important first step in the use of pharmacogenetics in complex traits, this model needs further prospective validation and refinements before it can be used in clinical practice.

Regarding MTX-induced toxicity, to date no associations exist between numerous polymorphisms in the purine and pyrimidine pathway enzymes, including thymidylate synthetase (*TYMS*), DHFR AMPD1, ITPA, MTHFD1, ABCB1, FPGS and RFC1 genes, and the occurrence of side-effects in patients with RA (Table 4.2). Only ATIC GG genotyped patients have been associated in three independent studies with toxicity, especially GI toxicity [33, 35, 37], although one group could not detect an association between ATIC and side-effects [49]. This discrepancy may be because of different ethnicities in these studies.

In addition, two groups found no relationship between *SHMT1* polymorphism and overall MTX-induced side-effects [35, 37], whereas Weisman *et al.* did establish an association between the CC genotype and specific side-effects such as MTX-induced alopecia and central nervous side-effects [37].

The results for the polymorphisms in the genes γ-glutamyl hydrolase (*GGH*), *MTR*, *MTRR* and *TSER* have been conflicting, with one study detecting a positive association between the polymorphism under study and toxicity, and at least one study finding no association [33, 35, 37, 40, 41]. Different methods and cut-off levels for the detection and definition of side-effects is probably the main reason for these disparate results.

In a number of reports, a combination of supposed risk genotypes in the purine and pyrimidine pathway were related to MTX efficacy and toxicity [34, 37]. These studies used a different approach to analyse the association of genetic variants with MTX toxicity. In these studies, composite mutation indexes were calculated via grouping of different risk genotypes. First, these authors use different outcome measures and different composite mutation indexes, which hamper the comparison of their results. Importantly, the calculation of the pharmacogenetic index is based on the assumption that the contribution of every polymorphism is small, but that every risk genotype affects the response in the same direction with an equal, additive value. However, to date there are no facts to support this assumption. Although polygenic analysis in relation to treatment outcome is advocated, it is difficult to imagine, with limited biological plausibility, that SNPs in different genes contribute to the same extent to treatment outcome.

Pharmacogenetic studies related to the complex biologic milieu in which MTX interacts involve studies with the human leucocyte antigen (HLA) genes. Many hypotheses have been proposed concerning the role of HLA alleles in RA. However, none of the hypotheses is accepted unanimously. The so-called shared epitope (SE) hypothesis proposes that a common peptide sequence (encoded by DRB1 0101, 0102, 0401, 0404, 0405, 0408, 1001, 1402) in the antigen presentation binding groove of HLA class II molecule is involved in the presentation of arthritogenic peptides. The presence of SE alleles has been associated with more severe RA and the SE is probably also a risk factor for anti-cyclic citrullinated peptide (anti-CCP)-positive RA [13, 52]. Since anti-CCP antibodies are highly specific for RA and have been associated with RA susceptibility and severity, it may be that anti-CCP positivity and/or SE positivity encode for a distinct group of patients with RA who may respond differently to treatment.

Only three groups have studied the contribution of the number of SE copies in relation to MTX outcome. No association of the number of SE copies with MTX efficacy as defined by a 50% disease activity reduction (ACR50, American College of Rheumatology [ACR] criteria) was found in one study [53]. In contrast, others showed that patients with MTX monotherapy were less likely to carry a SE allele when compared with patients requiring combination strategy [54]. In addition, patients were less likely to achieve 50% disease activity reduction (ACR50) if they were DR4/DR1 positive than if they were DR4/DR1-negative [55].

Recently, an association between MTX and HLA-G antigens, defined as non-classical major histocompatibility complex (MHC) class Ib molecules important for maintaining anti-inflammatory conditions, was found in an *ex vivo* study [56]. The HLA-G 14 basepair (bp) deletion is thought to increase HLA-G mRNA and protein stability, possibly leading to prolonged anti-inflammatory actions. Therefore, MTX may act synergistically with this deletion. It was shown that MTX induces soluble HLA-G, whereas a homozygous deletion of 14bp in this HLA gene was more frequently detected in patients with response to MTX.

So far, no convincing data are available to support the hypothesis that patients with poor prognostic genetic factors at disease onset such as DR4/DR1 positivity should not start with MTX monotherapy. However, we found that rheumatoid factor-positive patients are less likely to respond to MTX [51], and several studies show an association between rheumatoid factor positivity, anti-CCP positivity and SE positivity in patients with RA [52, 57]. Since these later factors distinguish patients with severe RA or even may distinguish patients with a different disease, it is currently unclear whether patients with these poor prognostic factors show less responsiveness to therapy because of poor pharmacogenetic factors or show a poor response because of a different underlying pathogenesis.

PHARMACOGENETICS OF BIOLOGICAL AGENTS

Infliximab, adalimumab and etanercept are currently available biologicals directed against TNF-α. This proinflammatory cytokine regulates monocyte and dendritic cell activation, endothelial cell adhesiveness, the organization of the lymphoid tissues, and collaboration in the induction of the acute-phase reaction. The anti-TNF-α blocker etanercept is a soluble TNF-α receptor fusion protein, whereas infliximab and adalimumab are antibodies directed against both membrane-bound and soluble TNF-α.

Surprisingly, several studies have revealed that failure to respond to TNF-α-blocking drugs is not a generic class effect in patients with RA, but instead is related to the individual drug [58, 59], which makes a general effect of anti-TNF-α blockers less likely. Therefore, pharmacogenetic results are presented in Table 4.3 with annotation of the specific anti-TNF-α blocking agent.

In theory, the cellular amount of TNF-α and, thus, the amount available for inhibition by anti-TNF-α drugs, might depend on the genotype on the *TNF* gene [60]. Therefore, owing to their mechanism of action, the dose of the anti-TNF-α agent should be considered when interpreting pharmacogenetic studies. However, most pharmacogenetic studies concerning anti-TNF-α agents were not performed in controlled trials and did not take into account in their analyses the potential role of TNF-α levels and the drug dose. Finally, the *TNF* gene has been mapped to the MHC class III region in the human genome, in the proximity to the *HLA-B* and the MHC Class II DR genes. Interestingly, this region has been associated with the susceptibility to RA and with the severity of RA disease. Notably, the association between several polymorphisms in this region has to be considered in interpreting anti-TNF-α treatment response associations. Given these facts, it may not be surprising that current pharmacogenetic studies with anti-TNF-α agents have yielded mixed results (Table 4.3).

The polymorphism in TNF promoter SNP −308A>G is one of the most broadly studied variations in *TNF* gene (Table 4.3). Most studies could not reveal an association between infliximab and etanercept efficacy with this polymorphism, whereas three studies have found a positive association between the GG genotype and infliximab efficacy [61–63]. In contrast, infliximab inefficacy has been related to IL-1 receptor antagonist and TNF-α soluble receptor type II polymorphisms [64, 65], whereas for etanercept only the association of TNF-α soluble receptor type II was associated with inefficacy (Table 4.3). Three studies have established positive associations with etanercept efficacy; TNF-α −857 T-allele carriers [66], HLA-DRB1 allele carriers [53] and patients with the IL-10 microsatellite R3 were likely to have more benefit from etanercept [67]. However, two additional independent studies could not detect associations between etanercept and other polymorphisms in the TNF promoter gene [53, 68]. In addition, the association of the HLA-DRB1 allele with efficacy has not been confirmed [66, 68] and one other group has found no association between the IL-10 gene −1087G>A polymorphism and etanercept efficacy [68].

Apart from anti-TNF-α neutralizing properties, anti-TNF-α blocking agents may, hypothetically, exert effects via their IgG1 Fc fragments, for example by complement activation and binding to cellular Fcγ receptors (FcγR) [69], or induction of apoptosis in synovial macrophages by ligation of the low-affinity FcγR type IIIA. However, Kastbom *et al.* [69] did not find any significant effects of FcγR IIIA −158V>F on the efficacy of infliximab and etanercept. In contrast, Tutuncu *et al.* [70] observed increased efficacy in patients with the −158 FF genotype.

In summary, there is no consensus on the role of polymorphisms in candidate or pathway genes on anti-TNF-α treatment response, and further studies are required in order to replicate and establish true associations [71]. From the studies that have been published, no conclusions can be made on the potential utility of genotyping for TNF, the HLA-DRB1 shared epitope or other genes to predict treatment outcome in patients with RA who are treated with these biological agents.

To date, genetic information has no established value with respect to RA treatment. Several studies showed that genetic variants affect treatment outcome. However, the understanding of the role of genes in response to therapy has only just begun. Unfortunately, currently available pharmacogenetic data are inconclusive and require more confirmation in controlled trials.

FUTURE RESEARCH PERSPECTIVES

The challenge for the coming years will be the identification of genes, polymorphisms and other biological markers that are relevant to the clinical response to DMARDs. In the near future, epidemiological research, gene expression analyses and proteomic methods (in target tissues) with developing statistical models are likely to be important for studies aiming to reveal multiple factors for drug response [20, 29].

The next step will be the prospective clinical replication and validation of factors linked to treatment outcome. These analyses require large multicentre clinical trials of uniformly treated and systematically characterized patients, with well-validated clinical readouts and sophisticated (bioinformatic) analyses. Only uniformly treated and systematically evaluated patients are suitable to detect factors and quantify drug response objectively, because effect sizes tend to be small in complex diseases [72]. In this respect, biobanks systematically collecting biological material, such as DNA, and information from a large number of people may represent an ideal resource [73].

Several recommendations can be made for conducting studies to develop polygenetic models for drug response [73, 74]. First, and most importantly, the SNPs in candidate genes should be documented as being functionally relevant through results from *in vitro* or animal studies. In addition, the genes under study should cover various aspects of the pharmacology of DMARDs and the complex biological environment in which these drugs interact – including receptors, enzymes, transporters and immunomodulators. If exploratory whole-genome analysis is applied, high-density arrays are preferred and single marker and at least haplotypes (the linkage between markers) should be tested for associations with the clinical phenotype. Since this approach is hypothesis generating, the detected association needs to be tested in a second independent group of patients. In such a study design, *P*-value cut-offs may be less strict than with the use of the Bonferroni correction, especially when biological plausibility of the candidate SNPs is obtained through gene expression and/or *in vitro* functionality analysis.

Second, a key step in any clinical pharmacogenetic study is the precise definition of responders, non-responders and toxic responders (or various clinical phenotypes). In such studies, clear validated clinical end-points to define groups of patients such as the DAS and radiographic progression (for example Sharp–van der Heijde score) are preferred over biomarkers and surrogate end-points such as CRP levels.

Third, neglecting the impact of non-genetic factors on drug response will lead to confounded associations. Therefore, disease characteristics and demographic and environmental factors should be considered as co-variates for response, as well as drug exposure and compliance, in order to reduce the 'noise' in the data [30]. Co-variates likely to influence RA treatment outcome are gender, smoking status, rheumatoid factor and the presence of anti-CCP antibodies.

Table 4.3 Pharmacogenetic association studies of anti-TNF-α agents and their efficacy of treatment in rheumatoid arthritis

Gene	Function	SNP	Postulated effect SNP	Clinical effects
TNF-α	TNF-α production and regulation	−308 G>A promoter region	May increase transcriptional activity; may increase TNF-α levels	GG associated with efficacy of INF [61–63]; no effect on efficacy of INF [64, 80]; no effect on efficacy of ETA [53, 66, 68]; GA associated with increased TNF-α levels after INF [80]
		−857C>T, promoter region	See above	T-allele associated with efficacy of ETA [66]
		−863C>A, promoter region	See above	No effect on efficacy of ETA [66]
		−238G>A, promoter region	See above	No effect on efficacy of ETA [53, 66]; no effect on efficacy of INF [64]
		−1031T>C promoter region	See above	No effect on efficacy of ETA [66]
		+488 intronic region	Unknown	No effect on efficacy of ETA [53]
		+2018	Unknown	No effect on efficacy of INF [64]
TNFRSF1	TNF-α soluble receptor type I	−609 −580 −383	May affect TNF-α binding	No effect on efficacy of ETA [53]
TNFRSF2	TNF-α soluble receptor type II	196G>T	May increase interleukin 6 production and affect TNF-α binding	No effect on efficacy of ETA [53]; GG associated with inefficacy of ETA and INF [65]
TNF-α/β microsatellites	Linked to TNF-α 308 polymorphism	A,b,c,d,e	May influence TNF-α levels; increased RA susceptibility risk	No effect on efficacy of ETA [53]; TNF-α11 and β4 haplotype associated with efficacy of INF [81]

Factor	Function	SNP/variant	Effect	Effect on efficacy
Lymphotoxin α (LTA)	Mediation of inflammatory actions	+177A>G, +319C>A, +249, +365, +720	Exhibits pro-inflammatory effects	No effect on efficacy of ETA [66]; No effect on efficacy of ETA [53]
HLA DRB1, DRQ1 alleles (SE)	Antigen-presenting molecules	See references	May affect anti-TNF-α efficacy; associated with increased susceptibility to and severity of RA	No effect on efficacy of INF [64, 81]; HLA-DBRB1 associated with efficacy of ETA [53]; no effect on efficacy of ETA [66, 68]
Fcγ receptor polymorphisms	Influence cell activation, apoptosis. Indirect target anti-TNF	131H/R (FcγRIIa), 176F/V (FcγRIIIa), NA1/NA2 (FcγRIIIb), -158V/F (FcγIIIa)	May affect IgG Fc binding affinity	No effect on efficacy of ETA [53]; No effect on efficacy of ETA and INF [69]; FF associated with efficacy of all three anti-TNF agents [70]
Interleukin 10 (IL-10)	Anti-inflammatory cytokine	-1087G>A, Several microsatellites, see reference	GG associated with increased anti-inflammatory response	No effect on efficacy of ETA [68]; IL-10-R3 and haplotype IL-10 R3-R9 associated with efficacy of ETA [67]
Interleukin 1 (IL-1)	Proinflammatory cytokine	IL-1β +3954C>T	May affect inflammatory response	No effect on efficacy of INF [64]
IL-1 receptor antagonist	Inhibits action of interleukin 1	IL-1-RN +2018T>C	May affect inflammatory response	C-allele associated with inefficacy of INF [64]

ETA, etancercept; HLA, human leucocyte antigen; IgG, immunoglobulin G; INF, infliximab; SNP, single nucleotide polymorphism; TNF, tumour necrosis factor.

Fourth, multicentre pharmacogenetic collaborations should lead to large patient populations with adequate power to detect small but significant differences, assuming that the method used to adjust for multiple testing can be agreed [30]. The interpretation of associations resulting from such larger collaborations needs to consider the genetic variation between racial and ethnic groups.

Given that genetic factors need to be put into perspective, the additional challenge is to assess the added clinical and economic value of genetic testing in drug therapy. Obviously, this added value is a complex question that relates not only to the cost of genetic testing itself but also to the costs such as the long-term effects of a patient with delayed successful treatment. General characteristics that will enhance cost- effectiveness of pharmacogenetic testing have already been defined [30, 73]. These critical factors are the avoidance of severe clinical or economic consequences through the use of a test, the difficulty in monitoring drug response with current methods, the lack of an alternative drug with equivalent therapeutic profile and price, the existence of a well-established association between genotype and clinical phenotype and a high prevalence of the relevant allelic variant in the target population. Clearly, a number of these characteristics apply to rheumatological disease. As a final point, the additional value of pharmacogenetic testing may only be present if other effective interventions are implemented as far as practicable. For example, it is essential to refer patients with inflammatory arthritis early for a rheumatological opinion in order to achieve optimal clinical outcome [75].

FUTURE CLINICAL IMPLICATIONS

Personalized therapy, even based on easily determined patient characteristics such as age or renal function, has not yet been widely embraced in medical care [28]. As a result, the choice of drug and course of therapy is currently made empirically for the majority of drugs. Pharmacogenetic testing is a new method to tailor therapy. Thus, even if there is indisputable evidence of allelic variants influencing DMARD response, introduction of pharmacogenetic testing in daily clinical practice may prove to be a challenge.

Furthermore, clinical pharmacogenetics requires an interpretation of genotypes, which will probably require education to apply this new knowledge in practice [20]. Information explaining the outcomes of the pharmacogenetic test and an agreed policy on further choices in drug therapy should be available for healthcare providers to assist them in making an informed choice with pharmacogenetic information [30, 73]. In addition, the genetic test itself needs to be widely available and the technique has to be reliable, simple, precise, valid and inexpensive to facilitate the clinical application and its usefulness in medical decision-making [74].

Improving and/or personalizing therapy involves complete 'patient profiling'. Therapy should aim to improve a patient's general well-being, meaning that co-morbidity also needs to be considered [76]. Accordingly, a clinical pharmacogenetic test should ideally provide information on numerous allelic variants for different DMARDs and should address the numerous relevant clinical conditions of the target population. For example, a pharmacogenetic test for the RA population may involve factors important for DMARD response in addition to factors contributing to drug responses in the treatment of pain, osteoporosis and cardiovascular disease.

Moreover, patients want to be informed about medications and alternative options in order to feel competent to participate in medical decisions [77, 78]. Although the reasons behind and the extent of patients' desire for information may differ among patients, patients' involvement in medical decisions ensures healthcare quality. Therefore, special attention to educating and informing patients regarding the use of pharmacogenetic information in order to choose or adjust therapy is necessary.

Even with these barriers to the clinical application of pharmacogenetics, in the future it may be considered unethical not to carry out a pharmacogenetic test to avoid exposing individuals to drugs or doses that could be ineffective or harmful to them [79].

CONCLUSION

Rheumatoid arthritis is a syndrome with a broad spectrum of clinical manifestations and no single therapeutic intervention is expected to provide the best answer for all patients [14]. As a consequence, it is important to consider subtle differences between patients with RA when conducting and interpreting pharmacogenetic studies.

The first steps have been taken to detect genetic variants that contribute to DMARD response, but currently available pharmacogenetic data are inconclusive, which does not allow us to draw clearcut conclusions about the relationship between genotype and treatment outcome. Therefore, genetic information as yet has no established value with respect to RA treatment. Nevertheless, current results hold the promise that pharmacogenetics has the potential to increase DMARD efficacy and to reduce adverse events. As discussed, the challenge in the future is to detect more factors that are important for DMARD treatment response, and to replicate and prospectively validate pharmacogenetics in large studies before the current results can be used in clinical practice.

Personalized medical care based on pharmacogenetic testing is, as yet, developing in common complex traits such as RA. However, in the near future its application might be of great clinical benefit for individual patients.

REFERENCES

1. Symmons DP. Epidemiology of rheumatoid arthritis: determinants of onset, persistence and outcome. *Best Pract Res Clin Rheumatol* 2002; 16:707–722.
2. Welsing PM, Landewe RB, van Riel PL, Boers M, van Gestel AM, van der LS *et al.* The relationship between disease activity and radiologic progression in patients with rheumatoid arthritis: a longitudinal analysis. *Arthritis Rheum* 2004; 50:2082–2093.
3. O'Dell JR. Drug therapy – therapeutic strategies for rheumatoid arthritis. *N Engl J Med* 2004; 350:2591–2602.
4. Mottonen T, Hannonen P, Korpela M, Nissila M, Kautiainen H, Ilonen J *et al.* Delay to institution of therapy and induction of remission using single-drug or combination-disease-modifying antirheumatic drug therapy in early rheumatoid arthritis. *Arthritis Rheum* 2002; 46:894–898.
5. Guidelines for the management of rheumatoid arthritis: 2002 update. *Arthritis Rheum* 2002; 46:328–346.
6. Cronstein BN. Low-dose methotrexate: a mainstay in the treatment of rheumatoid arthritis. *Pharmacol Rev* 2005; 57:163–172.
7. Aletaha D, Smolen JS. The rheumatoid arthritis patient in the clinic: comparing more than 1,300 consecutive DMARD courses. *Rheumatology* (Oxford) 2002; 41:1367–1374.
8. O'Dell JR, Haire CE, Erikson N, Drymalski W, Palmer W, Eckhoff PJ *et al.* Treatment of rheumatoid arthritis with methotrexate alone, sulfasalazine and hydroxychloroquine, or a combination of all three medications. *N Engl J Med* 1996; 334:1287–1291.
9. Mottonen T, Hannonen P, Leirisalo-Repo M, Nissila M, Kautiainen H, Korpela M *et al.* Comparison of combination therapy with single-drug therapy in early rheumatoid arthritis: a randomised trial. FIN-RACo trial group. *Lancet* 1999; 353:1568–1573.
10. Bathon JM, Martin RW, Fleischmann RM, Tesser JR, Schiff MH, Keystone EC *et al.* A comparison of etanercept and methotrexate in patients with early rheumatoid arthritis. *N Engl J Med* 2000; 343:1586–1593.
11. Keystone EC, Kavanaugh AF, Sharp JT, Tannenbaum H, Hua Y, Teoh LS *et al.* Radiographic, clinical, and functional outcomes of treatment with adalimumab (a human anti-tumor necrosis factor monoclonal antibody) in patients with active rheumatoid arthritis receiving concomitant methotrexate therapy: a randomized, placebo-controlled, 52-week trial. *Arthritis Rheum* 2004; 50:1400–1411.

12. Moreland LW, Baumgartner SW, Schiff MH, Tindall EA, Fleischmann RM, Weaver AL *et al.* Treatment of rheumatoid arthritis with a recombinant human tumor necrosis factor receptor (p75)-Fc fusion protein. *N Engl J Med* 1997; 337:141–147.

13. Wesoly J, Wessels JA, Guchelaar HJ, Huizinga TW. Genetic markers of treatment response in rheumatoid arthritis. *Curr Rheumatol Rep* 2006; 8:369–377.

14. Strand V, Kimberly R, Isaacs JD. Biologic therapies in rheumatology: lessons learned, future directions. *Nat Rev Drug Discov* 2007; 6:75–92.

15. Kremer JM, Westhovens R, Leon M, Di Giorgio E, Alten R, Steinfeld S *et al.* Treatment of rheumatoid arthritis by selective inhibition of T-cell activation with fusion protein CTLA4Ig. *N Engl J Med* 2003; 349:1907–1915.

16. Edwards JC, Szczepanski L, Szechinski J, Filipowicz-Sosnowska A, Emery P, Close DR *et al.* Efficacy of B-cell-targeted therapy with rituximab in patients with rheumatoid arthritis. *N Engl J Med* 2004; 350:2572–2581.

17. Breedveld FC, Weisman MH, Kavanaugh AF, Cohen SB, Pavelka K, van Vollenhoven R *et al.* The PREMIER study: a multicenter, randomized, double-blind clinical trial of combination therapy with adalimumab plus methotrexate versus methotrexate alone or adalimumab alone in patients with early, aggressive rheumatoid arthritis who had not had previous methotrexate treatment. *Arthritis Rheum* 2006; 54:26–37.

18. Maetzel A, Wong A, Strand V, Tugwell P, Wells G, Bombardier C. Meta-analysis of treatment termination rates among rheumatoid arthritis patients receiving disease-modifying anti-rheumatic drugs. *Rheumatology* 2000; 39:975–981.

19. Evans WE, McLeod HL. Pharmacogenomics – drug disposition, drug targets, and side effects. *N Engl J Med* 2003; 348:538–549.

20. Roden DM, Altman RB, Benowitz NL, Flockhart DA, Giacomini KM, Johnson JA *et al.* Pharmacogenomics: challenges and opportunities. *Ann Intern Med* 2006; 145:749–757.

21. Senn S. Individual response to treatment: is it a valid assumption? *BMJ* 2004; 329:966–968.

22. www.emea.europa.eu (Accessed 25 January 2007. Establish definitions for genomic biomarkers, pharmacogenomics, pharmacogenetics, genomic data and sample coding categories. ICH Topic E 15 (CHMP/ICH/437986/2006).http://www.hc-sc.gc.ca/dhp-mps/alt_formats/hpfb-dgpsa/pdf/prodpharma/e15_step2_etape2_e.pdf.

23. Stranger BE, Forrest MS, Dunning M, Ingle CE, Beazley C, Thorne N *et al.* Relative impact of nucleotide and copy number variation on gene expression phenotypes. *Science* 2007; 315:848–853.

24. Storey JD, Tibshirani R. Statistical significance for genome wide studies. *Proc Natl Acad Sci USA* 2003; 100:9440–9445.

25. Bland JM, Altman DG. Multiple significance tests: the Bonferroni method. *BMJ* 1995; 310:170.

26. Perneger TV. What's wrong with Bonferroni adjustments. *BMJ* 1998; 316:1236–1238.

27. Pfeiffer RM, Gail MH. Sample size calculations for population- and family-based case–control association studies on marker genotypes. *Genet Epidemiol* 2003; 25:136–148.

28. Evans WE, Relling MV. Moving towards individualized medicine with pharmacogenomics. *Nature* 2004; 429:464–468.

29. Eichelbaum M, Ingelman-Sundberg M, Evans WE. Pharmacogenomics and individualized drug therapy. *Annu Rev Med* 2006; 57:119–137.

30. Tucker G. Pharmacogenetics – expectations and reality. *BMJ* 2004; 329(7456):4–6.

31. Cutolo M, Sulli A, Pizzorni C, Seriolo B, Straub RH. Anti-inflammatory mechanisms of methotrexate in rheumatoid arthritis. *Ann Rheum Dis* 2001; 60:729–735.

32. Wessels JA, Vries-Bouwstra JK, Heijmans BT, Slagboom PE, Goekoop-Ruiterman YP, Allaart CF *et al.* Efficacy and toxicity of methotrexate in early rheumatoid arthritis are associated with single-nucleotide polymorphisms in genes coding for folate pathway enzymes. *Arthritis Rheum* 2006; 54:1087–1095.

33. Wessels JA, Kooloos WM, Jonge RD, Vries-Bouwstra JK, Allaart CF, Linssen A *et al.* Relationship between genetic variants in the adenosine pathway and outcome of methotrexate treatment in patients with recent-onset rheumatoid arthritis. *Arthritis Rheum* 2006; 54:2830–2839.

34. Dervieux T, Furst D, Orentas Lein D, Capps R, Smith K, Caldwell J *et al.* Pharmacogenetic and metabolite measurements are associated with clinical status in rheumatoid arthritis patients treated with methotrexate: results of a multicentred cross sectional observational study. *Ann Rheum Dis* 2005; 64:1180–1185.

35. Dervieux T, Greenstein N, Kremer J. Pharmacogenomic and metabolic biomarkers in the folate pathway and their association with methotrexate effects during dosage escalation in rheumatoid arthritis. *Arthritis Rheum* 2006; 54:3095–3103.

36. Dervieux T, Kremer J, Lein DO, Capps R, Barham R, Meyer G *et al.* Contribution of common polymorphisms in reduced folate carrier and gamma-glutamylhydrolase to methotrexate polyglutamate levels in patients with rheumatoid arthritis. *Pharmacogenetics* 2004; 14:733–739.

37. Weisman MH, Furst DE, Park GS, Kremer JM, Smith KM, Wallace DJ *et al.* Risk genotypes in folate-dependent enzymes and their association with methotrexate-related side effects in rheumatoid arthritis. *Arthritis Rheum* 2006; 54:607–612.

38. Berkun Y, Levartovsky D, Rubinow A, Orbach H, Aamar S, Grenader T *et al.* Methotrexate related adverse effects in patients with rheumatoid arthritis are associated with the A1298C polymorphism of the MTHFR gene. *Ann Rheum Dis* 2004; 63:1227–1231.

39. van Ede AE, Laan RF, Blom HJ, Huizinga TW, Haagsma CJ, Giesendorf BA *et al.* The C677T mutation in the methylenetetrahydrofolate reductase gene: a genetic risk factor for methotrexate-related elevation of liver enzymes in rheumatoid arthritis patients. *Arthritis Rheum* 2001; 44:2525–2530.

40. Kumagai K, Hiyama K, Oyama T, Maeda H, Kohno N. Polymorphisms in the thymidylate synthase and methylenetetrahydrofolate reductase genes and sensitivity to the low-dose methotrexate therapy in patients with rheumatoid arthritis. *Int J Mol Med* 2003; 11:593–600.

41. van der Straaten R, Wessels JA, Vries-Bouwstra JK, Goekoop-Ruiterman YP, Allaart CF, Bogaartz J *et al.* Exploratory analysis of four polymorphisms in human GGH and FPGS genes and their effect in methotrexate-treated rheumatoid arthritis patients. *Pharmacogenomics* 2007; 8:141–150.

42. Haagsma CJ, Blom HJ, van Riel PLCM, van't Hof MA, Giesendorf BAJ, Oppenraaij-Emmerzaal D *et al.* Influence of sulphasalazine, methotrexate, and the combination of both on plasma homocysteine concentrations in patients with rheumatoid arthritis. *Ann Rheum Dis* 1999; 58:79–84.

43. Ranganathan P, McLeod HL. Methotrexate pharmacogenetics: the first step toward individualized therapy in rheumatoid arthritis. *Arthritis Rheum* 2006; 54:1366–1377.

44. van Ede AE, Laan RF, Blom HJ, Boers GH, Haagsma CJ, Thomas CM *et al.* Homocysteine and folate status in methotrexate-treated patients with rheumatoid arthritis. *Rheumatology* (Oxford) 2002; 41:658–665.

45. Hughes LB, Beasley TM, Patel H, Tiwari HK, Morgan SL, Baggott JE *et al.* Racial/ethnic differences in allele frequencies of single nucleotide polymorphisms in the methylenetetrahydrofolate reductase gene and their influence on response to methotrexate in rheumatoid arthritis. *Ann Rheum Dis* 2006; 65:1213–1218.

46. Urano W, Taniguchi A, Yamanaka H, Tanaka E, Nakajima H, Matsuda Y *et al.* Polymorphisms in the methylenetetrahydrofolate reductase gene were associated with both the efficacy and the toxicity of methotrexate used for the treatment of rheumatoid arthritis, as evidenced by single locus and haplotype analyses. *Pharmacogenetics* 2002; 12:183–190.

47. Ranganathan P, Culverhouse R, Marsh S, Ahluwalia R, Shannon WD, Eisen S *et al.* Single nucleotide polymorphism profiling across the methotrexate pathway in normal subjects and patients with rheumatoid arthritis. *Pharmacogenomics* 2004; 5:559–569.

48. van Ede AE, Laan RF, Rood MJ, Huizinga TW, van de Laar MA, van Denderen CJ *et al.* Effect of folic or folinic acid supplementation on the toxicity and efficacy of methotrexate in rheumatoid arthritis: a forty-eight week, multicenter, randomized, double-blind, placebo-controlled study. *Arthritis Rheum* 2001; 44:1515–1524.

49. Takatori R, Takahashi KA, Tokunaga D, Hojo T, Fujioka M, Asano T *et al.* ABCB1 C3435T polymorphism influences methotrexate sensitivity in rheumatoid arthritis patients. *Clin Exp Rheumatol* 2006; 24:546–554.

50. Drozdzik M, Rudas T, Pawlik A, Kurzawski M, Czerny B, Gornik W *et al.* The effect of 3435C>T MDR1 gene polymorphism on rheumatoid arthritis treatment with disease-modifying antirheumatic drugs. *Eur J Clin Pharmacol* 2006; 62:933–937.

51. Wessels JA, van der Kooij SM, le Cessie S, Kievit W, Barerra P, Allaart CF *et al.* A clinical pharmacogenetic model to predict the efficacy of methotrexate monotherapy in recent-onset rheumatoid arthritis. *Arthritis Rheum* 2007; 56:1765–1775.

52. van der Helm-van Mil AH, Verpoort KN, Breedveld FC, Huizinga TW, Toes RE, de Vries RR. The HLA-DRB1 shared epitope alleles are primarily a risk factor for anti-cyclic citrullinated peptide antibodies and are not an independent risk factor for development of rheumatoid arthritis. *Arthritis Rheum* 2006; 54:1117–1121.

53. Criswell LA, Lum RF, Turner KN, Woehl B, Zhu Y, Wang J et al. The influence of genetic variation in the HLA-DRB1 and LTA-TNF regions on the response to treatment of early rheumatoid arthritis with methotrexate or etanercept. *Arthritis Rheum* 2004; 50:2750–2756.

54. Gonzalez-Gay MA, Hajeer AH, Garcia-Porrua C, Dababneh A, Thomson W, Ollier WE et al. Patients chosen for treatment with cyclosporine because of severe rheumatoid arthritis are more likely to carry HLA-DRB1 shared epitope alleles, and have earlier disease onset. *J Rheumatol* 2002; 29:271–275.

55. Ferraccioli GF, Gremese E, Tomietto P, Favret G, Damato R, Di Poi E. Analysis of improvements, full responses, remission and toxicity in rheumatoid patients treated with step-up combination therapy (methotrexate, cyclosporin A, sulphasalazine) or monotherapy for three years. *Rheumatology* (Oxford) 2002; 41:892–898.

56. Rizzo R, Rubini M, Govoni M, Padovan M, Melchiorri L, Stignani M et al. HLA-G 14-bp polymorphism regulates the methotrexate response in rheumatoid arthritis. *Pharmacogenet Genomics* 2006; 16:615–623.

57. Klareskog L, Stolt P, Lundberg K, Kallberg H, Bengtsson C, Grunewald J et al. A new model for an etiology of rheumatoid arthritis: smoking may trigger HLA-DR (shared epitope)-restricted immune reactions to autoantigens modified by citrullination. *Arthritis Rheum* 2006; 54:38–46.

58. Cohen G, Courvoisier N, Cohen JD, Zaltni S, Sany J, Combe B. The efficiency of switching from infliximab to etanercept and vice-versa in patients with rheumatoid arthritis. *Clin Exp Rheumatol* 2005; 23:795–800.

59. Nikas SN, Voulgari PV, Alamanos Y, Papadopoulos CG, Venetsanopoulou AI, Georgiadis AN et al. Efficacy and safety of switching from infliximab to adalimumab: a comparative controlled study. *Ann Rheum Dis* 2006; 65:257–260.

60. Bayley JP, Ottenhoff TH, Verweij CL. Is there a future for TNF promoter polymorphisms? *Genes Immun* 2004; 5:315–329.

61. Mugnier B, Balandraud N, Darque A, Roudier C, Roudier J, Reviron D. Polymorphism at position –308 of the tumor necrosis factor alpha gene influences outcome of infliximab therapy in rheumatoid arthritis. *Arthritis Rheum* 2003; 48:1849–1852.

62. Fonseca JE, Carvalho T, Cruz M, Nero P, Sobral M, Mourao AF et al. Polymorphism at position –308 of the tumour necrosis factor alpha gene and rheumatoid arthritis pharmacogenetics. *Ann Rheum Dis* 2005; 64:793–794.

63. Seitz M, Wirthmuller U, Moller B, Villiger PM. The –308 tumour necrosis factor-alpha gene polymorphism predicts therapeutic response to TNFalpha-blockers in rheumatoid arthritis and spondyloarthritis patients. *Rheumatology* (Oxford) 2007; 46:93–96.

64. Marotte H, Pallot-Prades B, Grange L, Tebib J, Gaudin P, Alexandre C et al. The shared epitope is a marker of severity associated with selection for, but not with response to, infliximab in a large rheumatoid arthritis population. *Ann Rheum Dis* 2006; 65:342–347.

65. Fabris M, Tolusso B, Di Poi E, Assaloni R, Sinigaglia L, Ferraccioli G. Tumor necrosis factor-alpha receptor II polymorphism in patients from southern Europe with mild-moderate and severe rheumatoid arthritis. *J Rheumatol* 2002; 29:1847–1850.

66. Kang CP, Lee KW, Yoo DH, Kang C, Bae SC. The influence of a polymorphism at position –857 of the tumour necrosis factor alpha gene on clinical response to etanercept therapy in rheumatoid arthritis. *Rheumatology* (Oxford) 2005; 44:547–552.

67. Schotte H, Schluter B, Drynda S, Willeke P, Tidow N, Assmann G et al. Interleukin 10 promoter microsatellite polymorphisms are associated with response to long term treatment with etanercept in patients with rheumatoid arthritis. *Ann Rheum Dis* 2005; 64:575–581.

68. Padyukov L, Lampa J, Heimburger M, Ernestam S, Cederholm T, Lundkvist I et al. Genetic markers for the efficacy of tumour necrosis factor blocking therapy in rheumatoid arthritis. *Ann Rheum Dis* 2003; 62:526–529.

69. Kastbom A, Bratt J, Ernestam S, Lampa J, Padyukov L, Soderkvist P et al. Fcgamma receptor type IIIA genotype and response to tumor necrosis factor alpha-blocking agents in patients with rheumatoid arthritis. *Arthritis Rheum* 2007; 56:448–452.

70. Tutuncu Z, Kavanaugh A, Zvaifler N, Corr M, Deutsch R, Boyle D. Fcgamma receptor type IIIA polymorphisms influence treatment outcomes in patients with inflammatory arthritis treated with tumor necrosis factor alpha-blocking agents. *Arthritis Rheum* 2005; 52:2693–2696.

71. Kooloos WM, de Jong DJ, Huizinga TW, Guchelaar HJ. Potential role of pharmacogenetics in anti-TNF treatment of rheumatoid arthritis and Crohn's disease. *Drug Discov Today* 2007; 12:125–131.

72. Burton PR, Tobin MD, Hopper JL. Key concepts in genetic epidemiology. *Lancet* 2005; 366(9489):941–951.

73. Davey SG, Ebrahim S, Lewis S, Hansell AL, Palmer LJ, Burton PR. Genetic epidemiology and public health: hope, hype, and future prospects. *Lancet* 2005; 366:1484–1498.
74. Hattersley AT, McCarthy MI. What makes a good genetic association study? *Lancet* 2005; 366:1315–1323.
75. Emery P, Breedveld FC, Dougados M, Kalden JR, Schiff MH, Smolen JS. Early referral recommendation for newly diagnosed rheumatoid arthritis: evidence based development of a clinical guide. *Ann Rheum Dis* 2002; 61:290–297.
76. Rupp I, Boshuizen HC, Roorda LD, Dinant HJ, Jacobi CE, van den Bos G. Poor and good health outcomes in rheumatoid arthritis: the role of comorbidity. *J Rheumatol* 2006; 33:1488–1495.
77. Ishikawa H, Hashimoto H, Yano E. Patients' preferences for decision making and the feeling of being understood in the medical encounter among patients with rheumatoid arthritis. *Arthritis Rheum* 2006; 55:878–883.
78. Kjeken I, Dagfinrud H, Mowinckel P, Uhlig T, Kvien TK, Finset A. Rheumatology care: involvement in medical decisions, received information, satisfaction with care, and unmet health care needs in patients with rheumatoid arthritis and ankylosing spondylitis. *Arthritis Rheum* 2006; 55:394–401.
79. Wolf CR, Smith G, Smith RL. Science, medicine, and the future: pharmacogenetics. *BMJ* 2000; 320:987–990.
80. Cuchacovich M, Ferreira L, Aliste M, Soto L, Cuenca J, Cruzat A *et al.* Tumour necrosis factor-alpha (TNF-alpha) levels and influence of –308 TNF-alpha promoter polymorphism on the responsiveness to infliximab in patients with rheumatoid arthritis. *Scand J Rheumatol* 2004; 33:228–232.
81. Martinez A, Salido M, Bonilla G, Pascual-Salcedo D, Fernandez-Arquero M, de Miguel S *et al.* Association of the major histocompatibility complex with response to infliximab therapy in rheumatoid arthritis patients. *Arthritis Rheum* 2004; 50:1077–1082.

5

Psoriatic arthritis

Eliza Pontifex, Oliver Fitzgerald

INTRODUCTION

Psoriatic arthritis (PsA) is a chronic systemic inflammatory disorder characterized by the association of arthritis with psoriasis. Although some patients with PsA have mild disease, in others the disease may be progressive despite treatment, with 47% of patients with early PsA showing erosive change after 2 years of follow-up [1]. In addition, recent studies have shown that PsA is associated with an increase in both morbidity and mortality. Thus, health treatment strategies aimed at the suppression of inflammatory joint and skin disease and with maintenance of good function may permit a good quality of life and a reduction in both disability and early mortality.

When considering treatment strategies for PsA it is important to stress that PsA is a complex, multifaceted disease, with some treatments having discordant effects on different disease features. The main disease features are shown in Table 5.1. Whereas some patients may present with predominant spinal disease, for example, with few or none of the other features demonstrated, other patients may present with a mixture of all of the features at the same time. Therefore, in considering treatment options, the physician should base the treatment decision on which feature appears to be predominant, as well as the published evidence for the efficacy of certain treatments for that particular disease manifestation. In order to aid the physician in this treatment decision and to develop a treatment algorithm for PsA, the Group for Research and Assessment of Psoriasis and Psoriatic Arthritis (GRAPPA) has recently undertaken a systematic review of treatments for PsA [2] and is in the process of developing treatment guidelines.

Considerable debate has also taken place recently regarding which outcome domains should be assessed in patients with PsA in clinical trials. The core outcome domains have now been approved [3], and the appropriate instruments to be used have been either validated or are the subject of ongoing research. There are additional domains, which can be included in clinical trials, but as yet they are not considered essential and more research is required. These include acute-phase reactants, nail disease, fatigue and dactylitis. The agreed core domains together with the appropriate instruments are shown in Table 5.2.

TREATMENT STRATEGIES

Treatment strategies in PsA may be considered under the following headings: non-steroidal anti-inflammatory drugs (NSAIDs), glucocorticosteroids, disease-modifying antirheumatic drugs (DMARDs) and biological agents.

Table 5.1 Main clinical features in psoriatic arthritis (PsA)

Peripheral joint disease
Often asymmetrical and polyarticular (more than four joints involved) but oligoarticular disease is not uncommon (20–30%). Involvement of the distal interphalangeal (DIP) joints is classic for PsA, and DIP involvement may be predominant in 5%

Axial disease
Up to 40% of patients with PsA may have clinical evidence of axial disease, and this percentage increases further when X-ray involvement is included. However, axial disease is the dominant feature in only 5%. Axial involvement in PsA on X-ray may be more asymmetrical, e.g. unilateral sacroiliitis

Psoriasis
Skin involvement in PsA may be fairly trivial, with only nail or minimal skin disease present. In the setting of typical PsA joint disease, a careful search for psoriasis is warranted

Dactylitis
The classic sausage-shaped swelling of toes or fingers may be found in 30%. Probably relates to both joint and adjacent teno-synovial involvement

Enthesitis
Inflammation at the point of insertion of ligament to bone is again one of the classic hallmarks of PsA. Found in up to 40% on clinical examination and more with ultrasound evaluation, entheseal disease may be severe and debilitating

---

NON-STEROIDAL ANTI-INFLAMMATORY DRUGS

There has been only one randomized controlled trial (RCT) in PsA which has compared an NSAID (nimesulide) with a placebo [4]. In this study, nimesulide significantly improved pain severity, morning stiffness, patient and investigator assessment of efficacy and both tender and swollen joint scores. There have been four RCTs in PsA which have compared different NSAIDs [5–8]. Three of these trials have involved indomethacin and one involved ibuprofen. All the clinical outcomes improved in these studies and there were no significant differences between any of the comparators. Despite the above lack of published evidence of a favourable therapeutic effect in PsA, NSAIDs are most often the agents first used, whatever the clinical disease pattern. Expert opinion supports this usage, although occasional exacerbations of psoriasis have been reported.

Table 5.2 Core outcome domains and instruments to be used in psoriatic arthritis clinical trials

Domain	*Instrument*
Peripheral joint inflammation	Tender/swollen joint count 68/66
Patient global assessment	Instrument under study
Skin assessment	PASI (BSA ≥3%)
	Lesion (erythema, induration, scale) + BSA
Pain	Visual Analogue Scale or Numeric Rating Scale
Physical function	HAQ/SF-36 PFC
HRQoL	Generic
	Disease specific (e.g. DLQI)

BSA, body surface area; DLQI, Dermatology Life Quality Index; HAQ, Health Assessment Questionnaire; HRQoL, health-related quality of life; PASI, Psoriasis Area and Severity Index; PFC, physical function component.

GLUCOCORTICOSTEROIDS

There have been no RCTs which have assessed systemic glucocorticosteroids in PsA. Systemic glucocorticosteroids are not advised in the treatment of psoriasis as its withdrawal can lead to an exacerbation of skin disease. Systemic glucocorticosteroids are, however, used frequently in PsA, with one study showing 24.4% of patients taking prednisolone [9]. As with systemic glucocorticosteroids, there have been no RCTs that have assessed the effects of intra-articular glucocorticosteroids. Intra-articular injections, however, are commonly used, particularly as a way of suppressing inflammation in patients with mono- or oligoarthritis. Expert opinion supports this usage.

DISEASE-MODIFYING ANTIRHEUMATIC DRUGS

In considering DMARDs in PsA, most of the studies which have examined their usage have confined their observations to the effects on peripheral joint disease. With the exception of psoriasis, there is a paucity of evidence that DMARDs are of benefit for any of the other features of PsA, including dactylitis, axial disease or enthesitis. This being the case, it is important to emphasize that the absence of evidence does not mean the absence of an effect. Other RCTs are required, in particular of DMARDs such as methotrexate (MTX), in which information is gathered on features such as dactylitis, axial disease or enthesitis.

Methotrexate. Most physicians would consider MTX as the DMARD of first choice in PsA. Expert opinion certainly supports this choice but there is very little published evidence which supports the usage of MTX in PsA. Only two small RCTs have compared MTX with placebo. In the first study, published in 1964, three intravenous (i.v.) MTX pulses (1–3 mg/kg body weight) resulted in a significant improvement compared with placebo [10]. There were a number of adverse events, however, and one patient died from marrow aplasia and haematemesis. The second study, published in 1984, showed that oral MTX in a range of doses between 7.5 and 15 mg weekly only reduced physician's global assessment at 12 weeks compared with placebo with other outcome measures not significantly different [11]. With the varying dose range used and the failure to increase MTX up to 20 or 25 mg, together with the small patient numbers, this study really fails to answer the question of treatment efficacy.

Two RCTs have compared the effects of MTX with other DMARDs. Spadaro *et al.* [12] compared MTX at 7.5–15 mg per week with ciclosporin at 3–5 mg/kg per day in 35 patients treated for 1 year. Both treatments were associated with a reduction in painful or swollen joints, decreased Ritchie score, a shorter duration of morning stiffness, improvement in grip strength, improvement in the psoriasis area and severity index (PASI) and improved patient and physician global assessments. The authors concluded that MTX was as effective as ciclosporin.

In a more recent RCT, 72 patients with active PsA and an incomplete response to MTX were randomized to receive, in addition, either ciclosporin or placebo [13]. Patients on combination therapy had a significant improvement from baseline in swollen joint count and in C-reactive protein (CRP) levels, which was not evident in those on the MTX–placebo group. In addition, synovitis detected by ultrasound and PASI scores were significantly better in patients treated with the combination as opposed to those who were treated with MTX alone.

There have been several uncontrolled retrospective studies which have reported clinical efficacy in patients treated with MTX. In one such study, the records of 87 patients with PsA who were treated with either MTX or intramuscular (i.m.) gold were reviewed; the likelihood of a clinical response was 8.9 times greater with MTX than i.m. gold [14]. In a more recent study of 10 patients receiving open-label MTX, there was a significant improvement in clinical scores after 3 months compared with baseline, and this was accompanied by significant reduction in synovial cellular infiltration, adhesion molecule expression, and proinflammatory cytokine mRNA expression, in particular interleukin 8 (IL-8) [15].

To date, a reduction in radiographic progression in patients treated with MTX has not been demonstrated. In the RCT of MTX plus ciclosporin described above, Larsen scores of radiographic damage increased in both groups [13]. A case–control study of 38 MTX-treated patients and 38 matched controls did not demonstrate any prevention of radiographic progression [16]. It is important to point out that the scores used for demonstration of radiographic change were developed for rheumatoid arthritis (RA) and to date have not been validated in PsA.

Adverse effects remain an important concern for patients with PsA treated with MTX. In one study of 104 patients, 165 adverse drug reactions were noted in 83 patients [17]. The most common side-effects were gastrointestinal including nausea and vomiting in 33%. Blood count changes were noted in 27% and serum liver enzyme increases in 27%. Other significant issues include pulmonary fibrosis, hair loss and the potential to affect pregnancy outcome. Assessment of possible liver toxicity remains controversial. A meta-analysis to evaluate the risk of liver toxicity from long-term administration of MTX concluded that patients with psoriasis were more likely than patients with RA to have advanced histological changes and to experience histological progression [18]. The rate of progression was associated with the cumulative dose of MTX. In psoriasis the probability of a normal liver biopsy dropped below 50% at a cumulative MTX dose between 3000 and 5800 mg [19]. Some dermatologists are advocating the serial evaluation of amino terminal propeptide of type III procollagen levels as a way of avoiding the need for repeat liver biopsies [20, 21]. Rheumatologists, however, continue to monitor blood biochemistry only as a means of predicting liver histopathological change. As it has been demonstrated that significant liver damage can occur without evidence of abnormal liver function tests, a prospective evaluation of liver histopathological change in patients with PsA is required.

Sulfasalazine. Six RCTs have compared sulfasalazine with placebo [22–27] and these have been the subject of a Cochrane review [28, 29]. These studies have shown that sulfasalazine has good clinical efficacy in PsA. A more recent multicentre study compared sulfasalazine with ciclosporin and standard therapy over 24 weeks [30]. Of the 99 patients with PsA studied, no significant differences were observed in clinical outcome measures between sulfasalazine and standard therapy alone. Furthermore, one case–control study of 20 patients treated with sulfasalazine compared with 20 controls showed that radiographic scores at 24 months were not statistically different [31]. In general, adverse effects with sulfasalazine are mild, with nausea and dizziness being the most common. However, in one RCT, adverse events were observed in up to one-third of patients receiving sulfasalazine [22].

Ciclosporin. No RCTs have compared ciclosporin with placebo. Three RCTs have compared ciclosporin with another DMARD: MTX in two and sulfasalazine in one [12, 13, 30]. In the first study of ciclosporin compared with MTX, both drugs appeared to be equally effective. In the second study the patients with an incomplete response to MTX were randomized to receive, in addition, either ciclosporin or placebo. Some improvements (as noted above) were noted in the MTX and ciclosporin group that were not evident in the MTX and placebo group. Finally, one small study of 15 patients with PsA addressed the question of radiographic progression and failed to show any reduction in the number of eroded joints in patients during a 24-month study period [32].

Adverse effects remain the prime concern in treating patients with PsA in the long term with ciclosporin. In particular, kidney dysfunction increases with the length of ciclosporin therapy and in some cases renal damage did not improve following discontinuation of therapy [9, 33].

Leflunomide. There has been one multicentre double-blind RCT of leflunomide in the treatment of active PsA and psoriasis [34]. In 190 patients, leflunomide was significantly superior to placebo in the number of patients who achieved the primary efficacy end-point, the Psoriatic Arthritis Response Criterion (PsARC) (59% vs. 30%). Individual scores, including joint pain/tenderness, joint swelling, tender joint count, swollen joint count, Health Assessment Questionnaire (HAQ) and Dermatology Life Quality Index (DLQI), also significantly improved. Serious adverse events occurred in 13.5% of patients treated with leflunomide compared with 5.4% of patients treated with placebo. Diarrhoea, an increase in liver enzymes, flu-like symptoms and headache were the most common adverse events experienced.

Gold salts. Two RCTs have compared gold salts with placebo [35, 36]. One compared oral gold and the other i.m. gold and oral gold with placebo. These trials have been included in a systematic review in which it was shown that gold salts were not statistically better than placebo for the treatment of PsA [28, 29]. A further study compared i.m. gold with oral gold and suggested that arthritis was better controlled in the i.m. gold group [37].

The main concern relating to the use of gold salts is the possibility that psoriasis may be exacerbated. Other adverse events include bone marrow suppression and the development of proteinuria.

Azathioprine. There has been one small RCT (12 patients) which has compared azathioprine with placebo [38]. Azathioprine appeared to show some effect but additional data are required.

Antimalarials. In one case–control study, a reduction in actively inflamed joint count was demonstrated in 24 patients taking chloroquine for at least 6 months [39]. A similar improvement, however, was seen in the control group taking no disease-modifying agents.

Antimalarials have been reported to cause an exacerbation of psoriasis. A review indicated that this may occur in up to 18% of patients with psoriasis treated with antimalarials [40].

BIOLOGICAL AGENTS

As in many other autoimmune diseases, the use of biological agents in PsA has set the scene for an exciting paradigm shift. From a patient's perspective, biological agents offer new treatment opportunities and the hope for better disease control, functional outcomes and quality of life. For the clinician or scientist, studying the immunological effects of biological agents gives us the opportunity to learn more about disease pathogenesis, predisposing factors and treatment targets.

As mentioned above, one of the great challenges of clinical studies in PsA has been the heterogeneity of disease presentation, and hence the recruitment of homogeneous populations for clinical trials. Organizations such as GRAPPA aim to develop evidence-based treatment guidelines, and help focus attention on non-articular as well as articular manifestations of the disease. Their research prioritization includes development of standardized instruments to report changes in outcome domains which have not previously been validated. It makes sense, therefore, that common articular and extra-articular manifestations of PsA are assessed separately in studies. Consistent with this concept, we shall also review the evidence for biological agents under the headings of the four major musculoskeletal manifestations (Table 5.1). This has been the approach undertaken recently in a GRAPPA-initiated systematic review of treatments in PsA [2].

Peripheral joint disease

All three currently available anti-tumour necrosis factor (TNF) antagonists are efficacious in peripheral joint disease in PsA (category A and B evidence) [41] when used either as monotherapy or when added to a DMARD (category A evidence) [41]. There is also a growing body of work investigating the efficacy of other classes of biological agents in PsA.

Infliximab. Infliximab is a human–mouse chimeric monoclonal antibody to TNF-α, a critical proinflammatory cytokine in the initiation and maintenance of synovial inflammation in RA and PsA. Two large RCTs have demonstrated the benefits of infliximab specifically in PsA – the Infliximab Multinational Psoriatic Arthritis Controlled Trials (IMPACT) 1 and 2 [42, 43]. Both trials administered infliximab as a monotherapy at 5 mg/kg dose or placebo at weeks 0, 2, 6 and 8 thereafter. In IMPACT 1, 104 patients with PsA with five or more involved joints were randomized, and, by week 16, 65% of treated patients had achieved ACR20 and 75% had a PsARC response, compared with 10% and 21%, respectively, of placebo-treated patients. No placebo-treated patient achieved ACR50 or ACR70 compared with 46% and 29%, respectively, of infliximab-treated patients. From week 16, all placebo patients crossed over to the treatment arm. By the end of 50 weeks, there was sustained clinical benefit in those receiving infliximab and evidence of equivalent inhibition of radiographic progression in both groups [44]. In the open-label extension to week 94, clinical improvement was sustained and radiographic progression was inhibited compared with the estimated baseline rate of progression [45]. IMPACT 2 involved 200 patients with PsA previously unresponsive to other therapies. By week 14, the number of ACR20 and PsARC responders was significantly higher in the treatment group than in the placebo group (58% vs. 11% and 77% vs. 27%, respectively). SF-36 outcomes [46] and productivity [47] were also improved in the treatment group compared with the placebo group. Treatment responses were maintained after 1 year of treatment, although some patients received higher drug doses as titrated by clinical response [48]. The 1-year radiographic data from IMPACT 2 were recently published [49]. At 24 weeks, those who received infliximab had significantly less radiographic progression than those who received placebo (Sharp–van der Heijde scoring method) and, despite the crossover design, this difference was maintained out to 54 weeks.

Etanercept. Two large RCTs have also demonstrated the effectiveness of etanercept, a soluble TNF receptor molecule, at 25 mg subcutaneously (s.c.) twice weekly in PsA. In the first, 60 patients were randomized to receive etanercept monotherapy or placebo. At 12 weeks, 87% of treated patients met the PsARC compared with 23% of patients on placebo [50]. A further RCT involving 205 randomized patients revealed that 59% of treatment-receiving patients versus 15% of placebo-receiving patients achieved ACR20 by 12 weeks. Quality-of-life measures also significantly improved in the treatment group [51]. From 24 weeks, patients could choose to continue open-label treatment. At 1 year, radiographic progression was inhibited in the treatment group but worsened in the placebo group [51]. By 2 years, similar ACR20 and PsARC responses were achieved and maintained in both groups, and radiographic progression was halted once patients began receiving treatment [52]. Results from the Psoriasis Randomized Etanercept Study in Subjects with Psoriatic Arthritis (PRESTA) study, which compared the effect of two dosing regimes of etanercept (50 mg twice weekly versus 50 mg once weekly) on the skin and articular and extra-articular manifestations of PsA, are awaited with interest.

Adalimumab. A total of 313 patients with PsA unresponsive to NSAID received adalimumab 40 mg s.c. fortnightly or placebo for 24 weeks in this RCT (ADEPT) [53]. Approximately half the patients in each group were also taking methotrexate (MTX) at the start of the trial. By week 24, ACR20 and PsARC were reached by 57% and 60%, respectively, of the treatment group, and 15% and 23%, respectively, of the placebo group. HAQ scores significantly improved and radiographic progression was significantly inhibited in the treatment group by 24 weeks. Scores of fatigue, pain, quality of life and physical and dermatological function also all improved after 24 weeks [54]. Patients could choose to receive open-label treatment from 24 weeks to 48 weeks. At 48 weeks, DAS20 responses and HAQ scores were maintained in the treatment arm and radiographic change did not progress from treatment versus placebo baseline-modified Sharp scores at 24 weeks [55]. Interestingly, concurrent use of MTX did not affect clinical or radiographic responses.

In a separate RCT, 100 patients with PsA unresponsive to DMARDs were treated with adalimumab monotherapy 40 mg s.c. fortnightly or placebo for 12 weeks, followed by an open-label treatment period [56]. By week 12, ACR20 was achieved by 39% versus 16% and

PsARC by 51% versus 24% of treatment versus placebo arm patients, respectively. Both results were statistically significant. After open-label switch, ACR20 was reached by 65% and 57% in both groups of patients. Psoriasis and disability scores also improved. Lastly, a large, open-label Phase IIIb study from Germany called STEREO for 442 enrolled patients with PsA, found that 75% of 376 previously biologically-naive patients with PsA who started adalimumab achieved ACR20 by 12 weeks [57].

Golimumab. This human anti-TNF alpha monoclonal antibody was studied in 405 patients with PsA in the GO-REVEAL (Golumimab – Randomized Evaluation of Safety and Efficacy in Subjects with Psoriatic Arthritis using a Human Anti-TNF Monoclonal Antibody) study [58]. Compared with placebo, more patients receiving golimumab achieved ACR20 by 14 weeks and this effect was maintained through to 24 weeks.

Use of second anti-TNF agent in PsA. Should an initially chosen anti-TNF agent prove to be ineffective, there is evidence that patients may achieve a response after switching to alternative anti-TNF agents in PsA. In an ongoing Italian longitudinal, observational study involving 165 patients with SpA (including ankylosing spondylitis [AS] and PsA) treated with anti-TNF antagonists, 22 patients switched from one anti-TNF antagonist to at least one other because of inefficacy or adverse events. Clinical response was observed in the majority of patients regardless of the anti-TNF antagonists involved [59]. In other studies, clinical response was observed in 19 patients with psoriasis and PsA who switched to adalimumab [60] and 11 of 15 patients with PsA who switched to etanercept [61] after failure of another biological agent. Furthermore, in the above-mentioned STEREO trial, 66 of 442 patients with PsA had discontinued infliximab or etanercept due to lack or loss of efficacy or intolerance. These 66 were switched to adalimumab, and by 12 weeks 67% had achieved ACR20, a figure similar to those who were biologically naive [57].

Alefacept. Alefacept is a fusion protein of soluble lymphocyte function antigen 3 (LFA-3) and IgG1 Fc fragments which has been studied more extensively in the treatment of psoriasis than in PsA. Alefacept blocks LFA-3–CD2 co-stimulation and hence reduces the number of pathogenic T cells. In a phase II RCT, 123 patients with PsA were treated with alefacept and MTX and 62 patients with PsA treated with placebo and MTX for 12 weeks, followed by MTX monotherapy for 12 weeks in both groups. At week 24, 54% of alefacept-treated patients versus 23% of placebo-treated patients achieved ACR20, suggesting that combination therapy may be an effective treatment strategy for PsA [62]. An additional 12 weeks of alefacept treatment with methotrexate led to an increase in the number of patients achieving ACR50 (American College of Rheumatology 50% improvement criteria) and ACR70, but not ACR20 [63].

Efalizumab. Efalizumab is a monoclonal IgG antibody to LFA-1, a T-cell adhesion molecule which inhibits cell migration and activation by binding to antigen-presenting cells. Following RCTs, it was approved for use in the treatment of moderate to severe plaque psoriasis. In a phase II RCT in 107 patients with PsA, 50% of patients received efalizumab and 50% placebo for 12 weeks, in addition to at least one of either NSAID, prednisolone, sulfasalazine or MTX. At week 12, there was no significant difference in ACR20 response between the two groups, implying that efalizumab is not an effective agent for PsA [64]. Furthermore, there are a number of reports which highlight the onset or worsening of arthritis in patients with psoriasis being treated with efalizumab [65, 66]. In 2009, efalizumab was voluntarily withdrawn from the US market and its marketing authorization withdrawn in Europe due to the potential risk of patients developing progressive multifocal leucoencephalopathy.

Anakinra. There are no RCT trials involving this IL-1 receptor antagonist in PsA. In our own experience of an open, pilot study in 12 patients with PsA treated with anakinra, only 50% of patients achieved an ACR20 response by 12 weeks and only one felt sufficiently improved to remain on therapy following completion of the study [67].

Rituximab. There are no reports in the literature of the use of anti-CD20 (rituximab) antibody specifically for PsA. A recently published case series, however, describes the development of psoriasis in three patients and of PsA in one patient treated with rituximab for other rheumatological diagnoses [68].

Abatacept. This drug is a CTLA-4/IgG Fc domain fusion protein which prevents CD28–CD80/86 co-stimulation on T cells and hence T-cell activation. Although abatacept is licensed for use in RA, there are no published studies to date on the use of abatacept in PsA. There is some support, however, for its effectiveness in psoriasis [69], and considering the evidence for T-cell involvement in the pathogenesis of PsA [70, 71] abatacept would seem a reasonable therapeutic approach to study. An RCT of abatacept in psoriasis and PsA has recently been completed and is expected to be reported shortly.

Ustekinumab. IL-12 and IL-23 are produced mostly by dendritic cells and share a common p40 subunit. Their presence activates a distinct T-cell lineage that expresses IL-17, which is implicated in the pathogenesis of psoriasis. A monoclonal antibody directed against the common p40 subunit has shown good efficacy in a phase II placebo-controlled randomized trial of 320 patients with psoriasis [72]. This same drug has also recently been shown to be effective in PsA. A total of 146 patients with active PsA were randomized to receive either ustekinumab as a weekly infusion for 4 weeks or placebo. By 12 weeks, 42% of those who received active drug achieved ACR20 compared with 14% of the placebo group [73].

Axial disease
The efficacy of anti-TNF therapies specifically in the subset of patients with axial PsA has not been studied. For this reason, until further studies are undertaken, GRAPPA decided to formulate its recommendations based on trial results incorporating biologicals in axial disease of PsA, ankylosing spondylitis (AS) and PsA. Apart from a small open-label study of anakinra, the anti-TNF antagonists are the only drug class to have demonstrated efficacy in axial PsA, with most evidence extrapolated from studies in AS. All three available anti-TNF antagonists have been assessed in double-blind RCT in AS (several for infliximab and etanercept, one for adalimumab) and, overall, approximately 80% of patients have responded to at least one of the drugs, with about 50% achieving 50% improvement in composite score measures such as <u>A</u>ssessmet in <u>A</u>nkylosing <u>S</u>pondylitis 50 (ASAS 50). Although magnetic resonance imaging (MRI)-detected sacroiliac joint inflammation significantly improves with infliximab or etanercept compared with placebo, it does not appear that plain radiographic progression is arrested out to 2 or 4 years [74, 75]. Clinical efficacy has been safely maintained for up to 5 years in the case of infliximab [76]. The ASAS working group has published guidelines for the use of anti-TNF agents in AS [77]. Until other specific information is available in PsA axial disease, as per the ASAS guidelines, anti-TNF antagonists are recommended in at least moderately to severely active axial disease, which has remained unresponsive to exercise and two NSAIDs [78].

Enthesitis
There are no tools for measuring changes in the presence of enthesopathy which have been validated in PsA. In both IMPACT trials, tenderness over two bilateral entheseal sites of the lower limbs was included as an outcome measure. There was a significant reduction in the number of tender entheseal sites in the infliximab compared with placebo groups in both trials. An RCT of 40 patients with AS and enthesitis used a modified Mander scale [79] to assess entheseal response following etanercept or placebo. In the treatment group, entheseal scores approached zero post treatment and were significantly different from the placebo group, despite wide standard deviations. The GO-REVEAL study used the PsA-modified Maastricht Ankylosing Spondylitis Enthesitis Score (MASES) index and found an improvement in enthesitis following golimumab treatment than with placebo [58]. The further development of validated enthesitis scoring systems and their use in RCTs in PsA is awaited.

Two RCTs comparing spinal enthesitis on MRI in patients with AS receiving infliximab or placebo have demonstrated significant improvement in the numbers of lesions in the treatment groups [80, 81].

Dactylitis

The effect of anti-TNF agents on this classic feature of PsA has been investigated in two RCTs of infliximab (IMPACT 1 and 2) and in one of adalimumab [53]. The same non-validated scoring method was used for dactylitis in IMPACT 1 and in the adalimumab trial. The mean baseline dactylitis scores were low and similar in both groups in IMPACT 1, such that the small change observed post treatment is difficult to interpret. No significant difference was noted between the groups following treatment in the adalimumab trial. In IMPACT 2, the percentage of patients who became dactylitis-free post treatment was 23% in the treatment group and 13% in the placebo group, which was significantly different. In this relatively evidence-free zone, only infliximab has shown modest efficacy and could be recommended for treatment. Results from the PRESTA study may allow the addition of etanercept to this list. Validated scoring methods and evidence for optimal dosing schedules hopefully await us in the future.

CONCLUSION

In general, DMARD studies in PsA are poorly controlled and have been conducted with small numbers. Additional clinical trials, in particular of MTX, are required in order to develop clear, evidence-based treatment guidelines. Anti-TNF efficacy has certainly been demonstrated but, to date, a comparison with MTX has not been undertaken. A large-scale clinical trial of patients with PsA incorporating all outcome measures and validated instruments and comparing the effectiveness of MTX alone versus anti-TNF alone versus both agents together is required. Additional agents showing promising results in RCTs include the novel IL-12/IL-23 common p40 subunit inhibitor, ustekinumab.

REFERENCES

1. Kane D, Stafford L, Bresnihan B, FitzGerald O. A prospective, clinical and radiological study of early psoriatic arthritis: an early synovitis clinic experience. *Rheumatology* 2003; 42:1460–1468.
2. Kavanaugh AF, Ritchlin CT. Systematic review of treatments for psoriatic arthritis: an evidence based approach and basis for treatment guidelines. *J Rheumatol* 2006; 33:1417–1421.
3. Gladman DD, Mease PJ, Strand V, Healy P, Helliwell PS, Fitzgerald O *et al.* Consensus on a core set of domains for psoriatic arthritis. *J Rheumatol* 2007; 34:1167–1170.
4. Sarzi-Puttini P, Santandrea S, Boccassini L, Panni B, Caruso I. The role of NSAIDs in psoriatic arthritis: evidence from a controlled study with nimesulide. *Clin Exp Rheumatol* 2001; 19(1 Suppl 22):S17–20.
5. Lassus A. A comparative pilot study of azapropazone and indomethacin in the treatment of psoriatic arthritis and Reiter's disease. *Curr Med Res Opin* 1976; 4:65–69.
6. Lonauer G, Wirth W. [Controlled double blind study on the effectiveness and adverse effects of acemetacin and indomethacin in the treatment of psoriatic arthritis]. *Arzneimittelforschung* 1980; 30:1440–1444.
7. Leatham PA, Bird HA, Wright V, Fowler PD. The run-in period in trial design: a comparison of two non-steroidal anti-inflammatory agents in psoriatic arthropathy. *Agents Actions* 1982; 12(1–2):221–224.
8. Hopkins R, Bird HA, Jones H, Hill J, Surrall KE, Astbury C *et al.* A double-blind controlled trial of etretinate (Tigason) and ibuprofen in psoriatic arthritis. *Ann Rheum Dis* 1985; 44:189–193.
9. Pipitone N, Kingsley GH, Manzo A, Scott DL, Pitzalis C. Current concepts and new developments in the treatment of psoriatic arthritis. *Rheumatology* (Oxford) 2003; 42:1138–1148.
10. Black RL, O'Brien WM, Vanscott EJ, Auerbach R, Eisen AZ, Bunim JJ. Methotrexate therapy in psoriatic arthritis; double-blind study on 21 patients. *Jama* 1964; 189:743–747.

11. Willkens RF, Williams HJ, Ward JR, Egger MJ, Reading JC, Clements PJ *et al.* Randomized, double-blind, placebo controlled trial of low-dose pulse methotrexate in psoriatic arthritis. *Arthritis Rheum* 1984; 27:376–381.

12. Spadaro A, Riccieri V, Sili-Scavalli A, Sensi F, Taccari E, Zoppini A. Comparison of cyclosporin A and methotrexate in the treatment of psoriatic arthritis: a one-year prospective study. *Clin Exp Rheumatol* 1995; 13:589–593.

13. Fraser AD, van Kuijk AW, Westhovens R, Karim Z, Wakefield R, Gerards AH *et al.* A randomised, double blind, placebo controlled, multicentre trial of combination therapy with methotrexate plus ciclosporin in patients with active psoriatic arthritis. *Ann Rheum Dis* 2005; 64:859–864.

14. Lacaille D, Stein HB, Raboud J, Klinkhoff AV. Longterm therapy of psoriatic arthritis: intramuscular gold or methotrexate? *J Rheumatol* 2000; 27:1922–1927.

15. Kane D, Gogarty M, O'Leary J, Silva I, Bermingham N, Bresnihan B *et al.* Reduction of synovial sublining layer inflammation and proinflammatory cytokine expression in psoriatic arthritis treated with methotrexate. *Arthritis Rheum* 2004; 50:3286–3295.

16. Abu-Shakra M, Gladman DD, Thorne JC, Long J, Gough J, Farewell VT. Longterm methotrexate therapy in psoriatic arthritis: clinical and radiological outcome. *J Rheumatol* 1995; 22:241–245.

17. Malatjalian DA, Ross JB, Williams CN, Colwell SJ, Eastwood BJ. Methotrexate hepatotoxicity in psoriatics: report of 104 patients from Nova Scotia, with analysis of risks from obesity, diabetes and alcohol consumption during long term follow-up. *Can J Gastroenterol* 1996; 10:369–375.

18. Whiting-O'Keefe QE, Fye KH, Sack KD. Methotrexate and histologic hepatic abnormalities: a meta-analysis. *Am J Med* 1991; 90:711–716.

19. Grismer LE, Gill SA, Harris MD. Liver biopsy in psoriatic arthritis to detect methotrexate hepatotoxicity. *J Clin Rheumatol* 2001; 7:224–227.

20. Zachariae H, Heickendorff L, Sogaard H. The value of amino-terminal propeptide of type III procollagen in routine screening for methotrexate-induced liver fibrosis: a 10-year follow-up. *Br J Dermatol* 2001; 144:100–103.

21. Saporito FC, Menter MA. Methotrexate and psoriasis in the era of new biologic agents. *J Am Acad Dermatol* 2004; 50:301–309.

22. Clegg DO, Reda DJ, Mejias E, Cannon GW, Weisman MH, Taylor T *et al.* Comparison of sulfasalazine and placebo in the treatment of psoriatic arthritis. A Department of Veterans Affairs Cooperative Study. *Arthritis Rheum* 1996; 39:2013–2020.

23. Farr M, Kitas GD, Waterhouse L, Jubb R, Felix-Davies D, Bacon PA. Treatment of psoriatic arthritis with sulphasalazine: a one year open study. *Clin Rheumatol* 1988; 7:372–377.

24. Fraser SM, Hopkins R, Hunter JA, Neumann V, Capell HA, Bird HA. Sulphasalazine in the management of psoriatic arthritis. *Br J Rheumatol* 1993; 32:923–925.

25. Dougados M, vam der Linden S, Leirisalo-Repo M, Huitfeldt B, Juhlin R, Veys E *et al.* Sulfasalazine in the treatment of spondylarthropathy. A randomized, multicenter, double-blind, placebo-controlled study. *Arthritis Rheum* 1995; 38:618–627.

26. Gupta AK, Grober JS, Hamilton TA, Ellis CN, Siegel MT, Voorhees JJ *et al.* Sulfasalazine therapy for psoriatic arthritis: a double blind, placebo controlled trial [see comments]. *J Rheumatol* 1995; 22:894–898.

27. Combe B, Goupille P, Kuntz JL, Tebib J, Liote F, Bregeon C. Sulphasalazine in psoriatic arthritis: a randomized, multicentre, placebo-controlled study. *Br J Rheumatol* 1996; 35:664–668.

28. Jones G, Crotty M, Brooks P. Psoriatic arthritis: a quantitative overview of therapeutic options. The Psoriatic Arthritis Meta-Analysis Study Group. *Br J Rheumatol* 1997; 36:95–99.

29. Jones G, Crotty M, Brooks P. Interventions for psoriatic arthritis. *Cochrane Database Syst Rev* 2000; (2):CD000212.

30. Salvarani C, Macchioni P, Olivieri I, Marchesoni A, Cutolo M, Ferraccioli G *et al.* A comparison of cyclosporine, sulfasalazine, and symptomatic therapy in the treatment of psoriatic arthritis. *J Rheumatol* 2001; 28:2274–2282.

31. Rahman P, Gladman DD, Cook RJ, Zhou Y, Young G. The use of sulfasalazine in psoriatic arthritis: a clinic experience. *J Rheumatol* 1998; 25:1957–1961.

32. Macchioni P, Boiardi L, Cremonesi T, Battistel B, Casadei-Maldini M, Beltrandi E *et al.* The relationship between serum-soluble interleukin-2 receptor and radiological evolution in psoriatic arthritis patients treated with cyclosporin-A. *Rheumatol Int* 1998; 18:27–33.

33. Korstanje MJ, Bilo HJ, Stoof TJ. Sustained renal function loss in psoriasis patients after withdrawal of low-dose cyclosporin therapy. *Br J Dermatol* 1992; 127:501–504.

34. Kaltwasser JP, Nash P, Gladman D, Rosen CF, Behrens F, Jones P et al. Efficacy and safety of leflunomide in the treatment of psoriatic arthritis and psoriasis: a multinational, double-blind, randomized, placebo-controlled clinical trial. Arthritis Rheum 2004; 50:1939–1950.

35. Carette S, Calin A, McCafferty JP, Wallin BA. A double-blind placebo-controlled study of auranofin in patients with psoriatic arthritis. Arthritis Rheum 1989; 32:158–165.

36. Palit J, Hill J, Capell HA, Carey J, Daunt SO, Cawley MI et al. A multicentre double-blind comparison of auranofin, intramuscular gold thiomalate and placebo in patients with psoriatic arthritis. Br J Rheumatol 1990; 29:280–283.

37. Bruckle W, Dexel T, Grasedyck K, Schattenkirchner M. Treatment of psoriatic arthritis with auranofin and gold sodium thiomalate. Clin Rheumatol 1994; 13:209–216.

38. KK Levy HP, EV Barnett A double-blind controlled evaluation of azathioprine treatment in rheumatoid arthritis and psoriatic arthritis. Arthritis Rheum 1972; 15:116–117.

39. Gladman DD, Blake R, Brubacher B, Farewell VT. Chloroquine therapy in psoriatic arthritis. J Rheumatol 1992; 19:1724–1726.

40. Wolf R, Ruocco V. Triggered psoriasis. Adv Exp Med Biol 1999; 455:221–225.

41. Soriano ER, McHugh NJ. Therapies for peripheral joint disease in psoriatic arthritis. A systematic review. J Rheumatol 2006; 33:1422–1430.

42. Antoni CE, Kavanaugh A, Kirkham B, Tutuncu Z, Burmester GR, Schneider U et al. Sustained benefits of infliximab therapy for dermatologic and articular manifestations of psoriatic arthritis: results from the infliximab multinational psoriatic arthritis controlled trial (IMPACT). Arthritis Rheum 2005; 52:1227–1236.

43. Antoni C, Krueger GG, de Vlam K, Birbara C, Beutler A, Guzzo C et al. Infliximab improves signs and symptoms of psoriatic arthritis: results of the IMPACT 2 trial. Ann Rheum Dis 2005; 64:1150–1157.

44. Kavanaugh A, Antoni CE, Gladman D, Wassenberg S, Zhou B, Beutler A et al. The Infliximab Multinational Psoriatic Arthritis Controlled Trial (IMPACT): results of radiographic analyses after 1 year. Ann Rheum Dis 2006; 65:1038–1043.

45. Antoni CE, Kavanaugh A, van der Heijde D, Beutler A, Keenan G, Zhou B et al. Two-year efficacy and safety of infliximab treatment in patients with active psoriatic arthritis: findings of the Infliximab Multinational Psoriatic Arthritis Controlled Trial (IMPACT). J Rheumatol 2008; 35:869–876.

46. Kavanaugh A, Antoni C, Krueger GG, Yan S, Bala M, Dooley LT et al. Infliximab improves health related quality of life and physical function in patients with psoriatic arthritis. Ann Rheum Dis 2006; 65:471–477.

47. Kavanaugh A, Antoni C, Mease P, Gladman D, Yan S, Bala M et al. Effect of infliximab therapy on employment, time lost from work, and productivity in patients with psoriatic arthritis. J Rheumatol 2006; 33:2254–2259.

48. Kavanaugh A, Krueger GG, Beutler A, Guzzo C, Zhou B, Dooley LT et al. Infliximab maintains a high degree of clinical response in patients with active psoriatic arthritis through 1 year of treatment: results from the IMPACT 2 trial. Ann Rheum Dis 2007; 66:498–505.

49. van der Heijde D, Kavanaugh A, Gladman DD, Antoni C, Krueger GG, Guzzo C et al. Infliximab inhibits progression of radiographic damage in patients with active psoriatic arthritis through one year of treatment: Results from the induction and maintenance psoriatic arthritis clinical trial 2. Arthritis Rheum 2007; 56:2698–2707.

50. Mease PJ, Goffe BS, Metz J, VanderStoep A, Finck B, Burge DJ. Etanercept in the treatment of psoriatic arthritis and psoriasis: a randomised trial. Lancet 2000; 356:385–390.

51. Mease PJ, Kivitz AJ, Burch FX, Siegel EL, Cohen SB, Ory P et al. Etanercept treatment of psoriatic arthritis: safety, efficacy, and effect on disease progression. Arthritis Rheum 2004; 50:2264–2272.

52. Mease PJ, Kivitz AJ, Burch FX, Siegel EL, Cohen SB, Ory P et al. Continued inhibition of radiographic progression in patients with psoriatic arthritis following 2 years of treatment with etanercept. J Rheumatol 2006; 33:712–721.

53. Mease PJ, Gladman DD, Ritchlin CT, Ruderman EM, Steinfeld SD, Choy EH et al. Adalimumab for the treatment of patients with moderately to severely active psoriatic arthritis: results of a double-blind, randomized, placebo-controlled trial. Arthritis Rheum 2005; 52:3279–3289.

54. Gladman DD, Mease PJ, Cifaldi MA, Perdok RJ, Sasso E, Medich J. Adalimumab improves joint-related and skin-related functional impairment in patients with psoriatic arthritis: patient-reported outcomes of the Adalimumab Effectiveness in Psoriatic Arthritis Trial. Ann Rheum Dis 2007; 66:163–168.

55. Gladman DD, Mease PJ, Ritchlin CT, Choy EH, Sharp JT, Ory PA *et al.* Adalimumab for long-term treatment of psoriatic arthritis: forty-eight week data from the adalimumab effectiveness in psoriatic arthritis trial. *Arthritis Rheum* 2007; 56:476–488.

56. Genovese MC, Mease PJ, Thomson GT, Kivitz AJ, Perdok RJ, Weinberg MA *et al.* Safety and efficacy of adalimumab in treatment of patients with psoriatic arthritis who had failed disease modifying antirheumatic drug therapy. *J Rheumatol* 2007; 34:1040–1050.

57. Burmester M RM, van den Bosch F, Kron M, Kary S, Kupper H. Effectiveness and Safety of Adalimumab (HUMIRA) After Failure of Etanercept or Infliximab Treatment in Patients With Rheumatoid Arthritits, Psoriatic Arthritis, or Ankylosing Spondylitis. *Arthritis Rheum* 2007; 56(9 Suppl):S393.

58. Kavanaugh A, McInnes I, Mease P, Krueger GG, Gladman D, Gomez-Reino J *et al.* Golimumab, a new human tumor necrosis factor alpha antibody, administered every four weeks as a subcutaneous injection in psoriatic arthritis: Twenty-four-week efficacy and safety results of a randomized, placebo-controlled study. *Arthritis Rheum* 2009; 60:976–986.

59. Conti F, Ceccarelli F, Marocchi E, Magrini L, Spinelli FR, Spadaro A *et al.* Switching tumour necrosis factor alpha antagonists in patients with ankylosing spondylitis and psoriatic arthritis: an observational study over a 5-year period. *Ann Rheum Dis* 2007; 66:1393–1397.

60. Papoutsaki M, Chimenti MS, Costanzo A, Talamonti M, Zangrilli A, Giunta A *et al.* Adalimumab for severe psoriasis and psoriatic arthritis: an open-label study in 30 patients previously treated with other biologics. *J Am Acad Dermatol* 2007; 57:269–275.

61. Delaunay C, Farrenq V, Marini-Portugal A, Cohen JD, Chevalier X, Claudepierre P. Infliximab to etanercept switch in patients with spondyloarthropathies and psoriatic arthritis: preliminary data. *J Rheumatol* 2005; 32:2183–2185.

62. Mease PJ, Gladman DD, Keystone EC. Alefacept in combination with methotrexate for the treatment of psoriatic arthritis: results of a randomized, double-blind, placebo-controlled study. *Arthritis Rheum* 2006; 54:1638–1645.

63. Mease PJ, Reich K. Alefacept with methotrexate for treatment of psoriatic arthritis: open-label extension of a randomized, double-blind, placebo-controlled study. *J Am Acad Dermatol* 2009; 60:402–411.

64. Papp KA, Caro I, Leung HM, Garovoy M, Mease PJ. Efalizumab for the treatment of psoriatic arthritis. *J Cutan Med Surg* 2007; 11:57–66.

65. Bang B, Gniadecki R. Severe exacerbation of psoriatic arthritis during treatment with efalizumab. A case report. *Acta Derm Venereol* 2006; 86:456–457.

66. Myers WA, Najarian D, Gottlieb AB. New-onset, debilitating arthritis in psoriasis patients receiving efalizumab. *J Dermatolog Treat* 2006; 17:353–354.

67. Pontifex EK, Gibbs A, Bresnihan B, Veale DJ, FitzGerald O. Clinical outcome measures in Psoriatic Arthritis: Comparing enrollment and response in a biologics study. *Arthritis and Rheumatism* 2007; 56(9 (Suppl)):S483.

68. Dass S, Vital EM, Emery P. Development of psoriasis after B cell depletion with rituximab. *Arthritis Rheum* 2007; 56:2715–2718.

69. Abrams JR, Lebwohl MG, Guzzo CA, Jegasothy BV, Goldfarb MT, Goffe BS *et al.* CTLA4Ig-mediated blockade of T-cell costimulation in patients with psoriasis vulgaris. *J Clin Invest* 1999; 103:1243–1252.

70. Turkiewicz AM, Moreland LW. Psoriatic arthritis: current concepts on pathogenesis-oriented therapeutic options. *Arthritis Rheum* 2007; 56:1051–1066.

71. Veale DJ, Ritchlin C, FitzGerald O. Immunopathology of psoriasis and psoriatic arthritis. *Ann Rheum Dis* 2005; 64 Suppl 2:ii26–29.

72. Krueger GG, Langley RG, Leonardi C, Yeilding N, Guzzo C, Wang Y *et al.* A human interleukin-12/23 monoclonal antibody for the treatment of psoriasis. *N Engl J Med* 2007; 356:580–592.

73. Gottlieb A, Menter A, Mendelsohn A, Shen YK, Li S, Guzzo C *et al.* Ustekinumab, a human interleukin 12/23 monoclonal antibody, for psoriatic arthritis: randomised, double-blind, placebo-controlled, crossover trial. *Lancet* 2009; 373:633–640.

74. van der Heijde D, Landewe, RDM, Ory, P *et al.* Two-year etanercept therapy does not inhibit radiographic progression in patients with ankylosing spondylitis. *Ann Rheum Dis* 2006; 65(Suppl 2):81.

75. Baraliakos X, Listing J, Brandt J, Haibel H, Rudwaleit M, Sieper J *et al.* Radiographic progression in patients with ankylosing spondylitis after 4 yrs of treatment with the anti-TNF-alpha antibody infliximab. *Rheumatology* (Oxford) 2007; 46:1450–1453.

76. Braun J, Baraliakos X, Listing J, Fritz C, Alten R, Burmester G *et al.* Persistent clinical efficacy and safety of anti-tumour necrosis factor alpha therapy with infliximab in patients with ankylosing spondylitis over 5 years: evidence for different types of response. *Ann Rheum Dis* 2008; 67:340–345.

77. Zochling J, van der Heijde D, Burgos-Vargas R, Collantes E, Davis JC, Jr., Dijkmans B *et al.* ASAS/EULAR recommendations for the management of ankylosing spondylitis. *Ann Rheum Dis* 2006; 65:442–452.

78. Nash P. Therapies for axial disease in psoriatic arthritis. A systematic review. *J Rheumatol* 2006; 33:1431–1434.

79. Gorman JD, Sack KE, Davis JC, Jr. Treatment of ankylosing spondylitis by inhibition of tumor necrosis factor alpha. *N Engl J Med* 2002; 346:1349–1356.

80. Braun J, Baraliakos X, Golder W, Brandt J, Rudwaleit M, Listing J *et al.* Magnetic resonance imaging examinations of the spine in patients with ankylosing spondylitis, before and after successful therapy with infliximab: evaluation of a new scoring system. *Arthritis Rheum* 2003; 48:1126–1136.

81. Marzo-Ortega H, McGonagle D, Jarrett S, Haugeberg G, Hensor E, O'Connor P *et al.* Infliximab in combination with methotrexate in active ankylosing spondylitis: a clinical and imaging study. *Ann Rheum Dis* 2005; 64:1568–1575.

6

Therapy of ankylosing spondylitis

Jurgen Braun

INTRODUCTION

Ankylosing spondylitis (AS) is the major subtype and a major outcome of an interrelated group of rheumatic diseases now named as spondyloarthritides (SpA) [1]. The most important clinical features of this group are inflammatory back pain (IBP); asymmetric peripheral oligoarthritis, predominantly of the lower limbs; enthesitis; and specific organ involvement such as anterior uveitis, psoriasis and chronic inflammatory bowel disease. Aortic root involvement and conduction abnormalities are rare complications of AS. For clinical purposes, five subgroups of SpA are differentiated: AS, psoriatic SpA (PsSpA), reactive SpA (ReSpA), SpA associated with inflammatory bowel disease (SpAIBD) and undifferentiated SpA (uSpA). The SpA are genetically linked – the strongest known contributing factor is the major histocompatibility complex (MHC) class I molecule human leucocyte antigen (HLA) B27; others are currently being identified [1].

Most frequently and characteristically, AS starts in the sacroiliac joints at a mean age of 26 years, affecting men only slightly more frequently than women. In about 80% of patients the disease spreads to the spine, where all three segments are affected, most frequently the thoracic spine. Osteodestructive structural changes such as erosions occur less frequently than osteoproliferative changes, which are pathognomonic for AS, being clinically impressive by their appearance as syndesmophytes and ankylosis. Vertebral fractures occur more frequently in patients with AS than in the general population.

Standard assessments for patients with AS are available and international recommendations for the management of AS have recently been published [2].

MANAGEMENT

Ten main recommendations for the management of AS have been proposed recently by a combined 'Assessment in Ankylosing Spondylitis' working group (ASAS)/European League Against Rheumatism (EULAR) task force [2] (Figure 6.1). Briefly, the treatment of AS should be tailored according to the current manifestations of the disease, the level of current symptoms and several other features including the wishes and expectations of the patient. The disease monitoring of patients with AS should include patient history, clinical parameters, laboratory tests and imaging. The frequency of monitoring should be decided on an individual basis depending on symptoms, severity and medication. The optimal treatment of AS requires a combination of non-pharmacological and pharmacological treatment modalities including patient education and physical therapy. Anti-tumour necrosis factor (TNF) therapy should be given according to the ASAS recommendations [3].

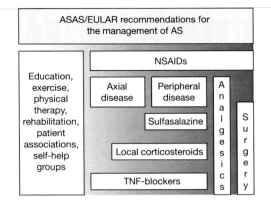

Figure 6.1 Assessment in Ankylosing Spondylitis working group/European League Against Rheumatism recommendations for the management of ankylosing spondylitis.

Joint replacement has to be considered in patients with radiographic evidence of advanced hip involvement who have refractory pain and disability. Spinal surgery is useful in selected patients with symptoms and disability due to disabilitating posture or unstable spine.

ASSESSMENTS

The main outcomes in AS are disease activity, which includes pain, morning stiffness and patient's global assessment; function; quality of life; and structural damage [4]. When assessing patients with AS, it is useful to think of measuring disease activity, physical function and structural damage as separate facets of the AS process: disease activity reflecting acute inflammation and rate of change, physical function reflecting the impact the disease has on the patient's ability to perform in his or her daily life, and structural damage being the end result of the AS process on anatomical structures. Accepted measurement domains within AS can be seen to cover one or more of these general concepts (Table 6.1).

The ASAS group, an international collaboration of clinicians, researchers and industry representatives with particular interest and expertise in AS, was established in 1995 with a goal to rationalize the assessment of this debilitating disease. ASAS has developed practical, concise core sets of concepts important for patient monitoring (Table 6.2), both in a clinical practice setting and for assessing treatment response in clinical trials [5]. The core sets were put together using a combination of expert consensus, research evidence and statistical approaches, and can be thought of as a standard framework for patient assessment. ASAS has subsequently reviewed the extensive literature on different outcome measures and instruments which have been used in AS clinical trials, and selected the most appropriate measures for each core set domain based on evidence of validity and consensus opinion [6].

The ASAS group recommends that the measures put forward in the core sets should be used in all research projects in AS to standardize outcome measurement, to ensure that meaningful patient outcomes are not overlooked, and to facilitate comparisons of response across studies. It is stressed that although the core sets describe the minimum set of domains that should be assessed and monitored in patients with AS, they are not exclusive or exhaustive; other concepts such as health-related quality of life can also add important information, and each situation should be individually assessed with regard to the specific aim of the assessment.

Table 6.1 Measurement domains in ankylosing spondylitis

Domain	Disease activity	Function	Damage
Patient global assessment	x	x	x
Spinal pain	x		x
Spinal stiffness	x	x	x
Spinal mobility	x	x	x
Physical function	x	x	x
Peripheral joints and entheses	x	x	
Fatigue	x		
Disease activity	x		
Quality of life	x	x	x
Acute-phase reactants	x		
Imaging	x		x

Table 6.2 Assessment in Ankylosing Spondylitis (ASAS) working group core sets for assessment in ankylosing spondylitis

Domain	Core set CR	SMARD/PT	DC-ART	Instruments
Patient global assessment	x	x	x	VAS in the last week
Spinal pain	x	x	x	VAS pain at night, average in the last week, and VAS, average in the last week
Spinal stiffness	x	x	x	VAS morning stiffness
Spinal mobility	x	x	x	Chest expansion, modified Schober index and occiput-to-wall distance
Physical function	x	x	x	Bath Ankylosing Spondylitis Functional Index or Dougados Functional Index
Peripheral joints and entheses	x		x	Number of swollen joints / No preferred instrument for entheseal disease
Fatigue			x	No preferred instrument
Acute-phase reactants	x		x	ESR
Imaging			x	AP and lateral X-rays lumbar spine, lateral cervical spine, pelvis (SI and hip joints)

AP, anteroposterior; CR, clinical record keeping; DC-ART, disease-controlling antirheumatic therapy; ESR, erythrocyte sedimentation rate; PT, physical therapy; SI, sacroiliac; SMARD, symptom-modifying antirheumatic drugs; VAS, visual analogue scale.

DISEASE ACTIVITY

Disease activity in AS is measured by the BASDAI [7], a composite index evaluating fatigue, axial and peripheral pain, stiffness and enthesopathy (Table 6.3). The self-administered instrument is made up of six questions, each to be answered on a visual analogue scale (VAS) (0–10 cm), where 0 = none (or 0 hours for morning stiffness) and 10 = very severe (or 2 or more hours for morning stiffness), regarding the patient's symptoms in the previous week. It is easy and quick to complete, the final score is a simple sum of its components, and the BASDAI has been extensively validated in clinical trials [18, 32] and translated into several

Table 6.3 Validated disease-specific instruments used for measurement in ankylosing spondylitis

Instrument	Abbreviation	Measures	Description
Bath Ankylosing Spondylitis Disease Activity Index [7]	BASDAI	Disease activity	A composite index made up of six questions, each measured on a 0–100 mm visual analogue scale (VAS): – fatigue – neck, back or hip pain – pain/swelling in other joints (not neck, back or hip) – overall discomfort from tender areas – overall level of morning stiffness (intensity) – duration of morning stiffness
Bath Ankylosing Spondylitis Functional Index [8]	BASFI	Function	A composite index made up of 10 questions, covering basic daily functions such as bending and standing, each measured on a 0–100 mm VAS
Bath Ankylosing Spondylitis Metrology Index [16]	BASMI	Function (spine and hip)	A composite index made up of five clinical measurements: – cervical rotation – tragus to wall distance – lumbar side flexion – modified Schober's test – intermalleolar distance
Bath Ankylosing Spondylitis Radiology Index [19]	BASRI	Structural damage	X-ray scoring system for the lateral cervical spine, AP and lateral lumbar spine and hips, using the New York system to grade the sacroiliac joints
Modified Stoke Ankylosing Spondylitis Spinal Score [18]	mSASSS	Structural damage	X-ray scoring system for the lateral cervical and lateral lumbar spine, score range 0–72

languages. A BASDAI score of > 4 is internationally accepted to indicate active disease, and most clinical trials of therapy in AS now require patients to have active disease as defined by a BASDAI > 4 before inclusion. The BASDAI is one of the most commonly used outcome measures in clinical trials, and is simple enough to be implemented in daily practice.

PHYSICAL FUNCTION

There is no single parameter that adequately measures the concept of physical function. A number of patient-assessed AS-specific instruments are available, which cover a range of physical functions and activities of daily living, in order to summarize how well a patient functions in daily life and to quantify 'disability' (Table 6.3). The most commonly used are the Bath Ankylosing Spondylitis Functional Index (BASFI; Table 6.3) [9], which has been shown to perform well in regards to reliability, validity and responsiveness across a range of settings [10, 11].

PERIPHERAL JOINTS AND ENTHESES

Peripheral joint involvement occurs in approximately 25% of patients with AS, usually in the form of oligoarticular, asymmetrical large joint involvement. The formal joint counts in use for rheumatoid arthritis (RA) are therefore not necessarily as useful in this setting. The ASAS group suggests using a 44-joint count, which includes the sternoclavicular joints, acromioclavicular joints, shoulders, elbows, wrists, knees, ankles, metacarpophalangeal and metatarsophalangeal joints, and the proximal interphalangeal joints of the hands. The core set advocates measuring only swollen joints in this way, although arguments can be made for recording painful joints also. Peripheral joint disease reflects both disease activity (acute inflammation) and physical function, but rarely progresses to significant structural damage.

There is no specific instrument recommended in the ASAS core sets for the assessment of enthesitis in AS. The Mander Enthesitis Index (MEI) was the first proposed, but is not feasible in clinical trials, whereas the Maastricht Ankylosing Spondylitis Enthesitis Score (MASES) includes only 13 entheses, and uses the dichotomous responses 'no pain' and 'painful' for each site, resulting in a score between 0 and 13 [12]. Another simplified enthesitis score has been developed in Berlin which requires the assessment of 12 different entheses for disease involvement concentrating on the clinically most relevant sites such as the heel and the trochanter, and is expressed as a simple score between 0 and 12 [13]; this method has not yet been formally validated.

FATIGUE

An important source of morbidity in patients with AS, fatigue seems to be associated with disease activity, functional ability and global well-being [14]. There are no specific disease-related measurement instruments for fatigue in AS. One question of the BASDAI [7] asks about the overall level of fatigue/tiredness in the past week (VAS, 0–100 mm), but none of the other composite instruments address this domain. This item has been recently shown to be sensitive and specific for fatigue in patients with AS with a cut-off of 70 mm [15], and is the recommended instrument for measuring fatigue in the ASAS core sets.

IMAGING

Structural changes of AS including syndesmophytes, erosions, sclerosis and ankylosis can be seen on spinal radiographs. Plain X-rays of the spine should include AP and lateral views of the lumbar spine and lateral views of the cervical spine. There are currently three validated scoring systems in use to assess spinal structural damage in clinical trials in AS: the original Stoke Ankylosing Spondylitis Spinal Score (SASSS [17]), a modified SASSS (mSASSS [18]) and the BASRI [19]. The mSASSS has been identified as the most reliable method [20].

Magnetic resonance imaging (MRI) of the sacroiliac joints and the spine is increasingly used to assess disease activity in AS. Although it has not been incorporated in the ASAS core set to date, it seems likely on the basis of recent data that MRI will have a role both in clinical trials and in daily care of the patients, because it is advantageous to have some objective evidence of spinal inflammation.

Although conventional radiography of the spine and the sacroiliac joints is mainly used to detect chronic structural changes in AS, MRI is indicated to detect active axial inflammation, including sacroiliitis, spondylitis and spondylodiscitis [21–24], which is not well seen with other imaging techniques. In clinical practice, a combination of X-rays and MRI appears most useful [24].

Ultrasonography can be a useful tool to detect enthesitis and bursitis in patients with spondyloarthritis [25, 26]. Ultrasound is much more sensitive than clinical examination for detecting these changes. In clinical practice it can assist in diagnosis and with ultrasound-directed aspiration or glucocorticosteroid injection.

LABORATORY TESTS

Whereas HLA-B27 is only useful for diagnosis, mainly in early disease, C-reactive protein (CRP) and erythrocyte sedimentation rate (ESR) are frequently used to assess disease activity, although their usefulness in this regard has been shown to be limited [27].

MEASURING TREATMENT RESPONSE

The ASAS group has taken the core sets and their respective measurement instruments to construct specific composite response criteria for measuring treatment response in AS trials (Table 6.4) [28]. Initially derived from five short-term trials of non-steroidal anti-inflammatory drugs (NSAIDs) in AS, the initial improvement criteria consist of four outcome domains: physical function, spinal pain, patient global assessment and inflammation. Improvement

Table 6.4 Assessment in Ankylosing Spondylitis (ASAS) working group response criteria

Instrument	Abbreviation	Description
ASAS improvement criteria [28]	ASAS-IC	Four domains, based on the discrimination between NSAID treatment and placebo – physical function, measured by the BASFI – spinal pain, measured on a 0–100 mm VAS – patient global assessment in the last week, on a 0–100 mm VAS – inflammation, measured as the mean of the last two BASDAI questions (intensity and duration of morning stiffness)
ASAS 20% response criteria [28]	ASAS20	Treatment response is defined as: – ≥20% and ≥10 mm VAS on a 0–100 scale in at least three of the four ASAS-IC domains, and – no worsening of ≥20% and ≥10 mm VAS on a 0–100 scale in the remaining fourth domain
ASAS 40% response criteria [30]	ASAS40	Treatment response is defined as: – ≥40% and ≥20 mm VAS on a 0–100 scale in at least three of the four ASAS-IC domains, and – no worsening of ≥40% and ≥20 mm VAS on a 0–100 scale in the remaining fourth domain
ASAS 5 out of 6 response criteria [30]	ASAS 5/6	Developed for use in trials of anti-TNF therapy, six domains were included: – pain – patient global assessment – function – inflammation – spinal mobility – C-reactive protein (acute phase reactant) Treatment response is defined as improvement in five of six domains without deterioration in the sixth domain, using predefined percentage improvements

is defined as a 20% improvement from baseline, or a 10-mm improvement from baseline for VAS measures on a 0–100 mm scale, in at least three of the four domains. There cannot be deterioration of 20% or more, or of 10 mm or more on a VAS scale, in the corresponding fourth domain. The response criteria show high specificity and moderate sensitivity [28], and have been validated in anti-TNF studies [29, 30].

BASIC PRINCIPLES OF TREATMENT

For decades the standard treatment of spinal symptoms of patients with AS has consisted of NSAIDs [31] and structured exercise programmes [32]. Whether, and to what extent, physical therapy and exercise are beneficial in every stage of the disease (e.g. in very active disease) is not known. Disease activity, especially the degree of spinal inflammation, function and damage, is likely to influence the outcome of physical therapy and regular exercise.

Besides physical therapy, non-pharmacological therapy comprises spa therapy, patient education and patient self-help groups. A recent Cochrane review [33] concluded that evidence-based medicine has difficulties ratifying that indication, but there is a strongly positive expert opinion; the effect size is probably small. However, intensive spa therapy has been shown to be more efficacious than standard prescriptions of exercises in an outpatient setting, for several months following treatment [34].

PHARMACOLOGICAL THERAPY WITH NON-STEROIDAL ANTI-INFLAMMATORY DRUGS

In general, NSAIDs work well in patients with AS. A good response to NSAIDs has even been identified as a diagnostic sign for SpA [35], and a state of non-responsiveness to NSAIDs may identify patients with a bad prognosis. Clinical experience suggests that active patients should be continuously treated with NSAIDs in a dosage sufficient to control pain and stiffness [36]. A recent study has even suggested that continuous dosing with NSAIDs rather than the usual on-demand prescription decelerates radiographic progression over 2 years [37]. However, NSAIDs, including coxibs, are known to have gastrointestinal, and potentially also cardiovascular, toxicity, which may limit their use in patients at risk [38]. Furthermore, about half of patients with AS report insufficient control of their symptoms by NSAIDs alone [39].

PHARMACOLOGICAL THERAPY WITH DISEASE-MODIFYING ANTIRHEUMATIC DRUGS

The use of disease-modifying antirheumatic drugs (DMARDs) for the treatment of axial disease in SpA has been rather disappointing. Therapies which are effective in suppressing disease activity and slowing disease progression in RA have notably failed to improve SpA, particularly for spinal disease [40]. Sulfasalazine has been shown to improve SpA-associated peripheral arthritis, but not spinal pain [41]. However, there are differences between the trials in relation to to disease duration and the proportion of patients with peripheral arthritis. Thus, the efficacy of sulfasalazine in earlier disease stages may be different. Indeed, in a recent controlled trial of sulfasalazine in uSpA and early AS, some efficacy on spinal pain was noted in patients with IBP, but no peripheral arthritis had a significantly larger improvement in disease activity than the placebo group, despite using fewer NSAIDs [42]. However, all patients improved, and definite conclusions are difficult.

Methotrexate (MTX) is commonly used in RA with good results, improving symptoms and slowing the progression of erosive disease. This is different in AS, suggesting another pathomechanism. In a systematic review on the use of MTX in AS [43], the conclusion was that there is no evidence for an effect on IBP and there is inconclusive evidence of efficacy for peripheral joint disease. The only randomized controlled trial of MTX in AS [44] failed to show a significant effect of 7.5 mg oral MTX weekly on spondylitis, but there was some improvement in peripheral arthritis. An open-label trial treating 20 active patients with AS with 20 mg MTX subcutaneously (s.c.) for 16 weeks also did not show any efficacy for axial and limited improvement of peripheral symptoms [45]. Many rheumatologists are still using MTX for AS because there were previously no other options. The differences in response between peripheral and axial symptoms may be because of the entheseal pathology.

Similarly, leflunomide (LFL) is effective in treating symptoms and slowing radiographic change in RA. In AS, LFL was not effective in treating axial manifestations [46], but patients with peripheral arthritis had some benefit [47]. LFL is effective in psoriatic arthritis [48].

Bisphosphonates may be useful in treating spinal symptoms of AS, as suggested by one study [49]. However, other studies with pamidronate failed to show a similar effect size in patients with AS [50].

Thalidomide has also been used with some success in patients with AS [51], but it is considered to be too toxic for widespread use.

TUMOUR NECROSIS FACTOR BLOCKERS

The introduction of TNF blockers has been the most substantial development in the treatment of AS and other SpA in recent years [1]. Three such agents are now approved for AS: the monoclonal chimeric antibody infliximab, which is given in a dosage of 3–5 mg/kg every 6–8 weeks intravenously (i.v.) (approved is the 5 mg/kg every 6–8 weeks regimen); the fully humanized monoclonal adalimumab, which is given in a dosage of 40 mg s.c. every other week; and the 75-kDa TNF receptor fusion protein etanercept given in a dosage of 50 mg s.c. once or 25 mg s.c. twice a week. The success of anti-TNF treatment is very likely to be a class effect. There is some evidence that this therapy works even better in SpA than in RA [52].

Large randomized controlled trials of infliximab [13, 53], etanercept [54, 55] and adalimumab [56] in AS have shown impressive short-term improvements in spinal pain, function and inflammatory markers with therapy compared with placebo. As shown by MRI, spondylitic changes are largely reduced with these therapies [23, 57–61]. As experience with these therapies grows out to 2- to 5-year trials now [61–64], it appears that efficacy may persist with ongoing treatment, and more than one-third of patients are in remission.

The trials show significant improvements in pain, function and disease activity in patients with AS with active disease compared with placebo. Indeed, all outcome measures, including BASDAI, BASFI, BASMI and the physical component of the SF-36, improved significantly after 24 and 102 weeks. The improvement usually starts within 2 weeks of therapy and CRP levels also tend to decrease rapidly.

Alongside the demonstrated long-term efficacy and safety of TNF blockers in AS, it is important to note the loss of response after cessation of continuous therapy with infliximab for 3 years [65], although re-administration was successful in gaining control. This was similar with etanercept [66].

The studies of infliximab in AS [13, 53] differ from etanercept and adalimumab [54–56] in that about 30% of patients were allowed to continue DMARD and glucocorticosteroid therapy because they were used to it.

Adalimumab also showed efficacy in AS in a pilot study [59], and in an RCT in which the pain of some patients with advanced spinal ankylosis also improved [56].

Although anti-TNF therapy was shown to decrease spinal inflammation as detected by MRI [57–61], no major inhibition of radiological progression of disease as assessed by the mSASSS [18] was seen in a small number of patients with AS treated with infliximab for 2 and 4 years [67, 68]. Bone mineral density was already shown to improve in patients on anti-TNF therapy after 6 months [69].

Clinical disease activity and spinal inflammation as detected by MRI are significantly reduced by TNF blockers, as shown after short- and long-term anti-TNF therapy. Whether anti-TNF treatment is capable of at least partly halting radiographic progression is as yet unclear; uncoupling of inflammation and new bone formation has been discussed as one possibility for why there could be a difference between AS and RA. However, structural damage may play a less important role in a disease with significant long-term functional disability which, although in part due to structural damage, is also due to persistent disease activity which may be effectively treated with anti-TNF agents.

The first pilot studies of infliximab and etanercept in undifferentiated SpA have been successful [70, 71]. The largest study with adalimumab in this indication showed that a high proportion of patients had major improvement of signs and symptoms.

Similarly, infliximab, etanercept and adalimumab have been shown to be effective for peripheral joint and skin symptoms in patients with psoriatic arthritis [72–75]. Etanercept is effective for rheumatic manifestations in inflammatory bowel disease (IBD), regarding both peripheral joint and spine, but not gut, symptoms [76]. In line with that, etanercept has no effect on IBD [77], and does not prevent flares of IBD [78]. This is in contrast to infliximab, which is approved for Crohn's disease (CD) [79] and ulcerative colitis (UC) [80]. Adalimumab is now also approved for CD. Thus, etanercept is not recommended for the comparatively small SpA subgroup with concomitant IBD. There may also be a difference in anti-TNF agents in the prevention and treatment of anterior uveitis [81–83].

Recommendations on which patients with AS should be treated with TNF-blockers are especially needed on the background of possible side-effects and the relatively high costs of these drugs. Thus, patients with the best risk–benefit ratio should be treated preferentially. An international ASAS consensus statement for the use of anti-TNF agents in patients with AS was published in 2003 and updated in 2006 [84]. A summary of these recommendations for the initiation of anti-TNF-α therapy is shown in Table 6.5. Prediction of response to anti-TNF therapy is difficult. Patients early in the course of their disease, with elevated CRP [85], positive MRI findings or less structural damage are more likely to respond, but, overall, all patient subgroups may benefit from this treatment.

Directed at a different cytokine in the inflammatory response than the TNF blockers, anakinra is a recombinant human interleukin 1 (IL-1) receptor antagonist. In contrast to TNF, it is unclear whether IL-1 is present in sacroiliac joints. Two recent open studies of anakinra in AS have been published, showing partly conflicting results [86, 87]. Other biologicals have not been tested so far – studies with rituximab, abatacept and tocilizumab are currently being planned.

SOCIOECONOMICS

Cost-effectiveness is an important issue when expensive therapies are considered. Despite the high costs, it was recently demonstrated that the clinical benefits and the improvements in quality of life in patients with AS treated with infliximab result in lower disease-associated costs than standard care, which translates to a short-term cost of approximately £35 000 per quality-adjusted life year (QALY) gained [88] – an amount society may be willing to pay. However, the calculated costs were higher in other analyses. When modelling for long-term therapy, using annual disease progression of 0.07 of the BASFI in the sensitivity analysis, the cost per QALY gained is reduced to < £10 000. It seems that the costs for anti-TNF therapy fall well inside what is considered to be 'cost-effective'. Much in line with this, it was recently shown that the daily productivity of patients with active AS which was significantly associated with functional impairment and disease activity greatly improved with infliximab, and this was associated with reduced workday loss among employed patients [89].

Table 6.5 Assessment in Ankylosing Spondylitis (ASAS) working group consensus for anti-tumour necrosis factor (TNF) therapy

Patient selection
Diagnosis
• Patients 'normally' fulfilling modified New York criteria for definitive AS [90]
• Modified New York criteria 1984 [90]
  – Radiological criterion
    • Sacroiliitis, grade >II bilaterally or grade III to IV unilaterally
  – Clinical criteria (two out of the following three)
    • Low back pain and stiffness for >3 months that improves with exercise but is not relieved by rest
    • Limitation of motion of the lumbar spine in both the sagittal and frontal planes
    • Limitation of chest expansion relative to normal values correlated for age and sex
Disease activity
• Active disease for >4 weeks
• BASDAI >4 (0–10) and an expert* opinion that anti-TNF treatment should be started†
Treatment failure
• All patients must have had adequate therapeutic trials of at least two NSAIDs. An adequate therapeutic trial is defined as:
  – Treatment for >3 months at maximal recommended or tolerated anti-inflammatory dose unless contraindicated
  – Treatment for <3 months where treatment was withdrawn because of intolerance, toxicity or contraindications
• Patients with symptomatic peripheral arthritis (normally having a lack of response to a local steroid injection for those with oligoarticular involvement) must have had adequate therapeutic trial of both NSAIDs and sulfasalazine‡
• Patients with symptomatic enthesitis must have had an adequate therapeutic trial of at least two local steroid injections unless contraindicated

Contraindications (as locally defined)

Assessment of disease
ASAS core set for daily practice
• Physical function (BASFI)
• Pain (VAS, past week, spine at night, because of AS and VAS, past week, spine because of AS)
• Spinal mobility (chest expansion and modified Schober test and occiput to wall distance and lateral lumbar flexion)
• Patient's global assessment (VAS, past week)
• Stiffness (duration of morning stiffness, spine, past week)
• Peripheral joints and entheses (number of swollen joints [44 joint count], enthesitis score such as developed in Maastricht, Berlin or San Francisco)
• Acute-phase reactants (ESR or CRP)
• Fatigue (VAS)
BASDAI
• VAS overall level of fatigue/tiredness past week
• VAS overall level of AS neck, back or hip pain past week
• VAS overall level of pain/swelling in joints other than neck, back or hips past week
• VAS overall discomfort from any areas tender to touch or pressure past week
• VAS overall level of morning stiffness from time of awakening past week
• Duration and intensity (VAS) of morning stiffness from time of awakening (up to 120 minutes)

Table 6.5 Continued

Assessment of response
Responder criteria
• BASDAI 50% relative change or absolute change of 2 (scale 0–10) and expert opinion: Continuation: yes/no
Time of evaluation
• Between 6 and 12 weeks

VAS, visual analogue scale; all VAS can be replaced by a numerical rating scale (NRS).

*The expert is a doctor, usually a rheumatologist, with expertise in inflammatory back pain and the use of biological agents. Experts should be locally defined.

†An expert opinion comprises clinical features (history and examination), serum acute phase reactant levels or imaging results, such as radiographs demonstrating rapid progression or MRI scans indicating inflammation.

‡Sulfasalazine: treatment for >4 months at standard target dose of 3 g/day, or maximum tolerated dose unless contraindicated or not tolerated. Treatment for <4 months, where treatment was withdrawn because of intolerance or toxicity or contraindicated.

REFERENCES

1. Braun J, Sieper J. Ankylosing spondylitis. *Lancet* 2007; 369:1379–1390.
2. Zochling J, van der Heijde D, Burgos-Vargas R, Collantes E, Davis JC Jr, Dijkmans B *et al.* ASAS/EULAR recommendations for the management of ankylosing spondylitis. *Ann Rheum Dis* 2006; 65:442–452.
3. Braun J, Davis J, Dougados M, Sieper J, van der Linden S, van der Heijde D. First update of the international ASAS consensus statement for the use of anti-TNF agents in patients with ankylosing spondylitis. *Ann Rheum Dis* 2006; 65:316–320.
4. Zochling J, Braun J. Assessments in ankylosing spondylitis. *Best Pract Res Clin Rheumatol* 2007; 21:699–712.
5. van der Heijde D, Bellamy N, Calin A, Dougados M, Khan MA, van der Linden S, Assessments in Ankylosing Spondylitis Working Group. Preliminary core sets for endpoints in ankylosing spondylitis. *J Rheumatol* 1997; 24:2225–2229.
6. van der Heijde D, Calin A, Dougados M, Khan MA, van der Linden S, Bellamy N, ASAS Working Group. Selection of instruments in the core set for DC-ART, SMARD, physical therapy and clinical record keeping in ankylosing spondylitis. Progress report of the ASAS Group. *J Rheumatol* 1999; 26:951–954.
7. Garrett S, Jenkinson T, Kennedy G, Whitelock H, Gaisford P, Calin A. A new approach to defining disease status in ankylosing spondylitis: The Bath Ankylosing Spondylitis Disease Activity Index (BASDAI). *J Rheumatol* 1994; 1:2286–2291.
8. Calin A, Nakache J-P, Gueguen A, Zeidler H, Mielants H, Dougados M. Defining disease activity in ankylosing spondylitis: is a combination of variables (Bath Ankylosing Spondylitis Disease Activity Index) an appropriate instrument? *Rheumatology* 1999; 38:878–882.
9. Calin A, Garrett S, Whitelock H, Kennedy LG, O'Hea J, Mallorie P, Jenkinson T. A new approach to defining functional ability in ankylosing spondylitis: the development of the Bath Ankylosing Spondylitis Functional Index. *J Rheumatol* 1994; 21:2281–2285.
10. Spoorenberg A, van der Heijde D, de Klerk E, Dougados M, de Vlam K, Mielants H, van der Tempel H, van der Linden S. A comparative study of the usefulness of the Bath Ankylosing Spondylitis Functional Index and the Dougados Functional Index in the assessment of ankylosing spondylitis. *J Rheumatol* 1999; 26:961–965.
11. Haywood KL, Garratt AM, Dawes PT. Patient-assessed health in ankylosing spondylitis: a structured review. *Rheumatology* 2005; 44:577–586.
12. Heuft-Dorenbosch L, Spoorenberg A, van Tubergen A, Landewe R, van ver Tempel H, Mielants H, Dougados M, van der Heijde D. Assessment of enthesitis in ankylosing spondylitis. *Ann Rheum Dis* 2003; 62:127–132.

13. Braun J, Brandt J, Listing J, Zink A, Alten R, Golder W, Gromnica-Ihle E, Kellner H, Krause A, Schneider M, Sorensen H, Zeidler H, Thriene W, Sieper J. Treatment of active ankylosing spondylitis with infliximab: a randomised controlled multicentre trial. *Lancet* 2002; 359:1187–1193.

14. Dagfinrud H, Vollestad NK, Loge JH, Kvien TK, Mengshoel AM. Fatigue in patients with ankylosing spondylitis: a comparison with the general population and associations with clinical and self-reported measures. *Arthritis Rheum* 2005; 53:5–11.

15. van Tubergen A, Coenen J, Landewé R, Spoorenberg A, Chorus A, Boonen A, van der Linden S, van der Heijde D. Assessment of fatigue in patients with ankylosing spondylitis: a psychometric analysis. *Arthritis Rheum* 2002; 47:8–16.

16. Jenkinson TR, Mallorie PA, Whitelock HC, Kennedy LG, Garrett SL, Calin A. Defining spinal mobility in ankylosing spondylitis (AS). The Bath AS Metrology Index. *J Rheumatol* 1994; 21:1694–1698.

17. Taylor HG, Wardle T, Beswich EJ, Dawes PT. The relationship of clinical and laboratory measurements to radiological change in ankylosing spondylitis. *Br J Rheumatol* 1991; 30:330–335.

18. Creemers MCW, Franssen MJAM, van't Hof MA, Gribnau FWJ, van de Putte LBA, van Riel PLCM. Assessment of outcome in ankylosing spondylitis: an extended radiographic scoring system. *Ann Rheum Dis* 2005; 64:127–129.

19. Calin A, Mackay K, Santos H, Brophy S. A new dimension to outcome: application of the Bath Ankylosing Spondylitis Radiology Index. *J Rheumatol* 1999; 26:988–992.

20. Wanders AJ, Landewe RB, Spoorenberg A, Dougados M, van der Linden S, Mielants H *et al.* What is the most appropriate radiologic scoring method for ankylosing spondylitis? A comparison of the available methods based on the Outcome Measures in Rheumatology Clinical Trials filter. *Arthritis Rheum* 2004; 50:2622–2632.

21. Baraliakos X, Landewe R, Hermann K-G, Listing J, Golder W, Brandt J *et al.* Inflammation in ankylosing spondylitis: a systematic description of the extent and frequency of acute spinal changes using magnetic resonance imaging. *Ann Rheum Dis* 2005; 64:730–734.

22. Braun J, Baraliakos X, Golder W, Hermann K-G, Listing J, Brandt J, Rudwaleit M, Zuehlsdorf S, Bollow M, Sieper J, van der Heijde D. Analysing chronic spinal changes in ankylosing spondylitis: a systematic comparison of conventional X rays with magnetic resonance imaging using established and new scoring systems. *Ann Rheum Dis* 2004; 63:1046–1055.

23. Braun J, Baraliakos X, Golder W, Brandt J, Rudwaleit M, Listing J, Bollow M, Sieper J, van der Heijde D. Magnetic resonance imaging examinations of the spine in patients with ankylosing spondylitis, before and after successful therapy with infliximab: evaluation of a new scoring system. *Arthritis Rheum* 2003; 48:1126–1136.

24. Heuft-Dorenbosch L, Landewe R, Weijers R, Wanders A, Houben H, van der Linden S *et al.* Combining information obtained from magnetic resonance imaging and conventional radiographs to detect sacroiliitis in patients with recent onset inflammatory back pain. *Ann Rheum Dis* 2006; 65:804–808.

25. Balint PV, Kane D, Wilson H, McInnes IB, Sturrock RD. Ultrasonography of entheseal insertions in the lower limb in spondyloarthropathy. *Ann Rheum Dis* 2002; 61:905–910.

26. D'Agostino MA, Said-Nahal R, Hacquard-Bouder C, Brasseur JL, Dougados M, Breban M. Assessment of peripheral enthesitis in the spondyloarthropathies by ultrasonography combined with power Doppler: a cross-sectional study. *Arthritis Rheum* 2003; 48:523–533.

27. Spoorenberg A, van der Heijde D, de Klerk E, Dougados M, de Vlam K, Mielants H, van der Tempel H, van der Linden S. Relative value of erythrocyte sedimentation rate and C-reactive protein in assessment of disease activity in ankylosing spondylitis. *J Rheumatol* 1999; 26:980–984.

28. Anderson JJ, Baron G, van der Heijde D, Felson DT, Dougados M. Ankylosing Spondylitis Assessment Group preliminary definition of short-term improvement in ankylosing spondylitis. *Arthritis Rheum* 2001; 44:1876–1886.

29. Stone MA, Inman RD, Wright JG, Maetzel A. Validation exercise of the ankylosing spondylitis assessment study (ASAS) group response criteria in ankylosing spondylitis patients treated with biologics. *Arthritis Rheum* 2004; 51:316–320.

30. Brandt J, Listing J, Sieper J, Rudwaleit M, van der Heijde D, Braun J. Development and preselection of criteria for short term improvement after anti-TNFα treatment in ankylosing spondylitis. *Ann Rheum Dis* 2004; 63:1438–1444.

31. Dougados M, Dijkmans B, Khan M, Maksymowych W, van der Linden S, Brandt J. Conventional treatments for ankylosing spondylitis. *Ann Rheum Dis* 2002; 61(Suppl. 3):iii40–50.

32. Kraag G, Stokes B, Groh J, Helewa A, Goldsmith C. The effects of comprehensive home physiotherapy and supervision on patients with ankylosing spondylitis – a randomized controlled trial. *J Rheumatol* 1990;17:228–233.

33. van Tubergen A, Landewe R, van der Heijde D, Hidding A, Wolter N, Asscher M *et al.* Combined spa-exercise therapy is effective in patients with ankylosing spondylitis: a randomized controlled trial. *Arthritis Rheum* 2001; 45:430–438.

34. Dagfinrud H, Kvien TK, Hagen KB. The Cochrane review of physiotherapy interventions for ankylosing spondylitis. *J Rheumatol* 2005; 32:1899–1906.

35. Amor B, Dougados M, Mijiyawa M. Criteria of the Classification of Spondylarthropathies. *Rev Rheum Mal Osteoartic* 1990; 57:85–89.

36. Dougados M, Behier JM, Jolchine I, Calin A, van der Heijde D, Olivieri I *et al.* Efficacy of celecoxib, a cyclooxygenase 2-specific inhibitor, in the treatment of ankylosing spondylitis: a six-week controlled study with comparison against placebo and against a conventional nonsteroidal antiinflammatory drug. *Arthritis Rheum* 2001; 44:180–185.

37. Wanders A, Heijde D, Landewe R, Behier JM, Calin A, Olivieri I *et al.* Nonsteroidal antiinflammatory drugs reduce radiographic progression in patients with ankylosing spondylitis: a randomized clinical trial. *Arthritis Rheum* 2005; 52:1756–1765.

38. Ward MM, Kuzis S. Medication toxicity among patients with ankylosing spondylitis. *Arthritis Rheum* 2002; 47:234–241.

39. Zochling J, Bohl-Buhler MH, Baraliakos X, Feldtkeller E, Braun J. Nonsteroidal anti-inflammatory drug use in ankylosing spondylitis-a population-based survey. *Clin Rheumatol* 2006; 25:794–800.

40. Dougados M, vam der Linden S, Leirisalo-Repo M, Huitfeldt B, Juhlin R, Veys E *et al.* Sulfasalazine in the treatment of spondylarthropathy. A randomized, multicenter, double-blind, placebo-controlled study. *Arthritis Rheum* 1995; 38:618–627.

41. Chen J, Liu C. Sulfasalazine for ankylosing spondylitis. Cochrane Database Syst Rev 2005(2):CD004800.

42. Braun J, Zochling J, Baraliakos X, Alten RH, Burmester GR, Grasedyck K *et al.* Efficacy of sulfasalazine in patients with inflammatory back pain due to undifferentiated spondyloarthritis and early ankylosing spondylitis: a multicentre randomized controlled trial. *Ann Rheum Dis* 2006; 65:1147–1153.

43. Chen J, Liu C. Methotrexate for ankylosing spondylitis. Cochrane Database Syst Rev 2004(3):CD004524.

44. Gonzalez-Lopez L, Garcia-Gonzalez A, Vazquez-Del-Mercado M, Munoz-Valle JF, Gamez-Nava JI. Efficacy of methotrexate in ankylosing spondylitis: a randomized, double blind, placebo controlled trial. *J Rheumatol* 2004; 31:1568–1574.

45. Haibel H, Brandt HC, Song IH, Brandt A, Listing J, Rudwaleit M *et al.* No efficacy of subcutaneous methotrexate in active ankylosing spondylitis: a 16-week open-label trial. *Ann Rheum Dis* 2007; 66:419–421.

46. Haibel H, Rudwaleit M, Braun J, Sieper J. Six months open label trial of leflunomide in active ankylosing spondylitis. *Ann Rheum Dis* 2005; 64:124–126.

47. Van Denderen JC, Van der Paardt M, Nurmohamed MT, De Ryck YM, Dijkmans BA, Van der Horst-Bruinsma IE. Double-blind, randomised, placebo-controlled study of leflunomide in the treatment of active ankylosing spondylitis. *Ann Rheum Dis* 2005; 64:1761–1764.

48. Kaltwasser JP, Nash P, Gladman D, Rosen CF, Behrens F, Jones P *et al.* Efficacy and safety of leflunomide in the treatment of psoriatic arthritis and psoriasis: a multinational, double-blind, randomized, placebo-controlled clinical trial. *Arthritis Rheum* 2004; 50:1939–1950.

49. Maksymowych WP, Jhangri GS, Fitzgerald AA, LeClercq S, Chiu P, Yan A *et al.* A six-month randomized, controlled, double-blind, dose–response comparison of intravenous pamidronate (60 mg versus 10 mg) in the treatment of nonsteroidal antiinflammatory drug-refractory ankylosing spondylitis. *Arthritis Rheum* 2002; 46:766–773.

50. Haibel H, Brandt J, Rudwaleit M, Soerensen H, Sieper J, Braun J. Treatment of active ankylosing spondylitis with pamidronate. *Rheumatology* (Oxford) 2003; 42:1018–1020.

51. Huang F, Gu J, Zhao W, Zhu J, Zhang J, Yu DT. One-year open-label trial of thalidomide in ankylosing spondylitis. *Arthritis Rheum* 2002; 47:249–254.

52. Heiberg MS, Nordvag BY, Mikkelsen K, Rodevand E, Kaufmann C, Mowinckel P *et al.* The comparative effectiveness of tumor necrosis factor-blocking agents in patients with rheumatoid arthritis and patients with ankylosing spondylitis: a six-month, longitudinal, observational, multicenter study. *Arthritis Rheum* 2005; 52:2506–2512.

53. van der Heijde D, Dijkmans B, Geusens P, Sieper J, DeWoody K, Williamson P et al. Efficacy and safety of infliximab in patients with ankylosing spondylitis: results of a randomized, placebo-controlled trial (ASSERT). *Arthritis Rheum* 2005; 52:582–591.

54. Davis JC Jr, Van Der Heijde D, Braun J, Dougados M, Cush J, Clegg DO et al. Recombinant human tumor necrosis factor receptor (etanercept) for treating ankylosing spondylitis: a randomized, controlled trial. *Arthritis Rheum* 2003; 48:3230–3236.

55. Calin A, Dijkmans BA, Emery P, Hakala M, Kalden J, Leirisalo-Repo M et al. Outcomes of a multi-centre randomised clinical trial of etanercept to treat ankylosing spondylitis. *Ann Rheum Dis* 2004; 63:1594–1600.

56. van der Heijde D, Kivitz A, Schiff M, Sieper J, Dijkmans B, Braun WE et al. Adalimumab therapy results in significant reduction of signs and symptoms in subjects with ankylosing spondylitis: the ATLAS trial. *Arthritis Rheum* 2006; 54:2136–2146.

57. Braun J, Landewe R, Hermann KG, Han J, Yan S, Williamson P et al. Major reduction in spinal inflam-mation in patients with ankylosing spondylitis after treatment with infliximab: results of a multicenter, randomized, double-blind, placebo-controlled magnetic resonance imaging study. *Arthritis Rheum* 2006; 54:1646–1652.

58. Baraliakos X, Davis J, Tsuji W, Braun J. Magnetic resonance imaging examinations of the spine in patients with ankylosing spondylitis before and after therapy with the tumor necrosis factor α receptor fusion protein etanercept. *Arthritis Rheum* 2005; 52:1216–1223.

59. Haibel H, Rudwaleit M, Brandt HC, Listing J, Grozdanovic Z, Kupper H et al. Adalimumab reduces spinal symptoms in active ankylosing spondylitis – clinical and magnetic resonance imaging results of a fifty-two week open label trial. *Arthritis Rheum* 2006; 54:678–681.

60. Sieper J, Baraliakos X, Listing J, Brandt J, Haibel H, Rudwaleit M et al. Persistent reduction of spinal inflammation as assessed by magnetic resonance imaging in patients with ankylosing spondylitis after 2 yrs of treatment with the anti-tumour necrosis factor agent infliximab. *Rheumatology* (Oxford) 2005; 44:1525–1530.

61. Baraliakos X, Brandt J, Listing J, Haibel H, Sörensen H, Rudwaleit M et al. Outcome of patients with active anklyosing spondylitis after 2 years of therapy with etanercept – clinical and magnetic resonance imaging data. *Arthritis Res Ther* 2005; 7:113.

62. Braun J, Baraliakos X, Brandt J, Listing J, Zink A, Alten R et al. Persistent clinical response to the anti-TNF-alpha antibody infliximab in patients with ankylosing spondylitis over 3 years. *Rheumatology* (Oxford) 2005; 44:670–676.

63. Davis JC, van der Heijde DM, Braun J, Dougados M, Clegg DO, Kivitz AJ et al. Efficacy and safety of up to 192 weeks of etanercept therapy in patients with ankylosing spondylitis. *Ann Rheum Dis* 2008; 67:346–352.

64. Braun J, Baraliakos X, Listing J, Fritz C, Alten R, Burmester G et al. Persistent clinical efficacy and safety of anti-TNFα therapy with infliximab in patients with ankylosing spondylitis over 5 years – evidence for different types of response. *Ann Rheum Dis* 2008; 67:340–345.

65. Baraliakos X, Listing J, Brandt J, Rudwaleit M, Sieper J, Braun J. Clinical response to discontinuation of anti-TNF therapy in patients with ankylosing spondylitis after 3 years of continuous treatment with infliximab. *Arthritis Res Ther* 2005; 7:R439–444.

66. Brandt J, Kariouzov A, Listing J, Haibel H, Sörensen H, Grassnickel L et al. Six months results of a German double-blind placebo controlled clinical trial of etanercept in active ankylosing spondylitis. *Arthritis Rheum* 2003; 48:1667–1675.

67. Baraliakos X, Listing J, Rudwaleit M, Brandt J, Sieper J, Braun J. Radiographic progression in patients with ankylosing spondylitis after 2 years of treatment with the TNF-α antibody infliximab. *Ann Rheum Dis* 2005; 64:1462–1466.

68. Baraliakos X, Listing J, Brandt J, Haibel H, Rudwaleit M, Sieper J, Braun J. Radiographic progression in patients with ankylosing spondylitis after 4 yrs of treatment with the anti-TNF-α antibody infliximab. *Rheumatology* (Oxford) 2007; 46:1450–1453.

69. Allali F, Breban M, Porcher R, Maillefert JF, Dougados M, Roux C. Increase in bone mineral density of patients with spondyloarthropathy treated with anti-tumour necrosis factor α. *Ann Rheum Dis* 2003; 62:347–349.

70. Brandt J, Haibel H, Reddig J, Sieper J, Braun J. Successful short term treatment of severe undifferenti-ated spondyloarthropathy with the anti-tumor necrosis factor-alpha monoclonal antibody infliximab. *J Rheumatol* 2002; 29:118–122.

71. Brandt J, Khariouzov A, Listing J, Haibel H, Sorensen H, Rudwaleit M et al. Successful short term treatment of patients with severe undifferentiated spondyloarthritis with the anti-tumor necrosis factor-alpha fusion receptor protein etanercept. *J Rheumatol* 2004; 31:531–538.
72. Feldman SR, Gordon KB, Bala M, Evans R, Li S, Dooley LT et al. Infliximab treatment results in significant improvement in the quality of life of patients with severe psoriasis: a double-blind placebo-controlled trial. *Br J Dermatol* 2005; 152:954–960.
73. Mease PJ, Kivitz AJ, Burch FX, Siegel EL, Cohen SB, Ory P et al. Etanercept treatment of psoriatic arthritis: safety, efficacy, and effect on disease progression. *Arthritis Rheum* 2004; 50:2264–2272.
74. Mease P, Gladman D, Ritchlin C, Ruderman E, Steinfeld D, Choy E et al. Adalimumab therapy in patients with psoriatic arthritis: 24-week results of a phase III study. *Arthritis Rheum* 2004; 50:4097.
75. Antoni C, Krueger GG, de Vlam K, Birbara C, Beutler A, Guzzo C et al. Infliximab improves signs and symptoms of psoriatic arthritis: results of the IMPACT 2 trial. *Ann Rheum Dis* 2005; 64:1150–1157.
76. Marzo-Ortega H, McGonagle D, O'Connor P, Emery P. Efficacy of etanercept for treatment of Crohn's related spondyloarthritis but not colitis. *Ann Rheum Dis* 2003; 62:74–76.
77. Braun J, Baraliakos X, Listing J, Davis J, van der Heijde D, Haibel H, Rudwaleit M, Sieper J. Differences in the incidence of flares or new onset of inflammatory bowel diseases in patients with ankylosing spondylitis exposed to therapy with anti-tumor necrosis factor alpha agents. *Arthritis Rheum* 2007; 57:639–647.
78. Sandborn WJ, Hanauer SB, Katz S, Safdi M, Wolf DG, Baerg RD et al. Etanercept for active Crohn's disease: a randomized, double-blind, placebo-controlled trial. *Gastroenterology* 2001; 121:1088–1094.
79. Hanauer SB, Feagan BG, Lichtenstein GR, Mayer LF, Schreiber S, Colombel JF et al. Maintenance infliximab for Crohn's disease: the ACCENT I randomised trial. *Lancet* 2002; 359(9317):1541–1549.
80. Rutgeerts P, Sandborn WJ, Feagan BG, Reinisch W, Olson A, Johanns J et al. Infliximab for induction and maintenance therapy for ulcerative colitis. *N Engl J Med* 2005; 353:2462–2476.
81. Braun J, Baraliakos X, Listing J, Sieper J. Decreased incidence of anterior uveitis in patients with ankylosing spondylitis treated with the anti-tumor necrosis factor agents infliximab and etanercept. *Arthritis Rheum* 2005; 52:2447–2451.
82. Guignard S, Gossec L, Salliot C, Ruyssen-Witrand A, Luc M, Duclos M et al. Efficacy of tumour necrosis factor blockers in reducing uveitis flares in patients with spondylarthropathy: a retrospective study. *Ann Rheum Dis* 2006; 65:1631–1634.
83. Lim LL, Fraunfelder FW, Rosenbaum JT. Do tumor necrosis factor inhibitors cause uveitis? A registry-based study. *Arthritis Rheum* 2007; 56:3248–3252.
84. Braun J, Davis J, Dougados M, Sieper J, van der Linden S, van der Heijde D. First update of the international ASAS consensus statement for the use of anti-TNF agents in patients with ankylosing spondylitis. *Ann Rheum Dis* 2006; 65:316–320.
85. Rudwaleit M, Listing J, Brandt J, Braun J, Sieper J. Prediction of a major clinical response (BASDAI 50) to tumour necrosis factor alpha blockers in ankylosing spondylitis. *Ann Rheum Dis* 2004; 63:665–670.
86. Tan AL, Marzo-Ortega H, O'Connor P, Fraser A, Emery P, McGonagle D. Efficacy of anakinra in active ankylosing spondylitis: a clinical and magnetic resonance imaging study. *Ann Rheum Dis* 2004; 63:1041–1045.
87. Haibel H, Rudwaleit M, Listing J, Sieper J. Open label trial of anakinra in active ankylosing spondylitis over 24 weeks. *Ann Rheum Dis* 2005; 64:296–298.
88. Kobelt G, Andlin-Sobocki P, Brophy S, Jonsson L, Calin A, Braun J. The burden of ankylosing spondylitis and the cost-effectiveness of treatment with infliximab (Remicade). *Rheumatology* (Oxford) 2004; 43:1158–1166.
89. van der Heijde D, Han C, Devlam K, Burmester G, van den Bosch F, Williamson P et al. Infliximab improves productivity and reduces workday loss in patients with ankylosing spondylitis: results from a randomized, placebo-controlled trial. *Arthritis Rheum* 2006; 55:569–574.
90. van der Linden S, Valkenburg HA, Cats A. Evaluation of diagnostic criteria for ankylosing spondylitis. A proposal for modification of the New York criteria. *Arthritis Rheum* 1984; 27:361–368.

7

Systemic lupus erythematosus

Tim Y.-T. Lu, Jose M. Pego-Reigosa, David A. Isenberg

INTRODUCTION

Systemic lupus erythematosus (SLE) is a chronic disease characterized by episodes of flares and remissions. Table 7.1 shows the 1997 revised American College of Rheumatology (ACR) criteria for the classification of SLE [1, 2]. The life expectancy of such patients has improved from an approximate 4-year survival rate of 50% in the 1950s [3] to a 15-year survival rate of 80% in the late 1990s [4], as a consequence of the use of traditional immunosuppressive agents, for example hydroxychloroquine, glucocorticosteroids, azathioprine (AZA) and cyclophosphamide (CYC), in conjunction with antihypertensive agents and improved management of renal complications of SLE through dialysis and renal transplantation [5]. With the advent of the biologicals era, there have been promising therapeutic advances in the treatment of SLE. These advances have led to randomized controlled trials which are currently in progress. In this chapter we will discuss mycophenolate mofetil (MMF), a relatively new therapeutic agent, and various targeted therapeutic approaches in the treatment of SLE.

MYCOPHENOLATE MOFETIL

The active metabolite of MMF inhibits purine synthesis and depletes lymphocytes and monocytes of guanosine triphosphate, thereby suppressing the proliferation of T and B lymphocytes [6]. The efficacy of MMF in the treatment of patients with lupus nephritis has been established in several open-label, randomized controlled trials.

In 2000, Chan *et al.* [7] published the results of a study designed to demonstrate the efficacy of MMF as an induction therapy in the treatment of 42 patients with diffuse proliferative lupus nephritis. In the two therapeutic regimes, prednisolone and MMF (1–2 g/day) administered for 12 months was compared with prednisolone and oral CYC (2.5 mg/kg/day) administered for 6 months, followed by prednisolone and AZA (1.5 mg/kg/day) for another 6 months. There were 21 patients in each group. Both regimes were found to be equally effective, with 81% of patients treated with MMF and prednisolone achieving complete remission, and 14% reaching partial remission, compared with 76% and 14%, respectively, of the patients treated with CYC and prednisolone followed by AZA and prednisolone. The improvements in the degree of proteinuria and the serum albumin and creatinine concentrations were similar in the two groups. The authors suggested that MMF is an appropriate therapeutic agent, given its better tolerability and lack of serious adverse effects compared with oral CYC. Limitations of this study included the small sample size, the short duration of follow-up and the lack of comparison to a standard intravenous CYC regime.

Table 7.1 1997 revised American College of Rheumatology criteria for the classification of systemic lupus erythematosus

Malar rash
Discoid lupus
Photosensitivity
Mucosal ulcers
Non-erosive arthritis
Serositis
Renal disorder
persistent proteinuria >0.5 g/day, cellular casts
Neurological disorder
seizures, psychosis
Haematological disorder
haemolytic anaemia, leucopenia, thrombocytopenia
Immunological disorder
antinuclear antibody in raised titre, anti-DNA antibodies, anti-Sm antibodies
antiphospholipid antibodies

For the purpose of identifying patients for clinical studies, a person has SLE if over 4 out of 11 features are present serially or simultaneously.

In 2005, Ong *et al.* [8] published the results of a trial comparing MMF (2 g/day) plus steroids for 6 months with pulse intravenous CYC (0.75–1.0 g/m²) monthly for 6 months plus steroids in the treatment of 44 patients with newly diagnosed proliferative lupus nephritis. Both regimes were found to be equally effective as induction therapy with a similar safety profile.

Ginzler *et al.* [9] reported on the results of a trial which randomized 140 patients with lupus nephritis (World Health Organization [WHO] class III, IV and V) to receive either MMF (1–3 g/day) plus steroids, or monthly intravenous CYC (0.5–1.0 g/m²) plus steroids as induction therapy. After 24 weeks of follow-up, 16 of the 71 patients (22.5%) receiving MMF and 4 of the 69 patients receiving CYC (5.8%) had complete remission, for an absolute difference of 16.7 percentage points (95% confidence interval [CI], 5.6–27.9 percentage points; $P = 0.005$), demonstrating the superiority of MMF to CYC. As noted in previous trials, MMF had fewer toxic effects and was better tolerated than CYC.

The role of MMF in maintenance therapy for patients with lupus nephritis was assessed by Contreras *et al.* [10] in a randomized trial involving 59 patients with lupus nephritis (WHO class III, IV, Vb). They were initially treated with an induction therapy consisting of monthly pulses of intravenous CYC (0.5–1.0 g/m²) plus steroids, and then assigned to receive one of the following maintenance regimes: 3-monthly intravenous CYC, AZA (1–3 mg/kg/day) or MMF (0.5–3 g/day) for 1–3 years. The 72-month event-free survival rate for the composite end-point of death or chronic renal failure was higher in the MMF and AZA groups than in the CYC group ($P = 0.05$ and $P = 0.009$, respectively). The rate of relapse-free survival was higher in the MMF group than in the CYC group ($P = 0.02$). The incidence of hospitalization, amenorrhoea, infections, nausea and vomiting was significantly lower in the MMF and AZA groups than in the CYC group.

It can be concluded from these open-label studies that MMF is an effective therapeutic option for treating patients with lupus nephritis, in both the induction and the maintenance phase of treatment. Its tolerability and lack of serious adverse effects is a major advantage in its use. Preliminary data from the Aspreva Lupus Management Study [11], which involved a greater number of patients and a longer follow-up period, suggested that MMF did not show superiority over CYC as an agent for inducing remission in lupus nephritis. However, there is a lack of evidence for the use of MMF in non-renal manifestation of SLE. Most of the available data are derived from case reports or case series involving patients with dermatological involvement and haematological disorders, and the results of these studies are inconclusive [12–14].

SPECIFIC TARGETED THERAPEUTIC AGENTS

As our understanding of the immune response and the clearance of apoptotic cell debris has increased, a variety of potential targets for intervention has emerged. A principle underlying the development of these targeted therapies is based on the premise that B cells play a central role in the pathogenesis of SLE through several functions, including antigen presentation, production of autoantibodies and communication with T cells. Therefore, B cells and cytokines which promote their survival and function present attractive targets for designing a specific biological agent. Figure 7.1 illustrates some of these targets.

B-CELL DEPLETION THERAPY

Anti-CD20 monoclonal antibody

Rituximab, a chimeric monoclonal antibody directed against the B-lymphocyte marker CD20, has been used with some success during the past 8 years in the treatment of patients with SLE. It is a non-selective inhibitor, in that all mature B cells which express the CD20 antigen are targeted, whether they are functionally normal, autoimmune or malignant. CD20 plays an important role in regulating the activation and differentiation of B cells [15]. The pharmacodynamic effect of rituximab results in the elimination of peripheral B cells without preventing the regeneration of B cells from stem cells and pro-B cells [16], as they do not express the CD20 antigen. Plasma cells are also spared from the effects of rituximab for the same reason. Treatment with rituximab induces a rapid depletion of CD20-expressing B cells in the peripheral blood with levels remaining low or undetectable for 2–6 months, followed by return to pretreatment levels generally within 12 months [17].

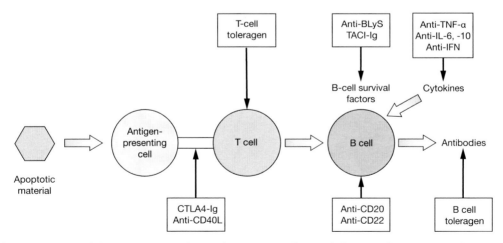

Figure 7.1 Targeted therapeutic approaches in the treatment of systemic lupus erythematosus. BLyS, B-lymphocyte stimulator; CTLA, cytotoxic T-lymphocyte antigen; IFN, interferon; Ig, immunoglobulin; IL, interleukin; TACI, transmembrane activator and calcium modulating cyclophilin ligand interactor; TNF-α, tumour necrosis factor alpha.

Several open-label, observational studies have demonstrated the efficacy of rituximab in treating patients with SLE, who were non- or poorly responsive to conventional immunosuppression. In 2002, Leandro et al. [18] published the results of a trial involving six women with refractory SLE treated with two intravenous infusions of 500 mg rituximab plus 750 mg CYC given 2 weeks apart, and with high-dose oral steroids. At 6 months, the five patients who had completed follow-up experienced a significant clinical improvement, as indicated by a reduction in the global British Isles Lupus Assessment Group (BILAG) [19] disease activity index scores. The mean duration of B-cell depletion was 4.4 months. No significant adverse effects were noted. The same authors performed an extension of this study in a longitudinal analysis of 24 patients with SLE treated with B-cell depletion therapy using two intravenous infusions of 1 g rituximab in conjunction with two intravenous infusions of 750 mg CYC and 250 mg methylprednisolone, given 2 weeks apart [20]. There was an improvement in the global BILAG scores, serum C3 levels and double-stranded DNA binding from the time of B-cell depletion to 6 months after this treatment was recorded. One patient failed to achieve B-lymphocyte depletion in the peripheral blood. Analysis of the regular BILAG assessments showed that improvements occurred in each of the eight organ systems. No major adverse events were reported, although one patient developed a severe infusion reaction related to rituximab, and another patient with very aggressive disease died of pancarditis 5 months after being treated (B-cell repopulation of the peripheral blood was already detectable at 4 months). Thirteen patients remained well without the need for further immunosuppressive therapy at a mean follow-up of 23 months. In another study involving seven subjects from the same cohort of patients, repeated treatment with B-cell depletion therapy was found to have similar efficacy [21]. Lastly, the same group of authors reported on the long-term clinical outcome and predictors of response of B-cell depletion therapy [22]. Baseline anti-extractable nuclear antigen antibody, notably the presence of anti-Sm, was the only identified independent predictor of disease flare after treatment from a multivariable analysis. Patients with low baseline serum C3 also had a shorter time to flare post B-cell depletion. These encouraging long-term results strongly suggest that removal of CD20-positive B cells is an effective therapy for treating patients with active SLE.

A phase I/II dose-escalation trial of rituximab was conducted by Looney et al. [23] in 2004 to assess its efficacy in the treatment of 18 patients with clinically active disease, as defined by a systemic lupus activity measure (SLAM) score of greater than five. Patients who were previously using CYC or bolus glucocorticosteroids were excluded from the study. Rituximab was administered as a single infusion of 100 mg/m^2 (low dose), a single infusion of 375 mg/m^2 (intermediate dose), or as four infusions (1 week apart) of 375 mg/m^2 (high dose), plus two 40-mg doses of oral steroids. At 12 months of follow-up, patients who achieved profound B-cell depletion (to < 5 CD19-positive B cells/μl) recorded a significant reduction in the mean SLAM scores compared with baseline. Manifestations such as rash, mucositis, alopecia and arthritis responded particularly well to this protocol. Rituximab was well tolerated in the majority of patients. However, there were four adverse events: one infusion-related bronchospasm of mild severity, one transient ischaemic attack and two infections. The same group of authors published further studies [24, 25] which highlighted important immunopathogenic features associated with the therapeutic action of rituximab. Firstly, the degree of B-cell depletion is related to the FcγRIIIa genotype, demonstrating the importance of antibody-dependent cell-mediated cytotoxicity and apoptosis induction as the mechanism of B-cell lysis by rituximab. Secondly, rituximab improves abnormalities in B-cell homeostasis and tolerance that are characteristic of this disease, and that the persistence of elevated autoantibody titres may reflect the presence of low levels of residual autoreactive memory B cells and/or long-lived autoreactive plasma cells.

Sfikakis et al. [26] established the clinical efficacy of rituximab in the treatment of active proliferative lupus nephritis in an open-label, prospective trial involving 10 patients.

They received four weekly intravenous infusions of $375\,mg/m^2$ rituximab combined with a tapering regime of oral steroids at a starting dose of $0.5\,mg/kg/day$ for 10 weeks. Five patients achieved complete remission, as defined by normal serum creatinine and albumin levels, inactive urinary sediment and urinary protein excretion of less than $500\,mg$ in 24 hours. At 12 months' follow-up, four patients remained free of active SLE without any immunosuppressive agents or with only low-dose oral steroids. No major adverse events were reported, other than one patient who developed a moderate hypersensitivity reaction which responded to intravenous hydrocortisone. The authors also observed that clinical remission of nephritis following B-cell depletion was preceded by downregulation of the T-cell co-stimulatory molecule CD40 ligand.

The efficacy of rituximab in the treatment of proliferative lupus nephritis was further demonstrated by Gunnarsson et al. [27] in a study involving seven patients with active proliferative lupus nephritis, using a combination protocol of rituximab and CYC. The outcome was assessed both clinically and histopathologically. At 6 months' follow-up, significant clinical improvement was noted, with a reduction in SLE disease activity index (SLEDAI) scores (from a mean of 15 to 3), anti-double-stranded DNA antibody levels (from a mean of $174\,IU/ml$ to $56\,IU/ml$) and anti-C1q antibody levels (from a mean of 35 units/ml to 22 units/ml). On repeat renal biopsy, improvement in the histopathological class of nephritis occurred in a majority of patients, and a decrease in the renal activity index was noted (from 6 to 3). A reduction in the number of CD3, CD4 and CD20 cells in the renal interstitium was noted in 50% of the patients on repeat biopsy.

Findings from these and other studies [28–42] (Table 7.2) strongly suggest that B-cell depletion therapy, based on rituximab, is effective in the treatment of patients with SLE. Although protocols differ, it appears that there is a synergistic effect in combining rituximab with CYC and glucocorticosteroids. The optimum regime, in terms of achieving the desired therapeutic effect while minimizing adverse events, has not been agreed. Disappointingly, Genetech (Genetech Inc., South San Francisco, CA, USA) have recently announced that double-blind control trials of non-renal and renal lupus have not found any advantage in using rituximab compared with a placebo. The full facts have yet to be published, but it seems likely that allowing patients to be treated with concomitant oral prednisolone of up to $1\,mg/kg$ may well have masked the ability of rituximab to show any benefit.

Anti-CD22 monoclonal antibody

Epratuzumab is a recombinant monoclonal antibody which has been recently developed to target CD22, a glycoprotein expressed in the cytoplasm of pro-B and pre-B cells and on the surface of mature B cells. It regulates B-cell activation and interaction with T cells [43]. CD22 is thus another potential target for therapy in SLE.

Dörner et al. [44] reported on the experience of an initial clinical trial of epratuzumab for immunotherapy of SLE in 2006. The authors conducted an open-label, prospective study to evaluate the efficacy, tolerance and safety of epratuzumab in 14 patients with active lupus (BILAG score 6–12) using four intravenous infusions of $360\,mg/m^2$ given 2 weeks apart. Total BILAG scores decreased by at least 50% in all 14 patients at some point during the study. Almost all patients (93%) experienced improvements in at least one BILAG B- or C-level disease activity at 6, 10 and 18 weeks. Additionally, three patients with multiple BILAG B involvement at baseline had completely resolved all B-level disease activities by 18 weeks. The drug was well tolerated with no adverse effects reported. Levels of B cells remained reduced at 6 months post treatment. A follow-up to this phase II trial was conducted by Jacobi et al. [45] to investigate the differential effects of epratuzumab on peripheral B cells of patients with SLE. They reported a marked reduction of CD27-positive B cells and CD22 surface expression on these cells, and a reduction of the enhanced activation and anti-Ig-induced proliferation of lupus B cells, respectively.

Table 7.2 Summary of clinical studies involving rituximab in systemic lupus erythematosus

Number of patients	Treatment regimes	Effects on activity	Serious adverse events	Reference
6	RTX – 2×1g 2 weeks apart	Median BILAG at baseline: 14; median BILAG at 6 months: 6 (in five patients)	None	18
2	RTX (four weekly infusions of 375 mg/m² plus prednis(ol)one; one patient additionally received CYC and CSA	'Partial' remission	–	28
18	RTX (phase I/II dose escalation study with single infusion of 100 mg/m² or 375 mg/m² or four weekly infusions of 375 mg/m² plus prednis(ol)one, AZA, MTX and/or MMF in individual cases)	Mean SLAM score at baseline: 8:4; mean SLAM score after 12 months: 5:5 (in 16 evaluable subjects)	Thigh abscess (n=1); transient ischaemic attack (n=1); necrotizing fasciitis (n=1)	23
13	RTX (one to four infusions of 375 mg/m²) plus methylprednis(ol)one, AZA HCQ, CSA, MMF, IVIg and/or plasmapheresis in individual cases	Mean SLEDAI at baseline: 11; mean SLEDAI after RTX: 5; 7 in CliR; 2 in PR; 2 in SD; 2 fatal outcomes	Neutropenia (n=2); deep vein thrombosis (n=1); serum sickness-like reaction (n=2); pulmonary embolism (n=1)	29
7	RTX (two infusions of 750 mg/m² 2 weeks apart) plus CYC plus prednis(ol)one; in individual cases additionally AZA or MMF	Median BILAG at baseline: 22; median BILAG at end of follow-up: 6	None	30
10	RTX (four weekly infusions of 375 mg/m² plus prednis(ol)one	Improvement of renal parameters; 5 in CliR; 3 in PR; 2 non-responders	Pneumococcal meningitis (n=1); hypersensitivity reaction (n=1)	26
24	RTX (two infusions of 500 mg and two infusions of 750 mg each 2 weeks apart or two infusions of 1000 mg 2 weeks apart) plus CYC and/or methylprednis(ol)one; in individual cases additionally HCQ or AZA	Mean BILAG at baseline: 13.9; mean BILAG after 6 months: 5.0	Fatal pancarditis (n=1); pancytopenia following second RTX infusion (n=1)	20
11	RTX (four weekly infusions of 375 mg/m²) plus CYC plus prednis(ol)one; in 10 patients additionally AZA or MMF	Median BILAG score at baseline: 14; median BILAG score after 6 months: 3; 6 in CliR; 5 in PR	Serum sickness-like reaction (n=1); pneumonia (n=2); subcutaneous abscess (n=1); herpes zoster (n=1); urinary tract infection (n=1)	31
5	RTX four weekly infusions of 375 mg/m² in three cases; 1 g×2, 2 weeks apart in two cases	SLEDAI average at baseline: 8; at 3 months: 2.6 (in four cases)	Not clarified	32

n	Treatment	Efficacy	Adverse events	Ref
22	RTX (two infusions of 500 mg or 1000 mg 2 weeks apart) plus glucocorticoids, AZA, MMF, MTX and/or CYC	Mean MEX-SLEDAI at baseline: 10.8; mean MEX-SLEDAI at 3 months: 6.8	Fatal pneumonia because of histoplasmosis and mucomycosis ($n=1$)	33
11	RTX (2–12 infusions of 350 to 400 mg/m²) plus prednis(ol)one; in six patients additionally AZA, MMF, MTX, CYC, CSA, IVIg and/or HCQ	8 in CliR or PR; 2 in SD; 1 in PD	Septicaemia ($n=2$); haematological toxicity ($n=4$)	34
10	RTX (four weekly infusions of 375 mg/m²) plus glucocorticosteroids plus CYC	Mean SLAM at baseline: 12.7; mean SLAM after 6 months: 7 (in 8 evaluable patients)	Not reported	35
10	RTX (1–4 weekly infusions of 375 mg/m² or 50 mg or 1000 mg) plus glucocorticoids; in one patient additionally AZA	Mean SLEDAI at baseline: 19.9; mean SLEDAI after 6 months: 6.2	Pneumonia ($n=2$); herpes zoster ($n=1$)	36
15	RTX (phase I/II study with four weekly infusions of 500 mg or two biweekly infusions of 1000 mg) plus prednis(ol)one >30 mg/day	Median BILAG at baseline: 12.5; median BILAG after 7 months: 7.1	Pneumonia ($n=1$); enteritis ($n=2$)	37
7	RTX (four weekly infusions of 375 mg/m²) plus methylprednis(ol)one plus CYC	Mean SLEDAI at baseline:15; mean SLEDAI after 6 months: 3	Herpes zoster ($n=1$); urinary tract infection ($n=1$)	27
32	RTX (2 × 500 mg or 1×1000 mg) and prednis(ol)one plus CYC (in 29 patients) and/or HCQ (in 24 patients) and/or AZA and/or MTX (in 4 patients)	Median BILAG at baseline: 13; median BILAG at 6 months: 5; mean time to flare: 10 months	Pneumococcal pneumonia and septicaemia ($n=1$); serum sickness-like reaction ($n=1$); fatal pancarditis ($n=1$); grand mal seizure related to hyponatraemia	22
9	RTX (4 × 375 mg/m² in weekly intervals) and prednis(ol)one plus AZA, CSA, HCQ, CYC, MMF and/or MTX	Mean ECLAM at baseline: 3.4; mean ECLAM at 6 months: 2.0; mean time to flare: not reported	Upper airway infection ($n=1$); fatal arrhythmia ($n=1$)	38
16	RTX (4 × 375 mg/m² in weekly intervals) plus CYC plus methylprednis(ol)one	Mean SLEDAI at baseline: 12.1; mean SLEDAI at 6 months: 4.7; 9 in CliR; 9 in PR	None reported	39

Continued overleaf

Table 7.2 Continued

Number of patients	Treatment regimes	Effects on activity	Serious adverse events	Reference
19	RTX (2 infusion of 750 mg/m² during a 2-week period) plus CYC (in 14 patients) plus prednis(ol)one; in individual cases additionally HCQ, AZA and/or MMF	Median BILAG at baseline:14; median BILAG at 1 month: 6; 9 in CliR; 4 in PR	No SAEs but herpes zoster ($n=5$)	40
18	RTX (2–4 applications in weekly intervals; first dose: 188 mg/m², thereafter 375 mg/m²) and glucocorticosteroids and HCQ and/or MMF or AZA; four patients received additional RTX courses	Mean SLEDAI-2K at baseline: 47; mean SLEDAI-2K after RTX (time-point not defined): 25	Fatal infectious endocarditis ($n=1$); cerebral vasculitis and seizures ($n=1$)	41
11	RTX (2×750 mg or 1g) plus CYC (2×500–750 mg), 2 weeks apart in nine patients; two patients received RTX (2×375mg/m²) alone	Median global BILAG reduction of 7.5 at 6 months; loss of all A and B scores by 7 months	Serum sickness-like reaction ($n=1$); infected pressure sores ($n=1$)	42

AZA, azathioprine; BILAG, British Isles Lupus Assessment Group score; CliR, clinical remission (healing of clinical manifestations but further treatment required); CR, complete remission (clinical remission and no further therapy needed); CSA, ciclosporine A; CYC, cyclophosphamide; ECLAM, European Consensus Lupus Activity Measurement; HCQ, hydrochloroquine; IVIg, intravenous immunoglobulin; MMF, myophenolate mofetil; MTX, methotrexate; PD, progressive disease (>25% more lesions or loss of muscle strength); PR, partial remission (healing of >50% of clinical manifestations); RTX, rituximab; SD, stable disease (<25% increase and <50% improvement); SLAM, Systemic Lupus Activity Measure; SLEDAI, Systemic Lupus Erythematosus Disease Activity Index.

B-CELL SURVIVAL FACTOR INHIBITORS

Research into B-cell biology in recent years has led to the understanding that the survival and maturation of B cells are dependent on several different factors. Two members of the TNF superfamily of ligands, namely the B-lymphocyte stimulator protein (BLyS), which is also called B-cell activating factor (BAFF), and a proliferation-inducing ligand (APRIL) have been found to play an important role in this process. Soluble forms of BLyS bind to three receptors on the surface of B cells: transmembrane activator and calcium-modulating cyclophilin ligand interactor (TACI), BAFF-receptor (BAFF-R) and B-cell maturation protein (BCMA), which mediates several cellular effects [46]. These include the differentiation and activation of B cells leading to antibody production, and the induction of a co-stimulatory response in T cells [47, 48].

A proliferation-inducing ligand also acts as a co-stimulator for T- and B-cell activation, as an inducer of tumour cell growth and as a proapoptotic factor [49]. It shares two receptors (TACI and BCMA) with BLyS but not BAAF-R, as it binds specifically to BLyS. The role of APRIL in SLE is unclear, although an inverse association between circulating APRIL levels and serological and clinical disease activity in patients with SLE has been found [50]. It has emerged from basic science studies that patients with SLE express elevated levels of BLyS in peripheral blood, which generally correlate with anti-dsDNA antibody titre, in comparison with the normal values in control subjects [51]. In addition, patients with active SLE demonstrate a higher receptor mRNA expression than patients with inactive SLE [52]. These observations suggest that inhibition of B-cell survival factors may be an effective method of achieving B-cell depletion. Indeed, therapeutic trials involving agents such as belimumb, a monoclonal antibody which inhibits the biological activity of BLyS, and atacicept, a fusion protein which blocks the TACI receptor, are currently being undertaken.

Furie *et al.* [53] assessed the safety, pharmacokinetic and pharmacodynamic effects of belimumab in a phase I dose-escalation study involving 57 patients with inactive SLE. The authors showed a significant reduction of B cells in peripheral blood without any effect on disease activity. Wallace *et al.* [54] performed a prospective, randomized, double-blind, placebo-controlled trial of belimumab (intravenous infusion of 1, 4 or 10 mg/kg on days 0, 14 and 28 then monthly for 52 weeks) in 449 patients with SLE. They did not find any significant statistical difference in the primary end-points in the whole sample, but the Safety of Estrogen in Lupus Erythematosus National Assessment – systemic lupus erythematosus disease activity index score [55] was significantly reduced at 52 weeks in patients who were antinuclear antibody (ANA) positive at entry (defined as titre $\geq 1:80$), or had a anti-dsDNA titre ≥ 30 IU. This study was unusual with respect to the high proportion of patients (28.5%) who were ANA negative. No clinically significant differences were found in safety in the belimumab arms versus placebo. Encouragingly, Human Genome Science and GlaxoSmithKline have announced that in two studies, BLISS-52 and BLISS-76, belimumab met its primary end-point. Detailed results are awaited.

A phase I study assessing the safety and tolerability of atacicept in patients with SLE and its biological effect on B-lymphocyte and immunoglobulin levels was undertaken by Dall'Era *et al.* [56] Atacicept is a TACI-Ig fusion protein that inhibits B-cell stimulation by binding to B-lymphocyte stimulator and a proliferation-inducing ligand. Biological activity of atacicept was demonstrated by dose-dependent reductions in immunoglobulin levels and in mature and total B-cell numbers. There were no changes in the numbers of T cells, natural killer cells or monocytes. Mild injection-site reactions occurred more frequently among the atacicept group than the placebo group. There were no differences in the frequency or type of adverse events and no severe or serious adverse events in patients treated with atacicept. A multicentre, phase II/III prospective trial is currently being undertaken.

ANTICYTOKINE THERAPY

The interaction between helper T cells and antigen-presenting cells, of which B cell is an example, stimulates the former to produce a number of cytokines, some of which act on the B cell to promote antibody formation. These cytokines include tumour necrosis factor (TNF)-α, interleukins (ILs) and interferons (IFNs).

Anti-TNF-α

The role of TNF-α in the immunopathogenesis of SLE is uncertain, as results from experimental murine models of autoimmune lupus nephritis are varied. This cytokine may be protective in patients with SLE, as the administration of TNF-α to lupus-prone mice delayed the development of lupus [57]. However, in some patients with rheumatoid arthritis who were treated with anti-TNF-α inhibitors, anti-dsDNA antibodies developed and clinical features of SLE became manifest in a few of these patients [58–60]. There is currently a lack of clinical data on the use of TNF-α inhibitors in patients with SLE. In 2004 Aringer *et al.* [61] reported on the safety and efficacy of TNF-α blockade (four intravenous infusions of 300 mg infliximab on day 0, weeks 2, 6 and 10, plus AZA or methotrexate) in six patients with SLE with arthritis and/or nephritis in an open-label study. None of the patients experienced an increase in disease activity while receiving infliximab or during the follow-up period. Resolution of joint swelling occurred in three patients with arthritis, and a reduction in proteinuria was noted in four patients with nephritis. These results were confirmed in a long-term follow-up study involving the same group of patients with an additional five subjects [62]. The use of anti-TNF-α agents in the treatment of patients with SLE cannot be recommended until results from larger and appropriately designed clinical trials become available.

Anti-IL-6 and -IL-10

Evidence from animal models and *in vitro* studies suggest that both IL-6 and IL-10 may play a role in the pathogenesis of SLE [63–66]. Administration of anti-IL-6 monoclonal antibody has been shown to inhibit autoimmune responses in a murine model of SLE [67]. In a trial involving 14 patients with SLE, tocilizumab, an anti-IL-6 receptor antibody, has been shown to cause a decrease in acute-phase reactants and activated lymphocytes [68]. Results from the clinical outcome are keenly awaited. In another open-label trial of anti-IL-10 antibody in six patients with SLE, a reduction in disease activity was reported at 6 months' follow-up [69].

Anti-interferons

Although there are controversial reports about the role of IFNs in murine models of lupus, serum levels of IFN-α are elevated in patients with active SLE [70]. Anti-IFN agents may therefore be another anticytokine therapy to be developed as treatment for patients with SLE.

TARGETING T CELLS

As mentioned previously, the interaction between helper T cells and antigen-presenting cells, of which B cell is an example, stimulates the former to produce a number of cytokines which act on the B cell. Activation of T cells requires not only the presentation of the antigen–major histocompatibility complex (MHC) to the T-cell receptor, but also a second molecular interaction [71]. Examples of co-stimulatory molecular pairs include the CD40–CD40 ligand and CD28–B7. Both interactions can generate the second signal required for T-cell activation.

The inhibition of these co-stimulatory molecules is a method of targeting the T cell within the cascade of T- and B-cell interaction and stimulation.

CTLA4-Ig

Cytotoxic T lymphocyte-associated protein 4 IgG1 (CTLA4-Ig), also known as abatacept, is a recombinant soluble fusion protein which blocks the CD28–B7 interaction, thereby inhibiting T-cell activation. This reduces the production of proinflammatory cytokines by activated T cells and also the subsequent generation of autoantibodies by B cells. Several studies of abatacept have demonstrated its therapeutic effect in murine models of lupus nephritis [72–74]. A major double-blind control trial in patients with SLE has been completed and the results are eagerly awaited.

Anti-CD40 ligand

Trials of monoclonal antibodies directed against CD40 ligand have been disappointing. A phase II randomized, double-blind, placebo-controlled study of IDEC-131 in patients with mild to moderate SLE failed to demonstrate any efficacy [75]. In a trial involving BG9588 in patients with proliferative lupus nephritis, the occurrence of thromboembolic complications in treated patients caused a premature termination of the study [76].

T- AND B-CELL TOLEROGENS

Abetimus sodium

Abetimus sodium is a conjugate of double-stranded oligonucleotide with polyethylene glycol. It binds to anti-dsDNA receptors on the surface of B cells, which undergo apoptosis rather than proliferation. Abetimus sodium also forms complexes with soluble anti-dsDNA antibodies, which are then removed from the circulation [77–79].

In a randomized, double-blind, placebo-controlled study, Alarcon-Segovia *et al.* [80] demonstrated the efficacy of abetimus sodium in delaying or preventing renal flares in 230 patients with SLE with lupus nephritis. Patients in the treatment arm also experienced an improvement in health-related quality of life as measured by SF-36 [81]. Sadly, IDEC Pharmaceuticals have recently abandoned other clinical trials of the compound, which were clearly not going to reach their end-point.

Edratide

This compound is a synthetic peptide based on the complementarity determining region 1 of a pathogenic anti-DNA antibody. It has been shown to modulate autoreactive responses of peripheral blood lymphocytes in patients with SLE [82], and to induce clinical amelioration of murine models of lupus [83]. Teva have recently announced, however, that a double-blind control trial (using improvement in SLEDAI scores as the primary end-point) failed to show any benefit compared with placebo.

COMPLEMENT BLOCKADE

Evidence from immunopathogenetic studies has confirmed the importance of complement activation in SLE. This downstream effect, which occurs after deposition of immune complexes, leads to an amplification of the inflammatory response. Bao *et al.* [84] have demonstrated that C5a promotes the development of lupus nephritis in a murine model, which can be blocked with a specific receptor antagonist. Eculizumab, a humanized anti-C5 monoclonal antibody, has been developed and is currently being investigated as a therapeutic agent for SLE and other autoimmune conditions.

IMMUNOABLATION

The ablation of abnormal cells with high-dose chemotherapeutic agents followed by the transplantation of healthy haematopoietic stem cells is an accepted therapeutic strategy in the management of haematological malignancies. The same concept can be applied to the treatment of autoimmune diseases. Indeed, there have been several reports of the successful use of immunoabalation in patients with refractory SLE complicated by life-threatening organ involvement [85–87]. However, this treatment should only be performed in centres with expertise in this area.

CONCLUSION

The regime of pharmacotherapy for patients with SLE should be tailored according to the severity of their disease. In the majority of patients who experience relatively minor symptoms, such as skin rash, photosensitivity, fatigue and arthralgia, the use of traditional immunosuppressive agents is appropriate. For the small proportion of patients with major organ involvement that is non-responsive to standard immunosuppression, targeted therapeutic agents may be considered. Currently, we favour the use of B-cell depletion with anti-CD20 monoclonal antibody as there are sufficient long-term clinical data, albeit only in open studies at present, on its efficacy and safety to justify its use. As cardiovascular disease is a significant co-morbidity in patients with SLE, treatment of associated risk factors such as raised cholesterol with diet and statins should also be considered. Antiplatelet agents and anticoagulants may be required for those who develop the antiphospholipid syndrome. However, a full discussion of this topic is beyond the remit of this chapter. Finally, frequent monitoring for adverse drug effects is an indispensable aspect of any pharmacotherapeutic regime.

DECLARATION OF INTEREST

The authors have no competing interests to declare.

REFERENCES

1. Tan EM, Cohen AS, Fries JF, Masi AT, McShane DJ, Rothfield NF et al. The 1982 revised criteria for the classification of systemic lupus erythematosus. Arthritis Rheum 1982; 25:1271–1277.
2. Hochberg MC. Updating the American College of Rheumatology revised criteria for the classification of systemic lupus erythematosus. Arthritis Rheum 1997; 40:1725.
3. Merrell M, Shulman LE. Determination of progress in chronic disease, illustrated by systemic lupus erythematosus. J Chronic Dis 1955; 1:12–32.
4. Abu-Shakra M, Urowitz MB, Gladman DD, Gough J. Mortality studies in systemic lupus erythematosus: results from a single center. II. Predictor variables for mortality. J Rheumatol 1995; 22:1265–1270.
5. Gladmann DD, Urowitz MB. Prognosis, mortality and morbidity in systemic lupus erythematosus. In: Wallace D, Hahn BH, eds. Dubois Lupus Erythematosus, 6th edn. Philadelphia: Lippincott, Williams, Wilkins; 2001. pp. 54–56.
6. Allison AC, Eugui EM. Purine metabolism and immunosuppressive effects of mycophenolate mofetil. Clin Transplant 1996; 10:77–84.
7. Chan TM, Li FK, Tang CS, Wong RW, Fang GX, Ji YL et al. Efficacy of mycophenolate mofetil in patients with diffuse proliferative lupus nephritis. N Engl J Med 2000; 343:1156–1162.

8. Ong LM, Hooi LS, Lim TO, Goh BL, Ahmad G, Ghazalli R *et al.* Randomized controlled trial of pulse intravenous cyclophosphamide versus mycophenolate mofetil in the induction therapy of proliferative lupus nephritis. *Nephrology* 2005; 10:504–510.

9. Ginzler EM, Dooley MA, Aranow C, Kim MY, Buyon J, Merrill JT *et al.* Mycophenolate mofetil or intravenous cyclophosphamide for lupus nephritis. *N Engl J Med* 2005; 353:2219–2228.

10. Contreras G, Pardo V, Leclercq B, Lenz O, Tozman E, O'Nan P *et al.* Sequential therapies for proliferative lupus nephritis. *N Engl J Med* 2004; 350:971–980.

11. Sinclair A, Appel G, Dooley MA, Ginzler E, Isenberg D, Jayne D *et al.* Mycophenolate mofetil as induction and maintenance therapy for lupus nephritis: rationale and protocol for the randomized, controlled Aspreva Lupus Management Study. *Lupus* 2007; 16:972–980.

12. Alba P, Karim MY, Hunt BJ. Mycophenolate mofetil as a treatment for autoimmune haemolytic anaemia in patients with systemic lupus erythematosus and antiphospholipid syndrome. *Lupus* 2003; 12:633–635.

13. Vasoo S, Thumboo J, Fong KY. Refractory immune thrombocytopenia in systemic lupus erythematosus: response to mycophenolate mofetil. *Lupus* 2003; 12:630–632.

14. Pisoni CN, Obermoser G, Cuadrado MJ, Sanchez FJ, Karim Y, Sepp NT *et al.* Skin manifestations of systemic lupus erythematosus refractory to multiple treatment modalities: poor results with mycophenolate mofetil. *Clin Exp Rheumatol* 2005; 23:393–396.

15. Tedder TF, Boyd AW, Freedman AS, Nadler LM, Schlossman SF. The B cell surface molecule B1 is functionally linked with B cell activation and differentiation. *J Immunol* 1985; 135:973–979.

16. Reff ME, Carner K, Chambers KS, Chinn PC, Leonard JE, Raab R *et al.* Depletion of B cells in vivo by a chimeric mouse human monoclonal antibody to CD20. *Blood* 1994; 83:435–445.

17. Kimby E. Tolerability and safety of rituximab. *Cancer Treat Rev* 2005; 31:456–473.

18. Leandro MJ, Edwards JC, Cambridge G, Ehrenstein MR, Isenberg DA. An open study of B lymphocyte depletion in systemic lupus erythematosus. *Arthritis Rheum* 2002; 46:2673–2677.

19. Hay EM, Bacon PA, Gordon C, Isenberg DA, Maddison P, Snaith ML *et al.* The BILAG index: a reliable and valid instrument for measuring clinical disease activity in systemic lupus erythematosus. *Q J Med* 1993; 86:447–458.

20. Leandro MJ, Cambridge G, Edwards JC, Ehrenstein MR, Isenberg DA. B-cell depletion in the treatment of patients with systemic lupus erythematosus: a longitudinal analysis of 24 patients. *Rheumatology* 2005; 44:1542–1545.

21. Ng KP, Leandro MJ, Edwards JC, Ehrenstein MR, Cambridge G, Isenberg DA. Repeated B cell depletion in treatment of refractory systemic lupus erythematosus. *Ann Rheum Dis* 2006; 65:942–945.

22. Ng KP, Cambridge G, Leandro MJ, Edwards JC, Ehrenstein M, Isenberg DA. B cell depletion therapy in systemic lupus erythematosus: long-term follow-up and predictors of response. *Ann Rheum Dis* 2007; 66:1259–1262.

23. Looney RJ, Anolik JH, Campbell D, Felgar RE, Young F, Arend LJ *et al.* B cell depletion as a novel treatment for systemic lupus erythematosus: a phase I/II dose-escalation trial of rituximab. *Arthritis Rheum* 2004; 50:2580–2589.

24. Anolik JH, Campbell D, Felgar RE, Young F, Sanz I, Rosenblatt J *et al.* The relationship of FcγRIIIa genotype to degree of B cell depletion by rituximab in the treatment of systemic lupus erythematosus. *Arthritis Rheum* 2003; 48:455–459.

25. Anolik JH, Barnard J, Cappione A, Pugh-Bernard AE, Felgar RE, Looney RJ *et al.* Rituximab improves peripheral B cell abnormalities in human systemic lupus erythematosus. *Arthritis Rheum* 2004; 50:3580–3590.

26. Sfikakis PP, Boletis JN, Lionaki S, Vigklis V, Fragiadaki KG, Iniotaki A *et al.* Remission of proliferative lupus nephritis following B cell depletion therapy is preceded by down-regulation of the T cell costimulatory molecule CD40 ligand: an open-label trial. *Arthritis Rheum* 2005; 52:501–513.

27. Gunnarsson I, Sundelin B, Jónsdóttir T, Jacobson SH, Henriksson EW, van Vollenhoven RF. Histopathologic and clinical outcome of rituximab treatment in patients with cyclophosphamide-resistant proliferative lupus nephritis. *Arthritis Rheum* 2007; 56:1263–1272.

28. Kneitz C, Wilhelm M, Tony HP. Effective B cell depletion with rituximab in the treatment of autoimmune diseases. *Immunobiology* 2002; 206:519–527.

29. Gottenberg JE, Guillevin L, Lambotte O, Combe B, Allanore Y, Cantagrel A *et al.* Tolerance and short term efficacy of rituximab in 43 patients with systemic autoimmune diseases. *Ann Rheum Dis* 2005; 64:913–920.

30. Marks SD, Patey S, Brogan PA, Hasson N, Pilkington C, Woo P *et al.* B lymphocyte depletion therapy in children with refractory systemic lupus erythematosus. *Arthritis Rheum* 2005; 52:3168–3174.
31. Smith KG, Jones RB, Burns SM, Jayne DR. Long-term comparison of rituximab treatment for refractory systemic lupus erythematosus and vasculitis: remission, relapse, and re-treatment. *Arthritis Rheum* 2006; 54:2970–2982.
32. Scheinberg M, Hame-Schlak N, Kutner JM, Ribeiro AAF, Ferreira E. Rituximab in refractory autoimmune diseases: Brazilian experiences with 29 patients (2002–2004). *Clin Exp Rheum* 2006; 24:65–69.
33. Vigna-Perez M, Hernandez-Castro B, Paredes-Saharopulos O *et al.* Clinical and immunological effects of Rituximab in patients with lupus nephritis refractory to convential therapy: a pilot study. *Arthritis Res Ther* 2006; 8:R83.
34. Willems M, Haddad E, Niaudet P, Koné-Paut I, Bensman A, Cochat P *et al.* Rituximab therapy for childhood-onset systemic lupus erythematosus. *J Pediatr* 2006; 148:623–627.
35. Risselada AP, Kallenberg CG. Therapy-resistent lupus skin disease successfully treated with rituximab. *Rheumatology* 2006; 45:915–916.
36. Tokunaga M, Saito K, Kawabata D, Imura Y, Fujii T, Nakayamada S *et al.* Efficacy of rituximab (anti-CD20) for refractory systemic lupus erythematosus involving the central nervous system. *Ann Rheum Dis* 2007; 66:470–475.
37. Tanaka Y, Yamamoto K, Takeuchi T, Nishimoto N, Miyasaka N, Sumida T *et al.* A multicenter phase I/II trial of rituximab for refractory systemic lupus erythematosus. *Mod Rheumatol* 2007; 17:191–197.
38. Chehab G, Sander O, Fischer-Betz R, Schneider M. [Anti-CD20 therapy for inducing and maintaining remission in refractory systemic lupus erythematosus]. *J Rheumatol* 2007; 66:328, 330–336.
39. Jonsdottir T, Gunnarsson I, Risselada A, Welin Henriksson E, Klareskog L, van Vollenhoven RF. Treatment of refractory SLE with rituximab plus cyclophosphomide: clinical effects, serological changes, and predictors of response. *Ann Rheum Dis* 2007; 67:330–334.
40. Podolskaya A, Stadermann M, Pilkington C, Marks SD, Tullus K. B-cell depletion therapy for 19 patients with refractory systemic lupus erythematosus. *Arch Dis Child* 2008; 93:401–406.
41. Nwobi O, Abitol CL, Chandar J, Seeherunvong W, Zilleruelo G. Rituximab therapy for juvenile-onset systemic lupus erythematosus. *Pediatr Nehprol* 2008; 23:413–419.
42. Reynolds J, Toescu V, Yee CS, Prabu A, Situnayake, Gordon C. Effects of rituximab on resistant SLE disease including lung involvement. *Lupus* 2009; 18:67–73.
43. Tedder TF, Tuscano J, Sato S, Kehrl JH. CD22, a B lymphocyte-specific adhesion molecule that regulates antigen receptor signaling. *Annu Rev Immunol* 1997; 15:481–504.
44. Dörner T, Kaufmann J, Wegener WA, Teoh N, Goldenberg DM, Burmester GR. Initial clinical trial of epratuzumab (humanized anti-CD22 antibody) for immunotherapy of systemic lupus erythematosus. *Arthritis Res Ther* 2006; 8:R74.
45. Jacobi AM, Goldenberg DM, Hiepe F, Radbruch A, Burmester GR, Dörner T. Differential effects of epratuzumab on peripheral blood B cells of patients with systemic lupus erythematosus versus normal controls. *Ann Rheum Dis* 2008; 67:450–457.
46. Thompson JS, Bixler SA, Qian F, Vora K, Scott ML, Cachero TG *et al.* BAFF-R, a newly identified TNF receptor that specifically interacts with BAFF. *Science* 2001; 293(5537):2108–2111.
47. Moore PA, Belvedere O, Orr A, Pieri K, LaFleur DW, Feng P *et al.* BLyS: member of the tumor necrosis factor family and B lymphocyte stimulator. *Science* 1999; 285(5425):260–263.
48. Huard B, Schneider P, Mauri D, Tschopp J, French LE. T cell costimulation by the TNF ligand BAFF. *J Immunol* 2001; 167:6225–6231.
49. Roschke V, Sosnovtseva S, Ward CD, Hong JS, Smith R, Albert V *et al.* BLyS and APRIL form biologically active heterotrimers that are expressed in patients with systemic immune-based rheumatic diseases. *J Immunol* 2002; 169:4314–4321.
50. Stohl W, Metyas S, Tan SM, Cheema GS, Oamar B, Roschke V *et al.* Inverse association between circulating APRIL levels and serological and clinical disease activity in patients with systemic lupus erythematosus. *Ann Rheum Dis* 2004; 63:1096–1103.
51. Stohl W, Metyas S, Tan SM, Cheema GS, Oamar B, Xu D *et al.* B lymphocyte stimulator overexpression in patients with systemic lupus erythematosus: longitudinal observations. *Arthritis Rheum* 2003; 48:3475–3486.
52. Ju S, Zhang D, Wang Y, Ni H, Kong X, Zhong R. Correlation of the expression levels of BLyS and its receptors mRNA in patients with systemic lupus erythematosus. *Clin Biochem* 2006; 39:1131–1137.

53. Furie J, Stohl W, Ginzler E, Becker M, Miuhra N, Chatham W. Safety, pharmacokinetic and phar-macodynamic results of a Phase I single and double dose escalation study of lymphostat-B (human monoclonal antibody to BLyS) in SLE patients. *Arthritis Rheum* 2003; 48:S377.
54. Wallace DJ, Stohl W, Furie R, Lisse JR, Mackey JD, Merrill J *et al*. A phase II, randomized, double-blind, placebo-controlled, dose-ranging study of belimumab in patients with active systemic lupus erythema-tosus. *Arthritis Rheum* 2009;61:1168–1178.
55. Petri M, Buyon J, Kim M. Classification and definition of major flares in SLE clinical trials. *Lupus* 1999; 8:685–691.
56. Dall'Era M, Chakravarty E, Wallace D, Genovese M, Weisman M, Kavanaugh A *et al*. Reduced B lymphocyte and immunoglobulin levels after atacicept treatment in patients with systemic lupus erythematosus: results of a multicenter, phase Ib, double-blind, placebo-controlled, dose-escalating trial. *Arthritis Rheum* 2007; 56:4142–4150.
57. Jacob CO, McDevitt HO. Tumour necrosis factor-alpha in murine autoimmune 'lupus' nephritis. *Nature* 1988; 331:356–358.
58. Charles PJ, Smeenk RJ, De Jong J, Feldmann M, Maini RN. Assessment of antibodies to double-stranded DNA induced in rheumatoid arthritis patients following treatment with infliximab. *Arthritis Rheum* 2000; 43:2383–2390.
59. Mohan AK, Edwards ET, Cote TR, Siegel JN, Braun MM. Drug-induced systemic lupus erythematosus and TNF-alpha blockers. *Lancet* 2002; 360:646.
60. Eriksson C, Engstrand S, Sundqvist K, Rantapää-Dahlqvist S. Autoantibody formation in patients with rheumatoid arthritis treated with anti-TNFα. *Ann Rheum Dis* 2005; 64:403–407.
61. Aringer M, Graninger WB, Steiner G, Smolen JS. Safety and efficacy of tumor necrosis factor alpha blockade in systemic lupus erythematosus: an open-label study. *Arthritis Rheum* 2004; 50:3161–3169.
62. Aringer M, Houssaiau FA, Graninger WB, Steiner G, Smolen JS. Open-label infliximab for systemic lupus erythematosus: long-term follow-up of 11 patients. *Arthritis Rheum* 2006; 54:S260–261.
63. Finck BK, Chan B, Wofsy D. Interleukin 6 promotes murine lupus in NZB/NZW F1 mice. *J Clin Invest* 1994; 94:585–591.
64. Houssiau FA, Lefebvre C, Vanden Berghe M, Lambert M, Devogelaer JP, Renauld JC. Serum interleu-kin 10 titers in systemic lupus erythematosus reflect disease activity. *Lupus* 1995; 4:393–395.
65. Park YB, Lee SK, Kim DS, Lee J, Lee CH, Song CH. Elevated interleukin-10 levels correlated with disease activity in systemic lupus erythematosus. *Clin Exp Rheumatol* 1998; 16:283–288.
66. Ripley BJ, Goncalves B, Isenberg DA, Latchman DS, Rahman A. Raised levels of interleukin 6 in systemic lupus erythematosus correlate with anaemia. *Ann Rheum Dis* 2005; 64:849–853.
67. Liang B, Gardner DB, Griswold DE, Bugelski PJ, Song XY. Anti-interleukin-6 monoclonal antibody inhibits autoimmune responses in a murine model of systemic lupus erythematosus. *Immunology* 2006; 119:296–305.
68. Shirota Y, Yarboro C, Sims G, Fritsch R, Ettinger R, Valencia X *et al*. The impact of in vitro anti-interleukin 6 receptor blockade on circulating T- and B-cell subsets in patients with systemic lupus erythematosus. *Arthritis Rheum* 2005; 52:S697.
69. Llorente L, Richaud-Patin Y, García-Padilla C, Claret E, Jakez-Ocampo J, Cardiel MH *et al*. Clinical and biologic effects of anti-interleukin-10 monoclonal antibody administration in systemic lupus erythema-tosus. *Arthritis Rheum* 2000; 43:1790–1800.
70. Ronnblom L, Alm GV. Systemic lupus erythematosus and the type 1 interferon system. *Arthritis Res Ther* 2003; 5:68–75.
71. Janeway CA, Bottomly K. Signals and signs for lymphocyte responses. *Cell* 1994; 76:275–285.
72. Finck BK, Linsley PS, Wofsy D. Treatment of murine lupus with CTLA4Ig. *Science* 1994; 265:1225–1227.
73. Daikh DI, Wofsy D. Cutting edge: reversal of murine lupus nephritis with CTLA4Ig and cyclophospha-mide. *J Immunol* 2001; 166:2913–2916.
74. Cunnane G, Chan OT, Cassafer G, Brindis S, Kaufman E, Yen TS, Daikh DI. Prevention of renal dam-age in murine lupus nephritis by CTLA-4Ig and cyclophosphamide. *Arthritis Rheum* 2004; 50:1539–1548.
75. Kalunian KC, Davis JC Jr, Merrill JT, Totoritis MC, Wofsy D; IDEC-131 Lupus Study Group. Treatment of systemic lupus erythematosus by inhibition of T cell costimulation with anti-CD154: a randomized, double-blind, placebo-controlled trial. *Arthritis Rheum* 2002; 46:3251–3258.
76. Boumpas DT, Furie R, Manzi S, Illei GG, Wallace DJ, Balow JE *et al.*; BG9588 Lupus Nephritis Trial Group. A short course of BG9588 (anti-CD40 ligand antibody) improves serologic activity and decreases hematuria in patients with proliferative lupus glomerulonephritis. *Arthritis Rheum* 2003; 48:719–727.

77. Jones DS, Hachmann JP, Osgood SA, Hayag MS, Barstad PA, Iverson GM *et al.* Conjugates of double-stranded oligonucleotides with poly(ethylene glycol) and keyhole limpet hemocyanin: a model for treating systemic lupus erythematosus. *Bioconjug Chem* 1994; 5:390–399.

78. Hartley SB, Cooke MP, Fulcher DA, Harris AW, Cory S, Basten A, Goodnow CC. Elimination of self-reactive B lymphocytes proceeds in two stages: arrested development and cell death. *Cell* 1993; 72:325–335.

79. Norvell A, Mandik L, Monroe JG. Engagement of the antigen-receptor on immature murine B lymphocytes results in death by apoptosis. *J Immunol* 1995; 154:4404–4413.

80. Alarcón-Segovia D, Tumlin JA, Furie RA, McKay JD, Cardiel MH, Strand V *et al.*; LJP 394 Investigator Consortium. LJP 394 for the prevention of renal flare in patients with systemic lupus erythematosus: results from a randomized, double-blind, placebo-controlled study. *Arthritis Rheum* 2003; 48:442–454.

81. Strand V, Aranow C, Cardiel MH, Alarcón-Segovia D, Furie R, Sherrer Y *et al.* Improvement in health-related quality of life in systemic lupus erythematosus patients enrolled in a randomized clinical trial comparing LJP 394 treatment with placebo. *Lupus* 2003; 12:677–686.

82. Sthoeger ZM, Dayan M, Tcherniack A, Green L, Toledo S, Segal R *et al.* Modulation of autoreactive responses of peripheral blood lymphocytes of patients with systemic lupus erythematosus by peptides based on human and murine anti-DNA autoantibodies. *Clin Exp Immunol* 2003; 131:385–392.

83. Sharabi A, Azulai H, Sthoeger ZM, Mozes E. Clinical amelioration of murine lupus by a peptide based on the complementary determining region-1 of an autoantibody and by cyclophosphamide: similarities and differences in the mechanisms of action. *Immunology* 2007; 121:248–257.

84. Bao L, Osawe I, Puri T, Lambris JD, Haas M, Quigg RJ. C5a promotes development of experimental lupus nephritis which can be blocked with a specific receptor antagonist. *Eur J Immunol* 2005; 35:2496–2506.

85. Burt RK, Traynor A, Statkute L, Barr WG, Rosa R, Schroeder J *et al.* Nonmyeloablative hematopoietic stem cell transplantation for systemic lupus erythematosus. *JAMA* 2006; 295:527–535.

86. Petri M, Jones RJ, Brodsky RA. High-dose cyclophosphamide without stem cell transplantation in systemic lupus erythematosus. *Arthritis Rheum* 2003; 48:166–173.

87. Gladstone DE, Prestrud AA, Pradhan A, Styler MJ, Topolsky DL, Crilley PA *et al.* High-dose cyclophosphamide for severe systemic lupus erythematosus. *Lupus* 2002; 11:405–410.

8

Antiphospholipid syndrome

Ann Scott-Russell, Christopher J. Edwards, Graham R. V. Hughes

INTRODUCTION

Antiphospholipid syndrome (APS) is a unique systemic prothrombotic disorder predisposing to recurrent pregnancy morbidity, thrombosis and, occasionally, thrombocytopenia. These features exist in conjunction with serum antibodies to proteins which bind phospholipids [1]. It may be a primary disorder or secondary to an autoimmune condition such as systemic lupus erythematosus (SLE). Antiphospholipid (aPL) antibodies are reported in up to 10% of healthy individuals, in 30–50% of patients with SLE [2], and up to 21% of those presenting with a thrombosis. Since 1983, when the syndrome was first described, it has become evident that the clinical manifestations can involve any organ or system (Table 8.1). It is being increasingly diagnosed in cases of neurological disease including memory loss, migraine, movement disorders and even multiple sclerosis. In addition, young cardiovascular and cerebrovascular disease is frequently due to APS.

The presence of antibodies against phospholipids is a cardinal feature of APS. They can be detected as anticardiolipin (aCL) antibodies, anti-β_2-glycoprotein 1 antibodies (anti-β_2GP1) and as lupus anticoagulant (LA). Positivity for more than one of these clinical tests has a higher predictive value for clinical events, the highest risk being positivity for all three assays [3]. Deep vein thrombosis and stroke are the major causes of morbidity and mortality among individuals with APS [4]. One of the reasons for the widespread interest in APS has been its revolutionary effect on approaches to therapy of autoimmune diseases. Before its recognition most features of SLE were attributed to inflammatory phenomena, requiring anti-inflammatory measures such as glucocorticosteroids and immunosuppressants. Now it is recognized that features as diverse as seizures, miscarriage, cardiovascular disease and hypertension may all be the result of a thrombotic process and in this case secondary prevention relies on anticoagulation. There are still unanswered questions around therapeutics in APS. There is also a general lack of randomized controlled trials. Controversy has also surrounded the correct intensity of anticoagulation needed in APS. There are also individuals who have aPL detected incidentally or following miscarriage. These individuals have not had a thrombosis but may be at risk. Recent trials have attempted to address the need for primary prevention in these cases.

This review will concentrate on the most recent publications pertaining to management and degree of warfarinization, primary prevention, trials of heparin in headache and memory loss, management of pregnancy, management of accelerated atheroma and the use of intravenous immunoglobulin. We will look to the future with development of new oral anticoagulants and the role of rituximab in the treatment of APS.

Table 8.1 Hughes syndrome (the antiphospholipid syndrome) [63]

General features	Both venous and arterial thrombosis
	Recurrent pregnancy loss
	Prominent neurological features
	Occasional thrombocytopenia
Cardiovascular	MI
	Syndrome X
	Accelerated atheroma
	Focal arterial stenotic lesions
CNS	Stroke and TIA
	Memory loss
	Movement disorders
	Seizures
	Visual disturbance
ENT	Balance problems
Renal	Microvascular thrombosis
	Renal artery stenosis (and hypertension)
	Renal vein thrombosis
	Transplant complications
Gastroenterology	Abdominal angina
	Bowel infarction
	Liver function abnormalities
	Budd–Chiari syndrome
Skin	Livedo reticularis
	Skin ulcers
Blood	Thrombocytopenia
	Marrow ischaemia
Endocrine	Addison's disease
	Pituitary infarction
Orthopaedic	Avascular necrosis
	Ischaemic fractures
Psychiatry	Memory loss
Surgery	Pro-thrombotic risk
Immunology	Related autoimmune diseases

MI, myocardial infarction; CNS, central nervous system; TIA, transient ischaemic attack; ENT, ear, nose and throat.

PRIMARY PREVENTION OF THROMBOSIS IN ANTIPHOSPHOLIPID SYNDROME

Predicting which individuals with aPL antibodies are likely to go on to develop thrombosis or other manifestations of APS is not easy. However, this information is needed to best assess the risk–benefit ratio of primary prophylaxis. The presence of co-existing SLE or previous miscarriages increases the likelihood of thrombotic events. The Johns Hopkins lupus cohort has shown a 50% chance of a thrombotic event for patients with SLE over a 20-year period who are LA positive [5]. Thrombosis is also a common cause of hospitalization for individuals with SLE [6]. A recent randomized control trial has been performed to assess the effect of using aspirin as primary prophylaxis for individuals who were aPL or LA positive on at least two occasions but who had not had a thrombosis [7]. The study suggested that thrombotic events in this group were rare but were not reduced by aspirin given daily at 80 mg. Despite this, it seems reasonable to suggest that aspirin might be used in individuals with aPL who have other risk factors for thrombosis, including SLE or previous miscarriage.

WARFARIN FOR SECONDARY PREVENTION OF ANTIPHOSPHOLIPID SYNDROME

It is becoming increasingly clear that APS can present in many ways. At one end of the spectrum there are those who have aPL antibodies yet never develop the clinical syndrome [8]. Then there are those patients who experience a severe arterial thrombosis such as a cerebrovascular accident or who repeatedly present with similar thrombotic episodes whilst taking warfarin. The most extreme manifestation of APS is the catastrophic APS, which is frequently fatal as a result of overwhelming thrombosis in multiple sites. Predicting the clinical phenotype and future disease course for any individual is difficult. However, the relationship between aPL antibodies and thrombosis strengthens as the titre increases and when antibodies of the immunoglobulin G (IgG) class are present. It is also stronger for the lupus anticoagulant than anticardiolipin antibodies [2]. In individuals with APS, thrombotic complications are the most common cause of death and serious morbidity, especially as a result of arterial thrombosis and recurrent thromboses [4]. In patients with APS who received no antithrombotic treatment after their first event, retrospective studies report recurrent thrombosis in the region of 52–69% [9, 10]. Interestingly, following a first thrombosis, patients often experience recurrence in the same vascular bed.

Long-term anticoagulation has dramatically improved the prognosis in APS and is the cornerstone of management following thrombosis. There is much debate about the level and duration of warfarinization needed for secondary prevention and a distinct lack of good-quality trial evidence to help in this area. A landmark retropective study described the history and response to anticoagulation of 147 individuals with APS with 62 individuals also having SLE or an SLE-like syndrome [10]. There were 186 further thrombotic events during follow-up and warfarin at an international normalized ratio (INR) of > 3.0 was necessary to prevent further events.

Susequently, some studies have suggested that a lower intensity of warfarin therapy (INR = 2–3) may be sufficient. A study of 114 patients with APS has found that high intensity (INR > 3) was not superior to low intensity (INR = 2–3) warfarin therapy [11]. However, this study enrolled individuals who had mainly had previous venous thrombosis and excluded individuals with recurrent thrombosis and those with recent stroke, and the high-intensity group did not achieve an INR > 3 for 40% of the time. A further randomized controlled trial looked at 109 patients with APS and randomized them to receive high-intensity warfarin therapy (INR = 3.0–4.5) or 'standard' therapy with either low-intensity warfarin (INR = 2.0–3.0) or aspirin alone (100 mg/day). They found that high-intensity warfarin was not superior to standard treatment in preventing recurrent thrombosis in patients with APS and was associated with an increased risk of haemorrhage [12]. Once again, the patients had predominantly venous thrombotic events, and those with recurrent thrombosis on warfarin were excluded. In addition, there were far fewer thrombotic events during follow-up than might have been expected.

A recent subgroup analysis of the WARSS (Warfarin Aspirin Recurrent Stroke Study) called the Antiphospholipid Antibody Stroke Study (APASS) was analysed [13]. The investigators looked at prevention of vascular recurrence in stroke patients comparing those on aspirin with those on warfarin. The subgroup analysis included all those with a single positive test for aPL antibodies (41% total population). There was no discernible difference found between aspirin and warfarin. However, it might not be possible to widely extrapolate these results to patients with APS. The patients were aPL antibody positive on one occasion at baseline with high-titre aCL antibodies, and/or aCL antibodies together with LA. It appears possible that most of the aPL antibody detected in these patients was transitory and not indicative of true APS. This study does suggest that, if aPL antibodies are detected post stroke, the test should be repeated in 6 weeks. If, at this time, no aPL antibody is detected, then treatment should be as for the general population.

Ruiz-Irastorza *et al.* [14] have studied the area using a systematic literature review. They looked at the published data on secondary prophylaxis of thrombosis in patients with APS. From this review they recommend that for individuals with APS a target INR of 2–3 can be used following a first venous thrombosis. However, an INR > 3 should be used for recurrent thrombosis or arterial events. They expressed concerns with the two published randomized controlled trials (RCTs) [11, 12]. They suggest that the results of these trials may only be extrapolated to those patients with APS at the less severe end of the spectrum.

In a number of cohort studies, patients with definite or probable APS were demonstrated to have a lower rate of thrombotic recurrence if on treatment and especially if this treatment was high-dose warfarin [9, 10, 15–17]. Furthermore, across all the studies reviewed, only 27% of recurrent thromboses occurred in those on warfarin. Of these, only 14% of events on warfarin occurred whilst the INR was > 3. This systematic review concluded that warfarin therapy at a target INR of 2.0–3.0 should be given to patients with APS after their first venous event. However, an INR > 3.0 should be the target in those with recurrent thrombotic events or an arterial thrombus [18] (Table 8.2). The problem of maintaining a high INR was highlighted especially in both RCTs, where there was considerable lack of achievement of target INRs in patients randomized to a target > 3.

TREATMENT OF HEADACHE AND MEMORY LOSS OF ANTIPHOSPHOLIPID SYNDROME

The brain features strongly in APS, with clinical features ranging from stroke to chorea and seizures. Teenage migraine, which returns in later life, is typical. Some have frequent, very

Table 8.2 Thrombosis rates [64]

Author/year	No.	Predominant type of thrombosis	Thrombosis rates (events per patient per year)		
			Untreated patients	Target INR 2.0–3.0	Target INR >3.0
Rosove *et al.* 1992 [9]	70	A/V	0.19	0.07	0
Khamashta *et al.* 1995 [10]	147	A/V	0.29	0.23	0.015
Krnic-Barrie *et al.* 1997 [17]	61	A/V	0.192(A) 0.11(V)	0.048(A)* 0(V)*	
Ruiz-Irastorza *et al.* 2002 [16]	66	A/V	–	–	0.06
Wittkowsky *et al.* 2006 [57]	36	A/V	–	0.096*	
Giron-Gonzalez *et al.* 2004 [58]	158	A/V	–	0.0005*	
Ames *et al.* 2005 [44]	67	V	–	0.04	0.1
Ginsberg *et al.* 1995 [59]	16	V	–	0	–
Prandoni *et al.* 1996 [60]	15	V	0.038	–	–
Rance *et al.* 1997 [61]	27	V	–	0	–
Schulman *et al.* 1998 [62]	68	V	0.1	0	–
Crowther *et al.* 2003 [11]	114	V	–	0.013	0.032
Finazzi *et al.* 2005 [12]	109	V	–	0.016	0.031

INR, international normalized ratio; A, arterial; V, venous.

*Includes all patients on oral anticoagulants.

severe, disabling headaches. Several case reports have shown the rapid disappearance of symptoms with adequate anticoagulation [19, 20]. Some individuals are very susceptible to small changes in the INR. This is illustrated by a reported case of a 36-year-old woman whose headaches and neurological symptoms recurred when INR < 2.8 and disappeared entirely at higher levels of anticoagulation [21]. Some experts have recommended a 'therapeutic trial' of low molecular weight (LMW) heparin following their published case series [19]. They reported improvement in all five of their patients with APS with intractable headache after a 7-day course of LMW heparin and return of the symptom after treatment cessation. A successful heparin trial may be an indicator that formal anticoagulation with warfarin is required. In addition, patients with APS treated with anticoagulants for thrombosis have noticed improvement in memory function. There are multicentre international trials currently in progress investigating memory loss and migraine treatment in APS [22].

ANTIPHOSPHOLIPID SYNDROME AND PREGNANCY

Antiphospholipid syndrome is now recognized as the commonest treatable cause of recurrent miscarriage. Other pregnancy complications such as intrauterine growth retardation, pre-eclampsia, prematurity and thrombosis are also reported. Advances in treatment and understanding mean that APS pregnancies have a successful outcome in 75–80% of cases. This is down to careful obstetric care and improved therapeutic intervention [23]. Obstetric care should start preconception with appropriate counselling of risks and ideally the introduction of aspirin. In one study amongst 687 aPL-positive women undergoing *in vitro* fertilization (IVF), birth rates were significantly higher when aspirin and heparin were administered than when no anticoagulation was given (46% vs. 17%), and this combination seemed particularly effective for those whose aPL was not directed to phosphatidylserine (PS) or phosphatidylethanolamine (PE). However, the addition of intravenous immunoglobulin (IVIg) to the regime enhanced the live birth rates among those whose aPL was directed to PS or PE from 17% to 41% [24].

In addition to close monitoring of blood pressure, proteinuria and fetal growth, Doppler blood flow analyses of the uterine and umbilical artery have useful predictive value for pregnancy outcome. Abnormal third trimester Doppler studies (with abnormal end-diastolic flow in either the umbilical artery or notched uterine arteries) in 18 women with APS predicted 13 who went on to experience obstetric complications. Conversely, 64 out of 72 APS women with normal third-trimester Doppler examination had uncomplicated pregnancies [25]. The Cochrane collaboration and a recent review by Petri and Qazi recommends aspirin plus heparin in those APS pregnant women with one fetal loss or multiple first-trimester losses [23, 26]. The only two RCTs to investigate whether combination therapy is superior to aspirin alone have produced conflicting results [27, 28]. Further research is required in this area, but most clinicians use combination therapy in APS pregnancy with an adverse obstetric history. Unfortunately, recurrent miscarriages despite this therapeutic approach are not uncommon, especially in pregnant women with previous thromboembolic episodes and triple aPL positivity. Case series have found that the combination of prophylactic plasma exchange, LMW heparin and IVIg therapy has been successful in high-risk pregnant APS women [29, 30]. Affinity-purified anti-aCL in a mouse model of APS has been shown to improve pregnancy success rates by 200-fold [31]. In addition to infarction, evidence of local inflammation in the placenta has recently been reported in patients with APS and it has been suggested that, in fact, heparin may inhibit complement and chemokines involved [3]. Additionally, heparin may compete with the binding of β2GPI to the placenta.

Women with APS and a previous thrombotic event, especially an arterial thrombosis, must be considered at high risk for a recurrent event or indeed for an obstetric complication when they become pregnant [32]. They, too, should receive low-dose aspirin and full-treatment-dose LMW heparin and sometimes, if recurrent thromboses occur (despite therapeutic heparin doses), warfarin may be needed as well. It appears safe to use warfarin, providing the INR is tightly controlled, after the first trimester when organogenesis is complete. Reports include 11 safely treated pregnant women with APS treated with warfarin between weeks 15 and 34 with no significant differences in pregnancy outcomes compared with 31 control subjects receiving enoxaparin [33].

NEW ORAL HEPARINS AND WARFARIN ALTERNATIVES

Warfarin is currently the standard anticoagulant used in the management of many conditions, including APS-related thrombosis. However, its use is cumbersome because of the need for frequent blood monitoring, bleeding complications, teratogenicity and slow 'on/off' effect. More importantly, many patients experience difficulty keeping their INR within their therapeutic range. Safer alternatives are needed and are currently under development. Fondaparinux, a pentasaccharide factor Xa inhibitor, does not require monitoring and does not pose any fetal risk in animal studies. Its successful use has been reported in the case of a 26-year-old female with APS secondary to SLE and recurrent thromboses [34]. LMW heparin used post surgery had caused thrombocytopenia, and she suffered pulmonary emboli whilst on this therapy instead of her normal warfarin. However, the use of fondaparinux proved to be successful.

Heparin displays a strong binding activity to β2GPI and is potentially able to compete with the binding of β2GPI to various structures including placental tissue. Furthermore, it also displays an inhibitory activity against complement and chemokines. In mice, heparin protected against pregnancy complications induced by aPL, whereas the other anticoagulants, fondaparinux and hirudin, were unable to do so [35]. Therefore, its therapeutic value probably goes beyond just straightforward anticoagulation. Currently, it is only available in an injectable form, and so out-of-hospital treatment is inconvenient. Combining unfractionated heparin with a carrier molecule to facilitate transport across the gastrointestinal epithelium is currently under development. This carrier molecule, sodium N-(8[2-hydroxybenzoyl]amino)caprylate, or SNAC, markedly increases gastrointestinal absorption of this drug, and clinical studies to date suggest that oral heparin-SNAC is clinically efficacious [36].

ANTIPHOSPHOLIPID SYNDROME AND ACCELERATED ATHEROMA

The primary cardiac manifestation of APS is accelerated atherosclerosis leading to cardiovascular disease and increased cardiac mortality, especially in secondary APS. aPL antibodies seem to be associated with accelerated atherosclerosis. It has been shown that aCL and anti-β2GPI antibodies are elevated in patients with coronary artery disease compared with controls [37]. Oxidation of low-density lipoprotein (LDL) is central to the formation of an atherosclerotic plaque by promoting the formation of macrophage-derived foam cells. Oxidized LDL binds to β2GPI and these complexes have been detected in many disease states including APS. In addition, autoantibodies to these complexes have been detected in SLE and patients with APS [38]. *In vitro* experiments show oxidized LDL–β2GPI complexes are internalized by macrophages via an anti-β2GPI antibody-mediated phagocytosis which may then lead to the development of foam cells and atherosclerotic plaques [39, 40]. Thus, there is evidence for immune-related atherogenesis involving aPL. *In vivo* experimental models show infusion of aPL leading to enhanced formation of atherosclerotic plaques [41]. However, in clinical practice the published studies have been conflicting or non-conclusive, with more work needing to be done in this area [42–44].

USE OF INTRAVENOUS IMMUNOGLOBULIN IN ANTIPHOSPHOLIPID SYNDROME

Intravenous immunoglobulin is used to treat a number of autoimmune diseases because of its immunomodulatory effect. IVIg is administered in APS for its anti-idiotypic properties in order to achieve short-term neutralization of aPLs, especially aCL and LA. There also appears to be a longer term reduction in autoantibody titres involving inactivation of idiotype bearing B-cell clones – another mechanism of action of IVIg. Animal models have been very useful in demonstrating the dramatic effects of IVIg. Here, IVIg has demonstrated a reduction in fetal resorptions compared with untreated mice and indeed complete clinical remission with decrease in autoantibody titre [24, 45].

Case reports and case series are found in the literature. Most relate to the use of IVIg for obstetric complications. Initial use was in those women with APS who had suffered recurrent abortion with successful pregnancy outcome following IVIg. A variety of different regimes have been used. A multicentre, randomized controlled trial has attempted to define the role of IVIg in preventing pregnancy complications in women with definite APS according to the Sapporo criteria [46]. All patients were treated with low-dose aspirin plus heparin. Women were randomized to receive additional 1 g/kg IVIg monthly or placebo. No pregnancy losses were observed in either group. In another multicentre placebo-controlled study, Vaquero et al. [47] compared the use of IVIg with prednisolone plus low-dose aspirin in terms of live birth rate and maternal and perinatal morbidity. This was a study of 82 recurrent APS aborters, 29 of whom were treated with aspirin and prednisolone, the remaining 53 with IVIg. Mean birth weight was higher in the IVIg group. Gestational hypertension and diabetes was significantly higher in the aspirin plus prednisolone group than in the IVIg group (14% vs. 5%). A 2003 randomized study compared IVIg and anticoagulation with LMW heparin plus low dose aspirin in a similar population. Those women treated with LMW heparin plus aspirin had a higher rate of live births than those treated with IVIg (84% vs. 57%) [48].

Catastrophic antiphospholipid syndrome (CAPS) is characterized by multiorgan failure due to systemic microcirculation thrombosis, and carries a mortality rate of almost 50%. As this condition is rare, evidence into the effectiveness of treatment is somewhat lacking. Most units treat with anticoagulation, steroids, plasma exchange or IVIg in a high-care setting to ensure the highest survival rate. This has reportedly improved survival rates to 70% [49]. Although plasma exchange and IVIg are both effective, it has not been shown whether one treatment is superior.

In future, a more targeted approach will be taken with smaller volume specific IVIg aimed at identified pathogenic antigens [50].

SELF-TESTING OF INTERNATIONAL NORMALIZED RATIO

Some patients, especially those with neurological manifestations, find that symptoms recur if their INR dips below a certain level. This level is individual for each patient. Using traditional hospital-based blood monitoring, subtherapeutic INR is a regular occurrence. In highly motivated patients with APS, self-testing has revolutionized symptom control [51].

THE EMERGING ROLE OF RITUXIMAB IN ANTIPHOSPHOLIPID SYNDROME

Several case reports have emerged in the last few years citing rituximab as a treatment for resistant APS. Firstly, it has been used by various teams to reduce aCL antibodies and consequently improve platelet count in difficult cases of thrombocytopenia resistant to conventional therapies [52–54]. Some reports suggest only a partial effect of rituximab on platelet count [55], whereas others have shown a reduction in IgM aCL co-existent with clinical improvement of refractory autoimmune haemolytic anaemia [56].

Rituximab has also been used in those with recurring thromboses despite high-dose warfarin, immunosuppressants, plasma exchange or IVIgs. Several authors have observed a dramatic resolution in symptoms ranging from 10 to 36 months' duration and there is now hope for a new potential therapy in CAPS with proven efficacy in CAPS and thrombocytopenia, after four infusions [46, 52, 54].

CONCLUSION

It is 25 years since APS was first fully described by Graham Hughes. During the last three decades huge advances have been made in detailing the clinical manifestations of this autoimmune disease and it is now recognized as being more systemic than SLE. Treatment strategies for the more common thrombotic manifestations are starting to be tested in randomized controlled trials, but therapies for the less recognized symptoms are still awaiting proper evaluation. As our knowledge increases around the exact mechanisms of aPL-induced thrombosis, pregnancy morbidity and cerebral symptoms, new therapies will be developed, such as rituximab, and existing therapies, such as heparin and IVIg, may be modified.

REFERENCES

1. Miyakis S, Lockshin MD, Atsumi T, Branch DW, Brey RL, Cervera R. International consensus statement on an update of the classification criteria for definite antiphospholipid syndrome (APS). *J Thromb Haemost* 2006; 4:295–306.
2. Galli M, Luciani D, Bertolini D, Barbui T. Lupus anticoagulants are stronger risk factors for thrombosis than anticardiolipin antibodies in the antiphspholipid syndrome: a systematic review of the literature. *Blood* 2003; 101:1827–1832.
3. Stone S, Pijnenborg R, Vercruysse L, Poston R, Khamashta MA, Hunt BJ, Poston L. The placental bed in pregnancies complicated by primary antiphospholipid syndrome. *Placenta* 2006; 27:457–467.
4. Cervera R, Piette JC, Font J, Khamashta MA, Shoenfeld Y, Camps MT et al. Antiphospholipid syndrome: clinical and immunologic manifestations and patterns of disease expression in a cohort of 1,000 patients. *Arthritis Rheum* 2002; 46:1019–1027.
5. Somers E, Madger L, Petri M. Antiphospholipid antibodies and incidence of venous thrombosis in a cohort of patients with systemic lupus erythematosus. *J Rheumatol* 2002; 29:2531–2536.
6. Edwards CJ, Lian TY, Badsha H, The CL, Arden N, Chng HH. Hospitalization of individuals with systemic lupus erythematosus: characteristics and predictors of outcome. *Lupus* 2003; 12:672–676.
7. Erkan D, Harrison M, Levy R, Peterson M, Petri M, Sammaritano L et al. Aspirin for primary thrombosis prevention in antiphospholipid syndrome: a randomized, double-blind placebo controlled trial in asymptomatic antiphospholipid antibody positive individuals. *Arthritis Rheum* 2007; 56:2382–2391.
8. Villa P, Hernandez MC, Lopez-Fernandez MF, Batlle J. Prevalence, follow-up and clinical significance of the anticardiolipin antibodies in normal subjects. *Thromb Haemostat* 1994; 72:209–213.
9. Rosovoe MH, Brewer PM. Antiphospholipid thrombosis: clinical course after the first thrombotic event in 70 patients. *Ann Intern Med* 1992; 117:303–308.
10. Khamashta MA, Cuadrado MJ, Mujic F, Taub MA, Hunt BJ, Hughes GR. The management of thrombosis in the antiphospholipid-antibody syndrome. *N Engl J Med* 1995; 332:993–997.
11. Crowther MA, Ginsberg JS, Julian J, Denburg J, Hirsch J, Douketis J et al. A comparison of two intensities of warfarin for the prevention of recurrent thrombosis in patients with the antiphospholipid syndrome. *N Engl J Med* 2003; 349:1133–1138.
12. Finazzi G, Marchioli R, Brancaccio V, Schinco P, Wilsoff F, Musial J et al. A randomized clinical trial of high-intensity warfarin vs. conventional antithrombotic therapy for the prevention of recurrent thrombosis in patients with the antiphospholipid syndrome (WAPS). *J Thromb Haemost* 2005; 3:848–853.
13. Levine SR, Brey RL, Tilley BC, Thompson JL, Sacco RL, Sciacca RR et al.; and the APASS Investigators. Antiphospholipid antibodies and subsequent thrombo-occlusive events in patients with ischemic stroke. *JAMA* 2004; 291:576–584.

14. Ruiz-Irastorza G, Hunt B, Khamashta M. A systematic review of secondary thromboprophylaxis in patients with antiphospholipid antibodies. *Arthritis Rheum* 2007; 57:1487–1495.
15. Munoz-Rodriguez FJ, Font J, Cervera R, Reverter JC, Tassies D, Espinosa G *et al.* Clinical study and follow-up of 100 patients with antiphospholipid syndrome. *Semin Arthrits Rheum* 1999; 29:182–190.
16. Ruiz-Irastorza G, Khamashta MA, Hunt BJ, Escudero A, Cuadrado MJ, Hughes GR. Bleeding and recurrent thrombosis in definite antiphopholipid syndrome: analysis of a series of 66 patients treated with oral anticoagulation to a target international normalized ration of 3.5. *Arch Intern Med* 2002; 162:1164–1169.
17. Krnic-Barrie S, O'Connor CR, Loony SW, Pierangeli SS, Harris EN. A retrospective review of 61 patients with antiphospholipid syndrome: analysis of factors influencing recurrent thrombosis. *Arch Intern Med* 1997; 157:2101–2108.
18. Guillermo R-I, Hunt BJ, Khamashta MA. A systemic review of secondary thromboprophylaxis in patients with antiphospholipid antibodies. *Arthritis Rheum* 2007; 57:1487–1495.
19. Cuadrado M, Khamashta MA, D'Cruz D, Hughes GRV. Migraine in Hughes syndrome – Heparin as a therapeutic trial? *QJM* 2001; 94:114–115.
20. Hughes GRV, Guadrado M, Khamashta MA, Sanna G. Headaches and memory loss: rapid response to heparin in the antiphospholipid syndrome. *Lupus* 2001; 10:778.
21. Letellier MD, Hughes GRV. 'Listen to the patient' – anticoagulation is critical in the antiphospholipid (Hughes) syndrome. *J Rheum* 2003; 30:897–899.
22. Hughes GRV. Migraine, memory loss and 'multiple sclerosis.' Neurological features of the antiphospholipid (Hughes') syndrome. *Postgrad Med J* 2003; 79:81–83.
23. Empson M, Lassere M, Craig J, Scott J. Prevention of recurrent miscarriage or women with antiphospholipid antibody or lupus anticoagulant. *Cochrane Database Syst Rev* 2005; 18:CD002859.
24. Sher G, Zouves C, Feiman M, Maassaran G, Matzner W, Chang P *et al.* A rational basis for the use of combined heparin/aspirin and IVIG immunotherapy in the treatment of recurrent IVF failure associated with antiphospholipid antibodies. *Am J Reprod Immunol* 1998; 39:391–394.
25. Le Thi Huong D, Wechsler B, Vauthier-Brouzes D, Duhaut P, Costedoat N, Andreu MR *et al.* The second trimester Doppler ultrasound examination is the best predictor of late pregnancy outcome in systemic lupus erythematosus and/or the antiphospholipid syndrome. *Rheumatology* 2006; 45:332–338.
26. Petri M, Qazi U. Management of antiphospholipid syndrome in pregnancy. *Rheum Dis Clin North Am* 2006; 32:591–607.
27. Rai R, Cohen H, Dave M, Regan l. Randomised controlled trial of aspirin and aspirin plus heparin in pregnant women with recurrent miscarriage associated with phospholipid antibodies (or antiphospholipid antibodies). *Br Med J* 1997; 314:253–257.
28. Farquharson RG, Quenby S, Greaves M. Antiphospholipid syndrome in pregnancy: a randomized controlled trial of treatment. *Obstet Gynecol* 2002; 10:408–413.
29. Ruffati A, Mason P, Pengo V, Favaro M, Tonello M, Bortolati M *et al.* Plasma exchange in the management of high risk pregnant patients with primary antiphospholipid syndrome. A report of 9 cases and a review of the literature. *Autoimm Rev* 2007; 6:196–202.
30. Stojanovich L, Mikovic Z, Mandic V, Popovich-Kuzmanovich D. Treatment of antiphospholipid syndrome in pregnancy with low doses of intravenous immunoglobulin. *Isr Med Assoc J* 2007; 9:555–556.
31. Blank M, Anafi L, Zandman-Goddard G, Krause I, Goldman S, Shalev E *et al.* The efficacy of specific IVIG anti-idiotypic antibodies in antiphospholipid syndrome (APS): trophoblast invasiveness and APS animal model. *Int Immunol* 2007; 19:857–865.
32. Ruiz-Irastorza G, Khamashta MA, Hughes GRV. Treatment of pregnancy loss in Hughes syndrome: a critical update. *Autoimmun Rev* 2002; 1:298–304.
33. Pauzner R, Dulitzki M, Lanevitz P, Livneh A, Kenett R, Many A *et al.* Low molecular weight heparin and warfarin in the treatment of patients with antiphospholipid syndrome during pregnancy. *Thromb Haemost* 2001; 86:1379–1384.
34. Holton SG, Knox SK, Tefferi A. Use of fondaparinux in a patient with antiphospholipid antibody syndrome and heparin-associated thrombocytopenia. *J Thromb Haemost* 2006; 4:1632–1634.
35. Girardi G, Redecha P, Salmon JE. Heparin prevents antiphospholipid antibody-induced foetal loss by inhibiting complement activation. *Nat Med* 2004; 10:1222–1226.
36. Arbit E, Goldberg M, Gomez-Oreliana I, Majuru S. Oral heparin: status review. *Thromb J* 2006; 4:6–15.
37. Sherer Y, Tenenbaum A, Praprotnik S, Shemesh J, Bank M, Fisman EZ *et al.* Coronary artery disease but not coronary calcification is associated with elevated levels of cardiolipin, beta-2-glycoprotein-I and oxidised LDL antibodies. *Cardiology* 2001; 95:20–24.

38. Kobayashi K, Kishi M, Atsumi T, Bertolaccini ML, Makino H, Sakairi N et al. Circulating oxidised LDL forms complexes with β2-glycoprotein I: implication as an atherogenic autoantigen. *J Lipid Res* 2003; 44:716–726.

39. Doria A, Sherer Y, Meroni PL, Shoenfeld Y. Inflammation and accelerated atherosclerosis: basic mechanisms. *Rheum Dis Clin North Am* 2005; 31:355–362.

40. Kobayashi K, Matsuura E, Liu Q, Furukawa J, Kaihara K, Inagaki J et al. A Specific ligand for β2 glycoprotein I mediates autoantibody-dependent uptake of oxidised low density lipoprotein by macrophages. *J Lipid Res* 2001; 42:697–709.

41. Yasuda S, Bohgaki M, Atsumi T, Koike T. Pathogenesis of antiphospholipid antibodies: impairment of fibrinolysis and monocyte activation via the p38 mitogen-activated protein kinase pathway. *Immunobiology* 2005; 210:775–780.

42. Matsura E, Kobayashi K, Tabuchi M, Lopez LR. Accelerated atheroma in the antiphospholipid syndrome. *Rheum Dis Clin North Am* 2006; 32:537–551.

43. Asanuma Y, Oeser A, Shintani AK, Turner E, Olsen N, Fazio S et al. Premature coronary artery atherosclerosis in systemic lupus erythematosus. *N Engl J Med* 2003; 349:2407–2415.

44. Ames PR, Margarita A, Sokoll KB, Weston M, Brancaccio V. Premature atherosclerosis in primary antiphospholipid syndrome: preliminary data. *Ann Rheum Dis* 2005; 64:315–317.

45. Bakimer R, Guilburd B, Zurgil N, Shoenfeld Y. The effect of intravenous γ-globulin on the induction of experimental antiphospholipid syndrome. *Clin Immunol Immunopathol* 1993; 69:97–102.

46. Branch DW, Peaceman AM, Druzin M, Silver RK, El Sayed Y, Silver RM et al. A multi-center placebo controlled pilot study of intravenous immune globulin treatment of antiphospholipid syndrome during pregnancy. The pregnancy loss study group. *Am J Obstet Gynaecol* 2000; 82(part1):122–127.

47. Vaquero E, Lazzarin N, Valensise H, Menghini S, Di Pierro G, Cesa F et al. Pregnancy outcome in recurrent spontaneous abortion associated with antiphospholipid antibodies: a comparative study of intravenous immunoglobulin versus prednisolone plus low dose aspirin. *Am J Reprod Immunol* 2001; 45:174–179.

48. Triolo G, Ferrante A, Ciccia F, Accardo-Palumbo A, Perino A, Castelli A et al. Randomized study of subcutaneous low molecular weight heparin plus aspirin versus intravenous immunoglobulin in the treatment of recurrent fetal loss associated with antiphospholipid antibodies. *Arth Rheum* 2003; 48:728–731.

49. Asherson RA, Cervera R, de Groot PG, Erkan D, Boffa MC, Piette JC et al. Catastrophic and antiphospholipid syndrome: international consensus statement on classification criteria and treatment guidelines. *Lupus* 2003; 12:530–534.

50. Blank M, Nur I, Toub O, Aron-Maor A, Shoenfeld Y. Toward molecular targeting with specific intravenous immunoglobulin preparation. *Clin Rev Allergy Immunol* 2005; 29:213–217.

51. Hughes GRV. Hughes syndrome.The antiphospholipid syndrome – a clinical overview. *Clin Rev Allergy Immunol* 2007; 32:3–11.

52. Trappe R, Loew A, Thuss-Patience P, Dorken B, Riess H. Successful treatment of thrombocytopenia in primary antiphospholipid antibody syndrome with the anti-CD20 antibody rituximab – monitoring of antiphospholipid and anti-GP antibodies: a case report. *Ann Haematol* 2006; 85:134–135.

53. Tomietto P, Gremese E, Tolusso B, Venturini P, De Vita S, Ferraccioli G. B cell depletion may lead to normalization of anti-platelet, anti-erythrocyte and antiphospholipid antibodies in systemic lupus erythematosus. *Thromb Haemost* 2004; 92:1150–1153.

54. Rubenstein E, Arkfeld D, Metyas S, Shinada S, Ehresmann S, Liebman HA. Rituximab treatment for resistant antiphospholipid syndrome. *J Rheumatol* 2006; 33:355–357.

55. Ames PRJ, Tommasino C, Fossati G, Scenna G, Brancaccio V, Ferrara F. Limited effect of rituximab on thrombocytopenia and anticardiolipin antibodies in a patient with primary antiphospholipid syndrome. *Ann Hematol* 2007; 86:227–228.

56. Erdozain JG, Ruiz-Irastorza G, Egurbide MB, Aguirre C. Sustained response to rituximab of autoimmune haemolytic anaemia associated with antiphospholipid syndrome. *Haematologica* 2004; 89:ECR34.

57. Wittowsky AK, Downing J, Blackburn J, Nutescu E. Warfarin related outcomes in patients with antiphospholipid antibody syndrome managed in an anticoagulation clinic. *Thromb Haemost* 2006;96:137–141.

58. Giron-Gonzalez JA, Garcia del Rio E, Rodriguez C, Rodriguez-Martorell J, Serrano A. Antiphospholipid syndrome and asymptomatic carriers of antiphosholipid antibody: prospective analysis of 404 individuals. *J Rheumatol* 2004;31:1560–1567.

59. Ginsberg JS, Wells PS, Brill-Edwards P, Donovan D, Moffatt K, Johnston M *et al.* Antiphospholipid antibodies and venous thromboembolism. *Blood* 1995; 10:3685–3691.

60. Pradoni P, Simioni P,Girolami A. Antiphospholipid antibodies, recurrent thromboembolism and intensity of warfarin anticoagulation. *Thromb Haemost* 1996; 75:859.

61. Rance A, Emmerich J, Fiessinger JN. Anticardiolipin antibodies and recurrent thromboembolism. *Thromb Haemost* 1997; 77:221–222.

62. Schulman S, Svenungsson E, Granqvist S and the Duration of Anticoagulation Study Group. Anticardiolipin antibodies predict early recurrence of thromboembolism and death among patients ith venousthromboembolism following anticoagulant therapy. *Am J Med* 1998; 104:332–338.

63. Hughes GRV. Hughes Syndrome (the antiphospholipid syndrome) .Ten clinical lessons. *Autoimmun Rev* 2008; 7:262–266.

64. Ruiz-Irastorza G, Khamashta M. The treatment of antiphospholipid syndrome: a harmonic contrast. *Best Prac Res Clin Rheum* 2007; 21:1079–1092.

9

Progress in the therapy of systemic sclerosis

Emma C. Derrett-Smith, Christopher P. Denton

INTRODUCTION

Systemic sclerosis (scleroderma; SSc) is a multisystem connective tissue disease in which skin and internal organ fibrosis are associated with an obliterative microvasculopathy and a degree of inflammation. These classically manifest as Raynaud's phenomenon, sclerodactyly, oesophageal dysmotility and a range of organ-specific complications. Despite its relative rarity, with prevalence in the UK estimated to be 1 in 10 000 [1], the high case-specific mortality and the similarities of SSc with more common organ-based fibrosis make it an important condition for clinicians and research scientists alike. It is the prototype fibrotic autoimmune disorder.

The pathogenesis underlying SSc involves the immune system, fibroblasts and the vasculature. All forms of SSc seem to involve these three processes, although their relative contributions vary. It seems likely from epidemiological data that a triggering event occurs in a genetically susceptible individual, with other factors, including autoantibody profile, determining the subset and complications which then result. A small number of recent studies have linked polymorphisms of candidate genes more strongly with the presence of specific autoantibodies than with systemic sclerosis itself, in some cases with suggested mechanisms linking the two. These are summarized in Table 9.1. Molecular biology techniques additionally suggest important roles for endothelin, the transforming growth factor (TGF)-β superfamily, the nitric oxide axis, tumour necrosis factor (TNF)-α, interleukin 4 (IL-4), IL-6 and platelet-derived growth factor (PDGF) within the interplay between the immune system and connective tissue.

In this chapter we focus on contemporary and future pharmacological therapies and discuss the importance of timely diagnosis of the critical complications and the importance of optimal pharmacological management based on current evidence.

THE ROLE OF INFLAMMATION IN SYSTEMIC SCLEROSIS: SHOULD ALL PATIENTS RECEIVE IMMUNOSUPPRESSION?

Models of pathogenesis in scleroderma focus on an initiating stimulus in a susceptible individual amplified by vascular, fibrotic and inflammatory processes, resulting in a final common pathway of fibrogenesis and extracellular matrix formation with disruption of tissue architecture and function. Broadly speaking, SSc can be subdivided into the limited and diffuse forms and a number of characteristics distinguish the two. Limited disease (limited cutaneous systemic sclerosis, LcSSc) typically presents with a long antecedent history of Raynaud's phenomenon, often severe enough to have caused digital ulceration

Table 9.1 Genetic associations with systemic sclerosis

Polymorphism	Clinical association	Reference
PTPN22 R620W	Anti-topoisomerase antibodies, anti-centromere antibodies	Gourh et al. 2006 [38]
ETRA	RNA polymerase antibodies	Fonseca et al. 2006 [39]
CTGF promoter	Systemic sclerosis	Fonseca et al. 2007 [40]
CXCR2	Systemic sclerosis	Renzoni et al. 2000 [41]
TNF-863A	Anticentromere antibodies	Sato et al. 2004 [42]
IL-10	Anticentromere antibodies	Hudson et al. 2005 [43]
SPARC	Systemic sclerosis	Zhou et al. 2002 [44]
SPARC	No association	Lagan et al. 2005 [45]
MCP-1	Systemic sclerosis	Karrer et al. 2005 [46]
MCP-1	No association	Carulli et al. 2008 [47]
TGF-β1	Systemic sclerosis	Crilly et al. 2002 [48]
TGF-β1	No association	Ohtsuka et al. 2002 [49]
TGF-β1	No association	Sugiura et al. 2003 [50]
ACE	Systemic sclerosis	Fatini et al. 2002 [51]
Fibrillin-1	Systemic sclerosis	Tan et al. 2001 [52]
COL1A2	Systemic sclerosis	Hata et al. 2000 [53]

and occasionally tissue infarction, with distal skin fibrosis progressing proximally over years. Calcinosis, telangiectasis and oesophageal involvement are seen commonly, as are the internal organ complications of mid-gut disease, pulmonary fibrosis and, notably, isolated pulmonary hypertension. Most patients carry anticentromere antibodies (sensitivity 60%, specificity 98%). Diffuse disease, in contrast, has a sudden onset with an early phase sometimes difficult to distinguish from an inflammatory arthritis and rapidly progressive skin fibrosis, which can be intensely pruritic and which is often accompanied by a catabolic state. Raynaud's phenomenon and oesophageal involvement will occur almost universally in this condition but may not be a presenting feature. Severe internal organ complications, in particular lung fibrosis and hypertensive renal crises, occur early in the course of disease. Hallmark antibodies are anti-topoisomerase-1 or scl-70 (sensitivity 38%, specificity 100%), anti-RNA polymerase I and III, anti-pm-scl, anti-fibrillarin and anti-nRNP. The clinical and immunological profiles of limited and diffuse disease are usually fairly distinct, but the major determinant required for a diagnosis of diffuse cutaneous SSc (DcSSc) remains the presence of significant skin fibrosis proximal to the elbows and knees.

Recently, the most obvious progress in therapy has been in the treatment of organ-based complications in SSc. Whether immunosuppression for the overall condition is appropriate is less clear. Treatments for SSc can be broadly discriminated into those modulating the immune system, antifibrotic and vascular therapies. In reality, these processes are closely linked and drugs may have effects on more than one of them. The degree of inflammation seen in LcSSc, both clinically and microscopically in affected skin, would not suggest that anti-inflammatory or immunomodulatory therapy was beneficial. Indeed, there is little evidence of improvement in modified Rodnan skin score (MRSS) in those patients treated with immunosuppression for organ-based complications, and general immunosuppression in patients with limited disease is not indicated. Patients with either subtype of SSc with late-stage skin disease again tend to have little ongoing inflammation and hence immunosuppression is not indicated.

In contrast, and excepting rare occurrences of paraneoplastic disease, the catabolic state experienced in the early development of DcSSc is indistinguishable from that seen in other connective tissue disease or inflammatory processes. This can comprise rapid weight loss with particular loss of muscle mass (in the absence of gut disease or proven myositis), fevers and profound fatigue. Serological markers of inflammation are elevated. Disease heterogeneity and the relative rarity of DcSSc mandate that each case is assessed individually but progressive skin disease in this context, even without further organ involvement, would generally be seen as an indication for systemic immunosuppressive therapy. Trials to assess the benefits of immunosuppression in this heterogeneous condition are, unfortunately, fraught with difficulty, not least because of the rarity of it, the difficulty in early diagnosis and because the natural history of the condition is one of rapidly progressive skin thickening over 1–3 years followed by gradual fibrosis then resolution. Differences in trial design, length and inclusion criteria therefore have a significant effect on outcome.

The initial decision on which immunosuppressive therapy to use in early diffuse cutaneous systemic sclerosis rests primarily on the presence of internal organ complications and to a lesser extent on autoantibody status. In a patient with severe skin disease in early dcSSc, an assessment of the presence of lung, renal, cardiac, muscle and joint disease will be made and the existence of any overlap syndromes will be considered. For instance a pulsed cyclophosphamide regime would be the immunosuppressive therapy of choice in this context if there is cardiac or respiratory involvement, or if overlap vasculitis is present. The use of low dose steroid would be considered but is likely to be avoided in the context of RNA polymerase antibody positivity. Methotrexate may be favoured if an associated inflammatory arthritis or myositis is a prominent feature. In severe early diffuse systemic sclerosis without internal organ involvement, there is evidence for the use of anti-thymocyte globulin induction followed by mycophenylate mofetil (MMF) maintenance [2]. Less severe skin disease would be treated with MMF alone. There is no overall consensus on gold-standard pharmacological management of this condition, and this is highlighted by the many National Institute of Health (NIH)-approved trials underway, which are directed at investigation of both new and existing treatment regimes in this cohort of early diffuse patients. These studies mainly use mortality and MRSS as the most objective primary end-points and variable secondary end-points [3]. Several of these are small scale open-label trials using drugs beneficial in other autoimmune diseases and we focus here on the larger, more robust trials or those in the later phases.

In the 1990s, high-dose immunosuppression with autologous haematopoietic stem cell transplantation (HSCT) had been reported anecdotally as showing benefit in various autoimmune diseases when being used as treatment for co-existing pathologies. The goal in autoimmune disease is to generate new self-tolerant lymphocytes after elimination of self- or autoreactive lymphocytes (lymphoablation) rather than ablation and reconstitution of the whole bone marrow compartment (myeloablation). The major problem faced when using this process has been the higher than expected transplant-related mortality. In addition, large-scale trials or meta-analyses have been difficult to compile because of differences in transplant procedure across centres as well as the variation within and between autoimmune diseases [4].

Despite this, there are three significant trials to assess the effect of this therapy compared with cyclophosphamide in early DcSSc, which are large scale given the rarity of this form of the presentation, and should provide good evidence of a benefit, if indeed one exists. They are based on an earlier open-label pilot study and a review of cases from the European Group for Blood and Marrow Transplantation (EBMT)/European League Against Rheumatism (EULAR) registry [5, 6] which suggested favourable outcome measures with acceptable transplant-related mortality (8.7%). The first of these, the European ASTIS (Autologous Stem Cell Transplantation International Scleroderma) trial, is a phase III prospective randomized controlled trial which will recruit 151 patients, and uses a conditioning regime of cyclophosphamide and rabbit ATG, along with CD34+ selection. The interim presentations show positive results with transplant-related mortality of 5.7% [7]. The American ASSIST

(American Scleroderma Stem Cell versus Immune Suppression Trial) is similar but does not select CD34+ cells. The second American SCOT (Scleroderma: Cyclophosphamide or Transplantation) trial differs from the others in that it uses a myeloablative regime and that regime includes total body irradiation. This has particular consequences as radiation is thought to exacerbate the pre-existing vasculopathy and fibrosis of SSc. Interim reports in 2004 suggested a benefit but with a mortality rate higher than that suggested by ASTIS. The trial is ongoing. In summary, although major trials are under way to determine whether the treatment benefit in those earlier studies was due to reparative effects of stem cells or the intense immune suppression required for the process, we do not have sufficient evidence so far to use this procedure except in the context of a clinical trial.

Intravenous pulsed cyclophosphamide (usually at a dose of $600\,mg/m^2$ monthly for 6 months in combination with low-dose oral steroid) is used in our centre when there is thought to be co-existent active alveolitis. Other centres use this as a standard induction therapy for early DcSSc and, again, there is a phase III safety/efficacy trial under way to help provide evidence for its use in this cohort, although, again, it is an open-label uncontrolled study. Double-blind, randomized, placebo-controlled evidence comes from a secondary end-point from the SLS (Scleroderma Lung Study) of scleroderma-related lung disease in which MRSS was measured at baseline, 6 and 12 months after treatment for 12 months with oral cyclophosphamide or placebo. Patients with DcSSc had a mean ± SD MRSS of 21 ± 10.1, falling to 15.9 ± 11.0 in the active group, versus minimal change in the placebo group, 20.2 ± 9.3, falling to 19.1 ± 11.2 ($P \le 0.01$) [8]. Ongoing analysis continuing to 12 months after the completion of the trial showed that this benefit was not sustained, supporting our current clinical practice of ongoing maintenance immunosuppression with drugs such as azathioprine or MMF. Reassuringly, there was no statistical difference in major adverse events or mortality.

Other therapies of interest undergoing clinical trials target different areas of scleroderma pathogenesis such as fibrosis and vascular disease and are discussed later.

THE ROLE OF INFLAMMATION IN SYSTEMIC SCLEROSIS: IMMUNOSUPPRESSION IN LUNG DISEASE IS BENEFICIAL

The early events in the development of fibrotic lung disease in SSc do seem to involve an inflammatory alveolitis. This complication affects about 25% of patients with LcSSc and up to 40% of patients with DcSSc. The most sensitive screening tool in current routine use is carbon monoxide diffusion capacity, with high-resolution computed tomography (HRCT) scanning warranted when there is a significant change, either symptomatically, or, more commonly, on routine testing. Serological markers such as KL-6 (a marker of epithelial cell injury) may provide prognostic information in the future [9]. Typical findings on HRCT are those of established fibrosis: reticular changes with traction bronchiectasis, or an amorphous ground-glass appearance which corresponds on lung biopsy to an inflammatory infiltrate amenable to immunosuppression, usually with steroid and cyclophosphamide. Unless there are atypical features to the CT appearance or clinical uncertainty, we do not advocate invasive procedures such as VATS-assisted biopsy. Two randomized controlled trials have now reported modest benefit of a cyclophosphamide regime over placebo in cases of active alveolitis due to scleroderma lung disease and this is the current treatment of choice. The first of these, the Fibrosing Alveolitis in Scleroderma Trial (FAST), differs from the Scleroderma Lung Study mentioned earlier by using a combination of low-dose oral steroid and monthly intravenous cyclophosphamide rather than oral dosing, and in addition used longer-term azathioprine as maintenance therapy [10]. Both studies reported in 2006, and although the outcomes are not directly comparable, both suggested a modest benefit in the forced vital capacity (FVC) in the treatment group compared with placebo ($P = 0.04$ in the FAST trial when corrected for body mass index [BMI], $P < 0.03$ in the SLS). Therapy stabilizes lung function without an increased incidence of serious adverse events. In our clinical practice, MMF is used as an alternative when other approaches are not appropriate in both early DcSSc and pulmonary fibrosis. A retrospective analysis of its use suggests it has equal efficacy when compared with other immunosuppressive agents [11]. There are no blinded randomized trials for MMF use for these indications. Treatments for SSc-related pulmonary fibrosis have understandably been guided by those for idiopathic fibrosis and hence those undergoing further evaluation currently include etanercept and acetylcysteine.

FIBROSIS IN SYSTEMIC SCLEROSIS: A BRIGHTER FUTURE FOR ANTIFIBROTIC THERAPIES?

The fibrotic complications of SSc are understandably widespread, but major problems develop in the lung and gastrointestinal tract as well as the skin. Lung fibrosis is, at present, best managed as an inflammatory process, as discussed above. Gastrointestinal involvement can occur anywhere from mouth to anus, with the most common complaint of oesophageal reflux due to failure of peristalsis and tertiary contractions in a fibrotic oesophagus. Mid-gut disease is complicated by bacterial overgrowth. These problems are managed supportively, with proton pump inhibitors, prokinetics and antibiotics where indicated. Large bowel disease can cause life-threatening pseudo-obstruction and perforation and is best managed conservatively if possible, whereas ano-rectal disease results in poor anal contractility and faecal incontinence, sometimes amenable to surgery by specialist ano-rectal surgeons. Overall, the incidence of gut disease of some description approaches 100% in our population, although very few require long-term total parenteral nutrition for absolute nutritional failure. Histologically, these consequences occur, once again, because of excess collagen and extracellular matrix deposition. Hence to treat the disease process, a pure antifibrotic agent would be ideal.

D-Penicillamine therapy, or more specifically, one of its consequences, cutis laxa, was considered to be one of the first potential antifibrotic therapies in SSc. D-Penicillamine chelates the intra- and intermolecular cross-linking of collagen and therefore has excellent antifibrotic potential. Although some patients noticed a marked benefit, the effect was by no means universal; results from a 24-month randomized controlled trial were disappointing [12] and hence the drug is no longer part of our repertoire of clinically useful therapies. Over the years, there have been several other potential antifibrotic therapies, but none has provided significant enough benefit to reach routine clinical use.

The advancement of molecular biology techniques coupled with the introduction of biological therapies may, however, provide us with some useful novel therapies. One area of interest in SSc research is the contribution TGF-β makes to the pathogenesis of systemic sclerosis. This cytokine is essential for the proliferation and differentiation of cells, embryonic development, wound healing and angiogenesis [13]. Within the context of SSc, TGF-β promotes fibrosis through multiple pathways. Both excess TGF-β1 and TGF-β receptor expression occurs in the skin of patients with active SSc, and serum levels of TGF-β1 are inversely correlated with skin score, suggesting sequestration in the active skin [14]. Abnormal TGF-β production is also associated with an activated and autonomous fibroblast profile, resulting in excess collagen synthesis [15]. However, it is likely that multiple cytokines have overlapping roles *in vivo* and the contribution of TGF-β1 alone is unknown. CAT-192, a recombinant human monoclonal antibody against active TGF-β1, provided an exciting insight into scleroderma pathogenesis, although there were several considerations before phase II trials could take place. In light of its numerous homeostatic functions, blocking TGF-β may have had serious adverse consequences and, furthermore, already autonomous scleroderma fibroblasts may have been resistant to blockade of TGF-β1. Nevertheless, a phase I/II trial for safety, tolerability and pharmacokinetics found this medication in a cohort of 45 early patients with DcSSc to be safe and well tolerated [16]. The study showed no evidence of efficacy, and although no further trials are planned for CAT-192, other, more potent, TGF-β blocking strategies are available.

Imatinib mesylate was initially developed as a PDGF receptor inhibitor and inhibits tyrosine kinase-mediated signalling pathways. These are common to many cells, and, currently, the major therapeutic uses for it are in certain leukaemias (due, in part, to its potent blockade of Abl family tyrosine kinases) and some rare gastrointestinal tumours. PDGF and TGF-β are both potent profibrotic cytokines, and hence the therapeutic potential to block PDGF-mediated fibrosis with imatinib was clear. The standard pathway of TGF-β signalling occurs through serine–threonine kinases (called Smads) and would be undisturbed. However, it is known that there are also Smad-independent signalling pathways which contribute to fibrosis, and, indeed, it appears that one of these uses c-Abl as a downstream mediator [17]. Hence, we can hypothesize that imatinib is capable of inhibiting the actions of two mediators of fibrosis. *In vitro*, it inhibits the growth of normal and scleroderma fibroblasts, and in animal models of pulmonary and hepatic fibrosis, imatinib has been shown to be an effective inhibitor of fibrosis [18, 19]. Less clearly defined are the benefits of using imatinib for the vasculopathic complications of SSc. There are case reports of dramatic improvements in end-stage pulmonary arterial hypertension responding to imatinib, with the likely mechanism of action related to PDGF-receptor blockade resulting in an antiproliferative effect on vascular smooth muscle (PDGF is a potent mitogen) [20]. The pilot studies and open-label trials currently under way for the use of this medication in SSc do hypothesize that the drug may act as both an antifibrotic and antivasculopathic agent in this condition. They are yet to report, although preliminary data are positive. This may become the most beneficial antifibrotic therapy available.

MODULATING VASCULOPATHY IN SYSTEMIC SCLEROSIS: ORAL THERAPIES CHANGE THE OUTLOOK IN SCLERODERMA-ASSOCIATED PULMONARY ARTERIAL HYPERTENSION

Vascular disease is responsible for the majority of the mortality and morbidity in SSc. All sizes of arterial vessel can be involved, but the microvasculopathy resulting in complications such as pulmonary arterial hypertension (PAH), scleroderma renal crisis (SRC), Raynaud's phenomenon and digital ulceration and infarction are the most commonly reported. Histological analysis of arterial vessels in the isolated PAH of SSc (that is, not occurring secondary to pulmonary fibrosis) reveals luminal narrowing due to increased intimal, medial and adventitial thickness and the pathognomonic plexiform lesion comprising proliferated endothelial and smooth muscle cells. Endothelial dysfunction is an early important factor in the development and progression of PAH, resulting in an important reduction of the vasodilators nitric oxide and prostacyclin and overproduction of the vasoconstrictor and mitogen endothelin-1 (ET-1). This all occurs in an environment of increased vascular resistance due to luminal narrowing, inflammation and thrombosis.

Historically, the survival after diagnosis in cases of scleroderma-associated PAH (SSc-PAH), which, depending on autoantibody positivity, can reach a prevalence of 10% of the total scleroderma population, was 47% at 2 years. Treatments included anticoagulants and diuretics and, with the advent of prostanoids (intravenous epoprostenol and inhaled iloprost are the currently licensed therapies), outcomes in both idiopathic and SSc-PAH improved [21]. Treprostinil is undergoing assessment as a prostanoid with both a longer half-life and choice of subcutaneous (s.c.) or inhaled administration options. A 12-week double-blind, placebo-controlled trial significantly favours s.c. treprostinil over placebo both in terms of symptoms using the Borg dyspnoea score and 6-minute walk distance (6MWD) and pulmonary haemodynamics, even in subgroup analysis of SSc-PAH [22, 23]. The added benefit of a longer-acting prostanoid is that it reduces the likelihood of rapid haemodynamic compromise if the drug not administered continuously.

The introduction of licensed 'oral therapies' in the 1990s dramatically improved patient outcomes in SSc-PAH. These comprise endothelin receptor antagonists and phosphodiesterase (PDE)-5 antagonists, the latter resulting *in vivo* in increased nitric oxide-mediated pulmonary vasodilation. ET-1 levels *in vivo* correlate closely in this population with pulmonary vascular resistance (PVR), mean pulmonary arterial pressure and 6MWD. A subgroup analysis of two pivotal trials comparing bosentan (an endothelin receptor A and B antagonist) with historical treatments looked specifically at the 66 patients in the studies with connective tissue disease-associated PAH. Although outcomes in the 44 actively treated patients did not reach statistical significance, there was a trend to stabilization in exercise capacity, delayed disease progression, increased time to lung transplantation, reduction in hospitalization for PAH, need to change to epoprostenol treatment or atrial septostomy [24]. A retrospective cohort study comparing survival rates between contemporary bosentan-treated patients and historical comparators showed improvement in mortality rate from 47% to 71% at 2 years [25]. Further studies have since also shown benefit in targeting both the ET-A and ET-B receptors, so that two licensed ET receptor antagonists are currently available – bosentan and sitaxsentan – the latter an endothelin A receptor antagonist. The PDE inhibitor sildenafil has been licensed for treatment of SSc-PAH after trials showed that sildenafil improves exercise capacity, World Health Organization (WHO) functional class and cardiac haemodynamics. Compared directly with bosentan, treatment over 12 weeks was not significantly different in terms of exercise capacity, right ventricular mass or *N*-terminal probrain natriuretic peptide (nt-proBNP) measurement, a reasonable serological surrogate marker of pulmonary hypertension [26]. Alternative PDE inhibitors, tadalafil and verdenafil, are also candidates for treatment.

Our current practice in patients with SSc-PAH is hence to treat initially with either bosentan or sitaxsentan. The drug is up-titrated over weeks, with serial measurements of nt-proBNP and 6MWD prior to a repeat cardiac catheterization at 3 months. The aim is to achieve a substantial reduction in PVR, which allows right ventricular remodelling and correlates with long-term survival [27]. If there is not a significant reduction in symptoms and PVR, the next step in the European Society of Cardiology (ESC) and American College of Chest Physicians (ACCP) guidelines recommends combination therapies of PDE inhibitors or prostanoids in addition to ET receptor antagonists [28, 29]. PDE inhibitors alone are used as an alternative in those unable to tolerate ET-receptor antagonists.

MODULATING VASCULOPATHY IN SYSTEMIC SCLEROSIS: DO THE SAME DRUGS WORK IN OTHER VASCULOPATHIC COMPLICATIONS?

Scleroderma renal crisis, which usually comprises acute renal failure, hypertension and a degree of proteinuria, again highlights the advances made in improving outcomes in SSc. The routine use of angiotensin-converting enzyme (ACE) inhibitors in this complication impressively reduced the mortality from 85% at 1 year to 24% [30]. The histological features seen on renal biopsy in the acute setting typically show accumulation of mucin in interlobular arteries, and fibrinoid necrosis of arterioles indistinguishable from the changes of accelerated hypertension. These are followed by more chronic changes of intimal thickening in arteries and hyalinosis in arterioles, and the typical onion-skin appearance (proliferation of intimal cells) reminiscent of vasculopathy in other organs such as the lung. Although the renin–angiotensin axis is clearly of importance here, immunohistochemical studies also suggest upregulation of the endothelin axis [31]. Patients with this complication are routinely treated with prostanoids (in our institution iloprost) and ACE inhibitors, and a trial is under way to assess the benefit of targeting the endothelin axis using bosentan in addition to the above standard therapy. Results in a cohort of six patients with SRC at one centre suggest beneficial blood pressure effects; short-term mortality and renal outcome data are not significantly different from historical control data [32].

Although digital ulceration, infarction and autoamputation may not usually be life-threatening, it is a complication which severely limits the hand function and therefore the independence of many of our patients, aside from the unwelcome cosmetic effects. At the microscopic level, the vessel changes seen in the peripheries mimic those seen elsewhere, with endothelial proliferation and thrombus formation late in the disease. Treatments are similar, comprising calcium channel antagonists to peripherally vasodilate, angiotensin receptor blockade, antiplatelet therapies, inhibitors of serotonin and, more recently, bystander benefits have been observed in patients using endothelin receptors antagonists and PDE-5 inhibitors for other organ-based indications. The use of bosentan in digital ulceration is the focus of previous and current trials, with treatment shown to reduce the frequency of formation of new digital ulcers and improve hand function, although the rate of healing of pre-existing ulcers was unchanged from the control group [33, 34]. Sildenafil significantly reduces the severity and frequency of Raynaud's attacks and may aid healing of chronic digital ulcers [35].

The use of prostanoids in treating digital ulcers is well described. Epoprostenol and iloprost are currently administered intravenously for this indication, which is expensive in terms of inpatient stay and inconvenient for patients. Improved delivery systems such as inhaled or oral prostanoids are far more attractive. Unfortunately, studies on oral iloprost have been disappointing, with doses high enough to allow significant benefit resulting in unacceptable side-effect profiles [36]. Further studies with sustained-release formulations are under way (Digital Ischemic Lesions in Scleroderma Treated with Oral Treprostinil Dithanolamine; DISTOL-1). A small open-label study of continuous s.c. treprostinil was beneficial, but at the cost of infusion site reactions [37]. The benefit of long-term home use of these efficacious drugs in those with refractory ischaemic ulcers is awaiting investigation.

CONCLUSION

Active investment in research, both laboratory based and clinical, has led to fruitful improvements in the understanding of the pathogenesis of fibrosis and vasculopathy in general, and in this prototypical disease in particular. Lessons learned from this condition have, and will continue to be, extrapolated in many different directions, and hence have implications in many areas of vascular biology and fibrosis research. We are now beginning to see the benefits of this labour with more targeted choices of therapies reaching clinical availability. Although there are still opportunities for significant improvements in therapy, the historical opinion that this disease is largely untreatable as well as incurable is unduly nihilistic. Outcomes in both scleroderma renal crisis and pulmonary arterial hypertension have improved dramatically, the diagnosis should be suspected early in any susceptible patient and investigated carefully to optimize outcomes.

Likely developments in this field in the next decade will include clarification of the roles of the therapies outlined above and continued discovery of the roles of mediators in the vasculopathic and fibrotic response to help design future therapies. International expert collaboration will aid the planning and administration of further high-quality trials to help investigate and manage patients in an evidence-based manner.

REFERENCES

1. Allcock RJ, Forrest I, Corris PA, Crook PR, Griffiths ID. A study of the prevalence of systemic sclerosis in northeast England. *Rheumatology* 2004; 43:596–602.

2. Stratton RJ, Wilson H and Black CM. Pilot study of anti-thymocyte globulin plus mycophenolate mofetil in recent-onset diffuse scleroderma. *Rheumatology* 2001; 40:84–88.
3. www.clinicaltrials.gov
4. Burt RK, Marmont A, Oyama Y *et al.* Randomized controlled trials of autologous hematopoietic stem cell transplantation for autoimmune diseases. *Arthritis Rheum* 2006; 54:3750–3760.
5. Nash RA, McSweeney PA, Crofford LJ *et al.* High-dose immunosuppressive therapy and autologous hematopoietic stem cell transplantation for severe systemic sclerosis: long-term follow-up of the US multicenter pilot study. *Blood* 2007; 110:1388–1396.
6. Vonk MC, Marjanovic Z, van den Hoogen FHJ *et al.* Long-term follow-up results after autologous haematopoietic stem cell transplantation for severe systemic sclerosis. *Ann Rheum Dis* 2008; 67:98–104.
7. van Laar JM, Farge D, Tyndall A. The ASTIS Trial. *Ann Rheum Dis* 2009; 68(Suppl3):462.
8. Tashkin DP, Elashoff R, Clements PJ *et al.* Cyclophosphamide versus placebo in scleroderma lung disease. *N Engl J Med* 2006; 354:2655–2666.
9. Hoyles RK, Sato H, Desai SR *et al.* Serum biomarkers in systemic sclerosis – associated pulmonary fibrosis: KL-6 correlates with disease severity. *Thorax* 2007; 62(Suppl. 3):A4–A63.
10. Hoyles RK, Ellis RW, Wellsbury J *et al.* A multicenter, prospective randomized, double-blind, placebo-controlled trial of corticosteroids and intravenous cyclophosphamide followed by oral azathioprine for the treatment of pulmonary fibrosis in scleroderma. *Arthritis Rheum* 2006; 54:3962–3970.
11. Nihtyanova SI, Brough GM, Black CM, Denton CP. Mycophenolate mofetil in diffuse cutaneous systemic sclerosis – a retrospective analysis. *Rheumatology* (Oxford) 2007; 46:442–445.
12. Clements PJ, Furst DE, Wong WK *et al.* High-dose versus low-dose D-penicillamine in early diffuse systemic sclerosis: analysis of a two-year, double-blind, randomized, controlled clinical trial. *Arthritis Rheum* 1999; 42:1194–1203.
13. Blobe GC, Schiemann WP, Lodish HF. Role of transforming growth factor β in human disease. *N Engl J Med* 2000; 342:1350–1358.
14. Dziadzio M, Smith RE, Abraham DJ *et al.* Circulating levels of active transforming growth factor β1 are reduced in diffuse cutaneous systemic sclerosis and correlate inversely with the modified Rodnan skin score. *Rheumatology* 2005; 44:1518–1524.
15. Varga J, Abraham D. Systemic sclerosis: a prototypic multisystem fibrotic disorder. *J Clin Invest* 2007; 117:557–567.
16. Denton CP, Merkel PA, Furst DE *et al.* Recombinant human anti-transforming growth factor β1 antibody therapy in systemic sclerosis: a multicenter, randomized, placebo-controlled phase I/II trial of CAT-192. *Arthritis Rheum* 2006; 56:323–333.
17. Wang S, Wilkes MC, Leof EB, Hirschberg R. Imatinib mesylate blocks a non-Smad TGF-β pathway and reduces renal fibrogenesis in vivo. *FASEB J* 2005; 19:1–11.
18. Distler JHW, Jüngel A, Huber LC *et al.* Imatinib mesylate reduces production of extracellular matrix and prevents development of experimental dermal fibrosis. *Arthritis Rheum* 2006; 56:311–322.
19. Daniels CE, Wilkes MC, Edens M *et al.* Imatinib mesylate inhibits the profibrogenic activity of TGF-β and prevents bleomycin-mediated lung fibrosis. *J Clin Invest* 2004; 114:1308–1316.
20. Ghofrani HA, Seeger W, Grimminger F. Imatinib for the treatment of pulmonary arterial hypertension. *N Engl J Med* 2005; 353:1412–1413.
21. Mclaughlin VV, Shillington A, Rich S. Survival in primary pulmonary hypertension: the impact of epoprostenol therapy. *Circulation* 2002; 106:477–482.
22. Simonneau G, Barst RJ, Galie N *et al.* Continuous subcutaneous infusion of treprostinil: a prostacyclin analogue, in patients with pulmonary arterial hypertension: a double-blind, randomized, placebo-controlled trial. *Am J Respir Crit Care Med* 2002; 165:800–804.
23. Oudiz RJ, Schilz RJ, Barst RJ *et al.* Treprostinil, a prostacyclin analogue, in pulmonary arterial hypertension associated with connective tissue disease. *Chest* 2004; 126:420–427.
24. Denton CP, Humbert M, Rubin L, Black CM. Bosentan treatment for pulmonary arterial hypertension related to connective tissue disease: a subgroup analysis of the pivotal clinical trials and their open-label extensions. *Ann Rheum Dis* 2006; 65:1336–1340.
25. Williams MH, Das C, Handler CE *et al.* Systemic sclerosis associated pulmonary hypertension: improved survival in the current era. *Heart* 2006; 92:926–932.
26. Wilkins MR, Paul GA, Strange JW *et al.* Sildenafil versus Endothelin Receptor Antagonist for Pulmonary Hypertension (SERAPH) study. *Am J Resp Crit Care Med* 2005; 171:1292–1297.
27. Hoeper M, Markevych I, Spiekerkoetter E, Welte T and Niedermeyer J. Goal-oriented treatment and combination therapy for pulmonary arterial hypertension. *Eur Respir J* 2005; 26:858–863.

28. www.escardio.org: Pulmonary Arterial Hypertension (Guidelines on Diagnosis and Treatment of) 2004.
29. Badesch DB, Abman SH, Simonneau G, Rubin LJ, McLaughlin VV. Medical therapy for pulmonary arterial hypertension: updated ACCP evidence-based clinical practice guidelines. *Chest* 2007; 131:1917–1928.
30. Steen VD, Costantino JP, Shapiro AP, Medsger TA. Outcome of renal crisis in systemic sclerosis: relation to availability of angiotensin converting enzyme (ACE) inhibitors. *Ann Intern Med* 1990; 113:352–357.
31. Kobayashi H, Nishimaki T, Kaise S *et al.* Immunohistological study of endothelin-1 and endothelin-a and b receptors in two patients with scleroderma renal crisis. *Clin Rheumatol* 1999; 18:425–427.
32. Penn H, Burns A, Black CM, Denton CP. An open-label trial of the Endothelin receptor antagonist bosentan in scleroderma renal crisis (BIRD-1). ACR/ARHP, Philadelphia 17-21st October 2009.
33. Korn JH, Mayes M, Matucci-Cerinic M *et al.* Digital ulcers in systemic sclerosis: prevention by treatment with bosentan, an oral endothelin receptor antagonist. *Arthritis Rheum* 2004; 50:3985–3993.
34. Seibold JR, Matucci-Cerinic M, Denton CP *et al.* Bosentan reduces the number of new digital ulcers in patients with systemic sclerosis. *Ann Rheum Dis* 2006; 65:S90.
35. Fries R, Shariat K, von Wilmowsky H, Böhm M. Sildenafil in the treatment of Raynaud's phenomenon resistant to vasodilatory therapy. *Circulation* 2005; 112:2980–2985.
36. Black CM, Halkier-Sørensen L, Belch JJ *et al.* Oral iloprost in Raynaud's phenomenon secondary to systemic sclerosis: a multicentre, placebo-controlled, dose-comparison study. *Br J Rheumatol* 1998; 37:952–960.
37. Chung L, Fiorentino D. A pilot trial of treprostinil for the treatment and prevention of digital ulcers in patients with systemic sclerosis. *J Am Acad Dermatol* 2006; 54:880–882.
38. Gourh P, Tan FK, Assassi S *et al.* Association of the PTPN22 R620W polymorphism with anti-topoisomerase i –and anticentromere antibody-positive systemic sclerosis. *Arthritis Rheum* 2006; 54:3945–3953.
39. Fonseca C, Renzoni E, Sestini P *et al.* Endothelin axis polymorphisms in patients with scleroderma. *Arthritis Rheum* 2006; 54:3034–3042.
40. Fonseca C, Lindahl GE, Ponticos M *et al.* A polymorphism in the CTGF promoter region associated with systemic sclerosis. *N Engl J Med* 2007; 357:1210–1220.
41. Renzoni E, Lympany P, Sestini P *et al.* Distribution of novel polymorphisms of the interleukin-8 and CXC receptor 1 and 2 genes in systemic sclerosis and cryptogenic fibrosing alveolitis. *Arthritis Rheum* 2000; 43:1633–1640.
42. Sato H, Lagan AL, Alexopoulou C *et al.* The TNF-863A allele strongly associates with anticentromere antibody positivity in scleroderma. *Arthritis Rheum* 2004; 50:558–564.
43. Hudson LL, Rocca KM, Kuwana M, Pandey JP. Interleukin-10 genotypes are associated with systemic sclerosis and influence disease-associated autoimmune responses. *Genes Immun* 2005; 6:274–278.
44. Zhou X, Tan FK, Reveille JD *et al.* Association of novel polymorphisms with the expression of SPARC in normal fibroblasts and with susceptibility to scleroderma. *Arthritis Rheum* 2002; 46:2990–2999.
45. Lagan AL, Pantelidis P, Renzoni EP *et al.* Single-nucleotide polymorphisms in the SPARC gene are not associated with susceptibility to scleroderma. *Rheumatology* 2005; 44:197–201.
46. Karrer S, Bosserhoff A, Weiderer P *et al.* The –2518 promoter polymorphism in the MCP-1 gene is associated with systemic sclerosis. *J Invest Dermatol* 2005; 124:92–98.
47. Carulli MT, Spagnolo P, Fonseca C *et al.* Single-nucleotide polymorphisms in CCL2 gene are not associated with susceptibility to systemic sclerosis. *J Rheumatol* 2008; 35; 839–844.
48. Crilly A, Hamilton J, Clark CJ *et al.* Analysis of transforming growth factor beta1 gene polymorphisms in patients with systemic sclerosis. *Ann Rheum Dis* 2002; 61:678–681.
49. Ohtsuka T, Yamakage A, Yamazaki S. The polymorphism of transforming growth factor-beta1 gene in Japanese patients with systemic sclerosis. *Br J Dermatol* 2002; 147:458–463.
50. Sugiura Y, Banno S, Matsumoto Y *et al.* Transforming growth factor beta1 gene polymorphism in patients with systemic sclerosis. *J Rheumatol* 2003; 30:1520–1523.
51. Fatini C, Gensini F, Sticchi E *et al.* High prevalence of polymorphisms of angiotensin-converting enzyme (I/D) and endothelial nitric oxide synthase (Glu298Asp) in patients with systemic sclerosis. *Am J Med* 2002; 112:540–544.
51. Tan FK, Wang N, Kuwana M *et al.* Association of fibrillin 1 single-nucleotide polymorphism haplotypes with systemic sclerosis in Choctaw and Japanese populations. *Arthritis Rheum* 2001; 44:893–901.
52. Hata R, Akai J, Kimura A *et al.* Association of functional microsatellites in the human type I collagen α2 chain (COL1A2) gene with systemic sclerosis. *Biochem Biophys Res Commun* 2000; 272:36–40.

10

Inflammatory myositis

David L. Scott

INTRODUCTION

Inflammatory myositis, which is often termed idiopathic inflammatory myositis, is a diverse group of diseases of skeletal muscle. Its three main forms comprise polymyositis, dermatomyositis and inclusion body myositis. There are several variants, including myositis associated with malignancy, childhood myositis and myositis occurring in the context of another connective tissue disease such as systemic lupus erythematosus (SLE). Inflammatory myositis and its variants are rare with fewer than eight per million new patients each year. This chapter reviews their classification and diagnosis, treatment and outcomes. The use of steroids, immunosuppressive treatments and biologicals, together with greater emphasis on exercise, has improved the outcome for patients with these disorders. Although treatment is not yet fully optimized, the overall outcome is favourable.

CLINICAL FEATURES

CLASSIFICATION

The two characteristic features of myositis are muscle weakness and evidence of muscle inflammation. Using clinical, histological and immunopathological criteria, myositis can be divided into three major groups:

- Dermatomyositis: affects children and adults and is commoner in women.
- Polymyositis: seen after the second decade of life.
- Sporadic inclusion-body myositis: more common in men over the age of 50.

Diagnostic criteria for myositis remain complex [1]. The most widely used criteria from Bohan and Peters [2] (Table 10.1) are of limited value as they were devised prior to current understanding of inclusion-body myositis. They also cannot differentiate myositis from some dystrophies.

A number of features should make the clinician reconsider whether myositis is the correct diagnosis. These include:

- disease onset before the age of 18;
- slow-onset myopathy that evolved over months to years;
- fatigue and myalgia, without muscle weakness, even if a transient rise in creatine kinase activity is seen; and
- no typical histological features of polymyositis.

Table 10.1 Bohan and Peters' diagnostic criteria

Features
1. Symmetrical proximal muscle weakness
2. Muscle biopsy evidence of myositis
3. Elevation in serum skeletal muscle enzymes
4. Characteristic electromyographic pattern of myositis
5. Typical rash of dermatomyositis

Polymyositis
Definite: all 1–4
Probable: any three of 1–4
Possible: any two of 1–4

Dermatomyositis
Definite: 5 plus any three of 1–4
Probable: 5 plus any two of 1–4
Possible: 5 plus any one of 1–4

EPIDEMIOLOGY

The annual incidence rate of polymyositis and dermatomyositis lies between 2 and 8 per million. One 20-year study from the USA found 6 per million between 1963 and 1982 [3]. Recent studies from Spain [4] also suggested an overall annual incidence of 8 per million. A study from North America focused on patients with myositis, rather than dermatomyositis, in Olmsted County, Minnesota, from 1981 to 2000 [5]. They found that for inclusion-body myositis the age- and sex-adjusted incidence rates were 8 per million and for polymyositis they were 4 per million. These were higher than previously reported. There are limited data on the prevalence of polymyositis and dermatomyositis. Retrospective studies from USA [6] and Japan [7] suggest that it is between 50 and 63 per million.

CLINICAL PRESENTATION

Dermatomyositis is characterized by a rash which accompanies or precedes muscle weakness. The dermatological features include:

- heliotrope rash on the upper eyelids;
- erythematosus rash on the face, neck and anterior chest;
- photosensitivity; and
- Gottron's papules (raised violaceous papules on the knuckles).

Weakness varies from mild to severe; in some patients muscle strength seems normal (amyopathic dermatomyositis). Dermatomyositis may be associated with cancer and can overlap with other connective tissue disease.

Polymyositis is usually a subacute myopathy that develops over weeks or months; there is weakness of the proximal muscles. Often its onset is indistinct. Polymyositis is often difficult to distinguish from other muscle diseases. It is essentially a diagnosis of exclusion.

Inclusion-body myositis is the commonest inflammatory myositis in patients aged over 50. It is characterized by a slow onset and progression and early involvement of finger flexors. It also responds poorly to treatment with steroids. There are several subsets including familial form and a retrovirus-associated form.

EXTRAMUSCULAR MANIFESTATIONS

A number of extramuscular features are common in myositis. These include:

- joint contractures, particularly in dermatomyositis;
- dysphagia, due to oropharyngeal muscles and upper oesophagus involvement;
- cardiac disease (conduction defects, tachyarrhythmias and myocarditis);
- lung disease due to weakness of the thoracic muscles or interstitial lung disease; and
- subcutaneous calcifications (only in dermatomyositis).

General symptoms include fever, malaise, weight loss and Raynaud's phenomenon.

INVESTIGATIONS

Three diverse investigations are needed to fully evaluate patients with a suspected inflammatory myositis. These comprise:

- muscle enzymes, particularly creatine kinase;
- an electromyography; and
- muscle biopsy.

Each investigation has its limitations. Muscle enzymes are usually raised in active myositis, but they are very non-specific. Elevated levels also occur in dystrophies, cardiac disease and many other disorders. In addition, the normal range differs across racial groups and normal levels are often high in some African and Afro-Caribbean patients.

An electromyography (EMG) provides valuable information but is highly subjective and its value is related to the skill and expertise of the clinician involved. A characteristic finding is the presence of positive sharp waves and fibrillation potentials, seen in over 90% of patients with acute disease. Complex repetitive discharges and pseudomyotonic discharges may also be seen.

Similarly, muscle biopsies require specific expertise in their interpretation, and are relatively subjective assessments. In addition, in many patients the disease is patchy and normal biopsies can be obtained from patients with overall serious disease. Frequent findings in dermatomyositis include decrease in the number of endomysial capillaries and perivascular inflammation in the perimysium. In polymyositis inflammation is primarily in the endomysium. The inflammatory response in inclusion body myositis is similar to that of polymyositis but there may also be rimmed vacuoles and an increase in ragged red fibres. Electron microscopy shows cytoplasmic and intranuclear tubulofilaments. Although rimmed vacuoles and tubulofilaments are fairly specific for inclusion-body myositis, they are sometimes absent in otherwise typical cases and so their absence does not exclude this diagnosis.

AUTOANTIBODIES

In common with other connective tissue diseases, inflammatory myositis is associated with the development of a range of autoantibodies to cellular constituents. Some are found specifically in patients with polymyositis and dermatomyositis; these are termed myositis-specific autoantibodies. Others are found in patients with a myositis overlap syndrome and are termed myositis-associated autoantibodies. The most recent classification is shown in Table 10.2, based on a review by Mimori *et al.* [8]. Recently identified autoantibodies include those linked to amyopathic dermatomyositis (anti-CADM-140 antibody) and malignancy-associated myositis (anti-p155 and anti-p155/p140 antibodies).

Table 10.2 Autoantibodies in myositis

Antibody	Antigen	Frequency
Myositis-specific autoantibodies		
Anti-Jo-1	Histidyl-tRNA synthetase	15–20%
Anti-PL-7	Threonyl-tRNA synthetase	5–10%
Anti-PL-12	Alanyl-tRNA synthetase	<5%
Anti-EL	Glcyl-tRNA synthetase	5–10%
Anti-OJ	Isoleucyl-tRNA synthetase	<5%
Anti-KS	Asparaginyl-tRNA synthetase	<5%
Anti-Zo	Phenylalanine-tRNA synthetase	<1%
Anti-YRS	Tyrosyl-tRNA synthetase	<1%
Anti-SRP	Signal recognition particle	5–10%
Anti-Mi2	218/240-kDa helicase family proteins	5–10%
Anti-CADM-140	Unknown 140-kDa protein	50% (C-ADM)
Anti-p155	Transcriptional intermediary factor 1γ	20% (dermatomyositis)
Anti-MJ	Unknown 140-kDa protein	<5%
Anti-PMS	DNA repair mismatch enzyme	<5%
Myositis-associated autoantibodies		
Anti-U1RNP	U1 small nuclear RNP	10%
Anti-Ku	70/80-kDa DNA-PK regulatory subunit	20–30%
Anti-OM-Scl	Nuclear protein complex of 11–16 proteins	8–10%

C-ADM, clinically amyopathic dermatomyositis.

IMAGING

Inflamed muscles can be assessed by a variety of imaging methods, particularly magnetic resonance imaging and ultrasound [9]. These indicate the extent of muscle disease and can be useful in identifying the optimal sites for muscle biopsy and for evaluating responses to treatment. Their use is limited at present as they are relatively non-specific.

ASSESSMENTS

As myositis affects not only the muscles, causing weakness, but also often damages many extramuscular components, there has been considerable interest in capturing the clinical effects of these disorders using standardized assessment methods. These include the Myositis Intention To Treat Index (MITAX) and the Myositis Disease Activity Assessment (MYOACT) visual analogue scale [10]. They have the ability to accurately and reproducibly assess patients; their use may be limited by both their relative complexity and the rarity of these diseases.

TREATMENTS

GLUCOCORTICOSTEROIDS

Glucocorticosteroids are the standard treatment for inflammatory myositis, although their effectiveness has not been subject to evaluation in a clinical trial [11]. There is an overwhelming consensus in favour of starting treatment with glucocorticosteroids in myositis [12]. The optimal dose remains uncertain; some physicians recommend a high initial dose such as prednisolone 60 mg/day. However, there is evidence that lower doses are equally effective and may limit adverse events [13]. For the foreseeable future, glucocorticosteroids will remain the mainstay of drug treatment.

IMMUNOSUPPRESSANTS

There is strong empirical evidence that immunosuppressive agents, especially azathioprine, methotrexate and ciclosporin, are beneficial in patients with polymyositis and dermatomyositis who are refractory to treatment with steroids. This is almost entirely based on clinical experience rather than randomized controlled trials (RCTs) [14].

Clinical experience based on retrospective reviews of treated cases suggested that up to 75% show a good response in retrospective reviews when treated with immunosuppressants [15]. A retrospective review of over 100 patients at a single centre suggested methotrexate may be superior to azathioprine or further steroid treatment in patients who do not respond completely to initial therapy with prednisolone [16]. Other immunosuppressive agents that are sometimes used include ciclosporin, cyclophosphamide and mycophenolate mofetil.

INTRAVENOUS IMMUNOGLOBULINS

Intravenous immunoglobulin has multiple mechanisms of actions and is the only treatment whose value is proven in RCTs (see below). The improvement with this treatment is noticeable by about 15 days. Repeated infusions may be required every 6–12 weeks to maintain improvement. As most patients with dermatomyositis respond to steroids, intravenous immunoglobulin is best reserved for steroid-resistant patients as a second-line therapy [17].

EVIDENCE-BASED IMMUNOSUPPRESSIVE TREATMENTS

As inflammatory myositis is both rare and includes a spectrum of diseases, there have been few RCTs that have defined effective treatment. A recent Cochrane review [18] identified seven potentially relevant RCTs of immunosuppressants. One of these was excluded because it was a reported follow-up data from an earlier RCT.

Three RCTs compared immunosuppressant with placebo control. These comprised trials of:

- High-dose intravenous immunoglobulin [19]: showing treatment was effective.
- Azathioprine [20]: showing no benefits of treatment.
- Plasma exchange and leucapheresis [21]: showing no benefits of treatment.

Three RCTs involved comparisons of different treatments, which comprised:

- Methotrexate and azathioprine [22]: showing no differences between groups.
- Ciclosporin and methotrexate [23]: showing no differences between groups.
- Intravenous methotrexate and oral methotrexate plus azathioprine [24]: showing no differences between groups.

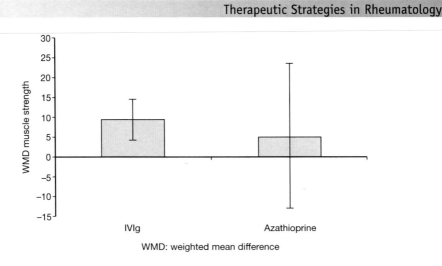

WMD: weighted mean difference

Figure 10.1 Comparison of active treatments with placebo from Cochrane review. WMD, weighted mean difference.

Key outcome data for the trials of intravenous immunoglobulin and azathioprine are shown in Figure 10.1. In all studies immunosuppressant therapy was associated with significant side-effects. Overall, there was minimal evidence that immunosuppressants are effective, mainly due to the relative dearth of RCTs.

TUMOUR NECROSIS FACTOR INHIBITORS

There is substantial evidence from studies of myositis pathogenesis that tumour necrosis factor (TNF) is involved and that inhibiting it might be effective [25]. However, in clinical practice its value appears questionable. A number of studies have now been reported, including two observational studies and an early RCT, and these give little indication of efficacy. The studies are as follows:

- A retrospective study of eight patients with dermatomyositis or polymyositis refractory to glucocorticosteroids and immunosuppressives were treated with TNF inhibitors between 1998 and 2004 [26]. Six patients were treated with etanercept alone, one with infliximab and one sequentially with both agents. Of the eight patients, six showed a favourable response with improved motor strength and decreased fatigue after 12 months. This study suggested potential benefit.
- An observational study of five patients with active dermatomyositis with lack of response to glucocorticosteroid and cytotoxic therapy were given etanercept for at least 3 months [27]. All patients experienced an exacerbation of disease, with increase of muscle weakness, elevation of muscle enzyme levels and unchanged rash.
- A multicentre open-label controlled trial [28] of infliximab in myositis was terminated prematurely because of a low inclusion rate and a high dropout rate due to disease progression. Although infliximab combined with weekly methotrexate might be safe and well tolerated in a small subgroup of patients with drug-naive recent-onset myositis, its use was not advocated because of the uncertainty about treatment response.

The balance of evidence from these studies is that TNF inhibition is not effective in myositis.

RITUXIMAB

A number of open-label trials have reported experience in treating myositis with rituximab, the biological that targets B cells. Three of these open-label pilot trials are particularly interesting, and all suggest a potential effect from targeting B cells. They are as follows:

- A study of seven adult patients with dermatomyositis reported that all six evaluable patients had major clinical improvements, with muscle strength increasing over baseline by 36–113% [29].
- A study of eight adult patients with dermatomyositis reported that three patients (38%) achieved partial remission by 6 months with improvements in muscle strength [30].
- A study of three patients with long-standing polymyositis or dermatomyositis poorly responsive to prednisone combined with immunosuppressants reported muscle strength improved in all, with strength returning to normal in two [31].

Rituximab infusions were invariably well tolerated, with no serious infection complications. The results are generally positive, but there is some uncertainty in their interpretation. The key need is for them to be confirmed in a definitive RCT; this will take some time to come to fruition.

DRUG TREATMENT OF INCLUSION-BODY MYOSITIS

Unlike polymyositis, which it closely mirrors, inclusion-body myositis invariably fails to respond to immunosuppressive treatment. Intravenous immunoglobulins have been of some benefit in occasional patients. However, glucocorticosteroids, immunosuppressants and biologicals all appear universally ineffective.

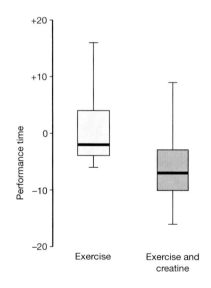

Figure 10.2 Improvements in performance time for four functional tasks in patients treated with creatine and exercise over 6 months.

EXERCISE

Until recently, patients with inflammatory myositis were discouraged from active exercise to avoid increasing muscle inflammation and were recommended to rest. Over the last two decades, a series of studies have shown that disability is reduced in patients with chronic polymyositis and dermatomyositis following resistive mild or intensive muscular training without signs of increased muscle inflammation. Patients with active, recent-onset disease also benefit from mild to moderate exercise without increased muscle inflammation [32].

A recent systematic review of exercise in a range of neuromuscular diseases identified seven trials that studied aerobic exercises for patients with muscle disorders [33]. Aerobic capacity benefited most; there were also improvements in muscle strength. A further three trials studied the combination of muscle strengthening and aerobic exercises and also showed evidence of benefit. Overall, this review concluded that strengthening exercises combined with aerobic exercises have positive effects on activities and participation in patients with muscle disorders and should be encouraged.

There is evidence that combining exercise with simple additional treatment to improve muscle strength increases performance. This has been shown in a recent RCT of creatine supplements, which increased performance in patients with myositis that had been treated with glucocorticosteroids and immunosuppressants [34]; all the patients had exercise but only those who had added creatine showed significant improvements. The extent of this improvement on an aggregated measure of performance (better performance reduces time involved) is shown in Figure 10.2.

OUTCOMES

Myositis had a poor prognosis in the presteroid era. After glucocorticosteroids became available in the 1950s, outcomes improved considerably. A UK study from Sultan and colleagues [35] assessed long-term outcome in 46 patients with idiopathic myositis diagnosed from 1978 to 1999 by assessing cumulative survival probability over 20 years. During the course of the disease, seven patients (15%) went into full remission, eight (17%) had monophasic illness, nine (20%) had a relapsing–remitting course, 16 (35%) had chronic progressive illness and six (13%) died. The 5-year survival rate was 95% and the 10-year survival rate was 84%. A similar study from Finland [36] evaluated 176 patients with polymyositis and 72 patients with dermatomyositis diagnosed from 1969 to 1985. Their 5-year survival rate for polymyositis was 75% and for dermatomyositis was 63%; respective 10-year survival rates were 55% and 53%.

The most recent overall outcome data come from Bronner and colleagues [37]. They reviewed the clinical data and muscle biopsy specimens at presentation of 268 adult patients with 'myositis' or 'possible myositis' diagnosed from 1977 to 1998. Over 100 patients were excluded because of diagnostic uncertainty, leaving 165 considered to have definite myositis; these were followed for a mean of 5 years. During this time, 157 patients (95%) were treated with glucocorticosteroids and 94 (57%) were subsequently treated with one immunosuppressive or immunomodulating drug. Thirty-four (21%) patients died; in 18 patients death was related to their myositis. These associated deaths included cancer (in seven patients), pulmonary complications (in four patients) and adverse reactions to drugs (in four patients). Subsequently, 110 of 131 surviving patients (84%) were re-examined after 5 years' follow-up. This showed 24% had considerable disability and 25% of the patients had muscle weakness (MRC sum score < 128); 41% were using prednisone or immunosuppressive treatment at follow-up. The relation of outcome to autoantibody categorization is shown in Figure 10.3.

The relation between myositis and malignancy is complex. A study from Hungary by András *et al.* [38] evaluated 309 patients with myositis; 37 of these had a malignancy. Thirty

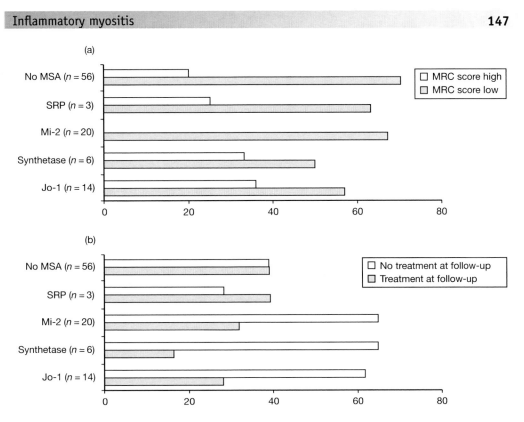

Figure 10.3 Muscle strength and treatment needs by antibody subtype in myositis patients. (a) Muscle strength. (b) Treatment at follow-up. MRC, Medical Research Council; SRP, signal recognition particle [37]. *Ann Rheum Dis* 2006; 65:1456–1461.

patients had dermatomyositis and seven had polymyositis. In 65% the malignancy and myositis appeared within 1 year. The overall survival rate was 92% at 5 years and 89% at 10 years; it was considerably worse in patients with malignancy and myositis, and 32% of these patients died.

CONCLUSION

Most patients with dermatomyositis and polymyositis respond to treatment with glucocorticosteroids; the optimal dose is uncertain, but the benefits of high doses are probably overstated. Added immunosuppressants such as methotrexate or azathioprine will help most patients who show an incomplete response to steroids. Intravenous immunoglobulins should be reserved for patients who show an incomplete response to these approaches. Biologicals such as rituximab are likely to be more widely used in the future and have the potential to be highly effective. All patients will benefit from exercise. There is a need to increase the inclusion of patients with rare diseases of this sort in large RCTs and mechanisms need to be found to achieve this so that there is a firm evidence base for treatment.

REFERENCES

1. Dalakas MC. The future prospects in the classification, diagnosis and therapies of inflammatory myopathies: a view to the future from the 'bench-to-bedside'. *J Neurol* 2004; 251:651–657.

2. Bohan A, Peter JB. Polymyositis and dermatomyositis. *N Engl J Med* 1975; 292:344–347.
3. Oddis CV, Conte CG, Steen VD, Medsger TA Jr. Incidence of polymyositis–dermatomyositis: a 20-year study of hospital diagnosed cases in Allegheny County, PA 1963–1982. *J Rheumatol* 1990; 17:1329–1334.
4. Vargas-Leguás H, Selva-O'Callaghan A, Campins-Martí M, Hermosilla Pérez E, Grau-Junyent JM, Martínez Gómez X, Vaqué Rafart J. Polymyositis–dermatomyositis: incidence in Spain (1997–2004). *Med Clin* (Barc) 2007; 129:721–724.
5. Wilson FC, Ytterberg SR, St Sauver JL, Reed AM. Epidemiology of sporadic inclusion body myositis and polymyositis in Olmsted County, Minnesota. *J Rheumatol* 2008; 35:445–447.
6. Kurland LT, Hauser WA, Ferguson RH, Holley KE. Epidemiologic features of diffuse connective tissue disorders in Rochester, Minn., 1951 through 1967, with special reference to systemic lupus erythematosus. *Mayo Clin Proc* 1969; 44:649–663.
7. Koh ET, Seow A, Ong B, Ratnagopal P, Tija H, Chang HH. Adult onset polymyositis/dermatomyositis: clinical and laboratory features and treatment response in 75 patients. *Ann Rheum Dis* 1993; 52:857–861.
8. Mimori T, Imura Y, Nakashima R, Yoshifuji H. Autoantibodies in idiopathic inflammatory myopathy: an update on clinical and pathophysiological significance. *Curr Opin Rheumatol* 2007; 19:523–529.
9. Scott DL, Kingsley GH. Use of imaging to assess patients with muscle disease. *Curr Opin Rheumatol* 2004; 16:678–683.
10. Isenberg DA, Allen E, Farewell V, Ehrenstein MR, Hanna MG, Lundberg IE *et al.*; International Myositis and Clinical Studies Group (IMACS). International consensus outcome measures for patients with idiopathic inflammatory myopathies. Development and initial validation of myositis activity and damage indices in patients with adult onset disease. *Rheumatology* (Oxford) 2004; 43:49–54.
11. Dalakas MC. Current treatment of the inflammatory myopathies. *Curr Opin Rheumatol* 1994; 6:595–601.
12. Oddis CV. Therapy for myositis. *Curr Opin Rheumatol* 1993; 5:742–748.
13. Nzeusseu A, Brion F, Lefebvre C, Knoops P, Devogelaer JP, Houssiau FA. Functional outcome of myositis patients: can a low-dose glucocorticoid regimen achieve good functional results? *Clin Exp Rheumatol* 1999; 17:441–446.
14. Dalakas MC. Inflammatory disorders of muscle: progress in polymyositis, dermatomyositis and inclusion body myositis. *Curr Opin Neurol* 2004; 17:561–567.
15. Ramirez G, Asherson RA, Khamashta MA, Cervera R, D'Cruz D, Hughes GR. Adult-onset polymyositis–dermatomyositis: description of 25 patients with emphasis on treatment. *Semin Arthritis Rheum* 1990; 20:114–120.
16. Joffe MM, Love LA, Leff RL, Fraser DD, Targoff IN, Hicks JE *et al.* Drug therapy of the idiopathic inflammatory myopathies: predictors of response to prednisone, azathioprine and methotrexate and a comparison of their efficacy. *Am J Med* 1993; 94:379–387.
17. Dalakas MC. Therapeutic targets in patients with inflammatory myopathies: present approaches and a look to the future. *Neuromuscul Disord* 2006; 16:223–236.
18. Choy EH, Hoogendijk JE, Lecky B, Winer JB. Immunosuppressant and immunomodulatory treatment for dermatomyositis and polymyositis. *Cochrane Database Syst Rev* 2005; 3:CD003643.
19. Dalakas MC, Illa I, Dambrosia JM, Soueidan SA, Stein DP, Otero C *et al.* A controlled trial of high-dose intravenous immune globulin infusions as treatment for dermatomyositis. *N Engl J Med* 1993; 329:1993–2000.
20. Bunch TW, Worthington JW, Combs JJ, Ilstrup MS, Engel AG. Azathioprine with prednisone for polymyositis. *Ann Intern Med* 1980; 92:365–369.
21. Miller FW, Leitman SF, Cronin ME, Hicks JE, Leff RL, Wesley R *et al.* Controlled trial of plasma exchange and leukapheresis in polymyositis and dermatomyositis. *N Engl J Med* 1992; 326:1380–1384.
22. Miller J, Walsh Y, Saminaden S, Lecky BRF, Winer JB. Randomised double blind controlled trial of methotrexate and steroids compared with azathioprine and steroids in the treatment of idiopathic inflammatory myopathy. *J Neurol Sci* 2002; 199(Suppl. 1):S53.
23. Vencovsky J, Jarosova K, Machacek S, Studynkova J, Kafkova J, Bar-tunkova J *et al.* Cyclosporine A versus methotrexate in the treatment of polymyositis and dermatomyositis. *Scand J Rheumatol* 2000; 29:95–102.
24. Villalba L, Hicks JE, Adams EM, Sherman JB, Gourley MF, Leff RL *et al.* Treatment of refractory myositis: a randomized crossover study of two new cytotoxic regimens. *Arthritis Rheum* 1998; 41:392–399.
25. Efthimiou P. Tumor necrosis factor-alpha in inflammatory myopathies: pathophysiology and therapeutic implications. *Semin Arthritis Rheum* 2006; 36:168–172.

26. Efthimiou P, Schwartzman S, Kagen LJ. Possible role for tumour necrosis factor inhibitors in the treatment of resistant dermatomyositis and polymyositis: a retrospective study of eight patients. *Ann Rheum Dis* 2006; 65:1233–1236.

27. Iannone F, Scioscia C, Falappone PC, Covelli M, Lapadula G. Use of etanercept in the treatment of dermatomyositis: a case series. *J Rheumatol* 2006; 33:1802–1804.

28. Hengstman GJ, De Bleecker JL, Feist E, Vissing J, Denton CP, Manoussakis MN, Slott Jensen H, van Engelen BG, van den Hoogen FH. Open-label trial of anti-TNF-alpha in dermato- and polymyositis treated concomitantly with methotrexate. *Eur Neurol* 2008; 59:159–163.

29. Levine TD.Rituximab in the treatment of dermatomyositis: an open-label pilot study. *Arthritis Rheum* 2005; 52:601–607.

30. Chung L, Genovese MC, Fiorentino DF. A pilot trial of rituximab in the treatment of patients with dermatomyositis. *Arch Dermatol* 2007; 143:763–767.

31. Noss EH, Hausner-Sypek DL, Weinblatt ME. Rituximab as therapy for refractory polymyositis and dermatomyositis. *J Rheumatol* 2006; 33:1021–1026.

32. Alexanderson H, Lundberg IE. The role of exercise in the rehabilitation of idiopathic inflammatory myopathies. *Curr Opin Rheumatol* 2005; 17:164–171.

33. Cup EH, Pieterse AJ, Ten Broek-Pastoor JM, Munneke M, van Engelen BG, Hendricks HT, van der Wilt GJ, Oostendorp RA. Exercise therapy and other types of physical therapy for patients with neuromuscular diseases: a systematic review. *Arch Phys Med Rehabil* 2007; 88:1452–1464.

34. Chung YL, Alexanderson H, Pipitone N, Morrison C, Dastmalchi M,Ståhl-Hallengren C, Richards S, Thomas EL, Hamilton G, Bell JD, Lundberg IE, Scott DL. Creatine supplements in patients with idiopathic inflammatory myopathies who are clinically weak after conventional pharmacologic treatment: six-month, double-blind, randomized, placebo-controlled trial. *Arthritis Rheum* 2007; 57:694–702.

35. Sultan SM, Ioannou Y, Moss K, Isenberg DA. Outcome in patients with idiopathic inflammatory myositis: morbidity and mortality. *Rheumatology* (Oxford) 2002; 41:22–26.

36. Airio A, Kautiainen H, Hakala M. Prognosis and mortality of polymyositis and dermatomyositis patients. *Clin Rheumatol* 2006; 25:234–239.

37. Bronner IM, van der Meulen MF, de Visser M, Kalmijn S, van Venrooij WJ, Voskuyl AE, Dinant HJ, Linssen WH, Wokke JH, Hoogendijk JE. Long-term outcome in polymyositis and dermatomyositis. *Ann Rheum Dis* 2006; 65:1456–1461.

38. András C, Ponyi A, Constantin T, Csiki Z, Szekanecz E, Szodoray P, Dankó K. Dermatomyositis and polymyositis associated with malignancy: a 21-year retrospective study. *J Rheumatol* 2008; 35:438–444.

11

Disease-modifying drugs in osteoarthritis

Alexandra N. Colebatch, Nigel K. Arden

INTRODUCTION

Osteoarthritis (OA) is the most common joint disorder in the Western world and the fourth most common cause of disability in women worldwide. It is the principal indication for arthroplasty, at 90% at the knee and 70% at the hip. In the UK, around 550000 people have moderate to severe knee OA and 210000 moderate to severe hip OA. Approximately 2 million people consult their GP and 115000 are admitted to hospital in the UK each year because of OA [1].

Despite the prevalence of OA, the pathogenesis of the disease remains unclear. Current treatments are aimed at symptomatic and supportive measures, such that a significant proportion of patients eventually require joint replacement surgery for severely damaged joints. In the UK, approximately 52048 total hip replacements and 44645 total knee replacements were performed by the NHS in 2002.

Osteoarthritis is a disease of the whole joint including loss of hyaline articular cartilage, sclerosis of the underlying bone and involvement of soft-tissue structures such as the synovium, ligaments and muscles [2]. This process results in reduced joint function and pain. Catabolic cytokines and anabolic growth factor pathways are also known to control destruction and repair in OA.

Drug treatment of OA can, therefore, be targeted towards any of these affected structures. Interfering with the anatomical progression of OA is a potential means to preserve normal joint function. Drugs providing cartilage protection in OA are chondoprotective drugs, whereas disease-modifying osteoarthritis drugs (DMOADs) have been sought to intervene in the disease process and halt radiographic progression [3]. Painful joints in OA are thought to be secondary to the anatomical changes, including inflammatory events in the synovium, as well as subchondral intraosseous hypertension caused by venous congestion. As there is a poor correlation between radiographic changes and symptoms [4], outcome may be better assessed through correlation with symptomatic and functional benefit.

The various potential DMOADs that have published evidence are addressed below.

GLUCOSAMINE AND CHONDROITIN

Glucosamine is an aminosaccharide which plays an essential role in the synthesis of cartilage. Glucosamine also inhibits both anabolic and catabolic gene expression of OA cartilage, the latter of which is thought to be important for its therapeutic role [5]. Glucosamine sulphate is a stronger inhibitor of gene expression than glucosamine hydrochloride, which may explain the differences in action of these two drugs, as discussed below [6].

Studies into the use of glucosamine and chondroitin have looked at the effect on symptoms, as well as on structural modification. These have resulted in variable results, whether given in combination or separately. Differences in results are also seen with variations in preparations, study designs and study populations.

A recent Cochrane review analysed data from 20 glucosamine studies, which included over 2500 patients, and concluded that outcome from 2 to 3 months of treatment with glucosamine depended on the type of preparation used [7]. This review found improvement in pain in those taking Rotta preparations of 1500 mg glucosamine sulphate (crystalline glucosamine sulphate), but no such improvement was found in those taking non-Rotta preparations, which are often esterified.

Two randomized controlled trials (RCTs) showed that the Rotta preparation was also able to slow radiographic progression of knee OA over a 3-year period [8, 9]. These studies showed no significant progression of cartilage loss in those treated with glucosamine sulphate, which suggests a potential role of glucosamine as a disease-modifying drug.

Studies have also looked at the efficacy of glucosamine hydrochloride versus glucosamine sulphate, again resulting in mixed results. Qiu *et al.* [10] found no difference between safety and efficacy when comparing these drugs in a multicentre RCT. Both were found to result in improvement in symptoms after just 4 weeks of treatment. The Glucosamine/Chondroitin Arthritis Intervention Trial (GAIT) [11] compared 1500 mg of glucosamine hydrochloride daily with 1200 mg chondroitin sulphate daily, 200 mg celecoxib daily and placebo for 24 weeks. In this study, glucosamine hydrochloride and chondroitin sulphate, alone or in combination, were found not to have a significant effect on reducing pain when compared with placebo. These findings were consistent with those from an earlier study by Houpt *et al.* [12].

Although there is conflicting evidence regarding the efficacy of glucosamine, it is inexpensive (2008 price about £2.50/month, 1500 mg glucosamine sulphate daily) and has very few side-effects, and appears to be as safe as placebo [7]. Therefore, a reasoned case can be made to include glucosamine sulphate in the management of OA. However, largely because of the heterogeneity of RCTs, NICE does not recommend its use (www.nice.org.uk).

Chondroitin sulphate has also been well studied, and meta-analyses have shown it to be effective in reducing pain in OA. This effect, although slow in onset, has been shown to last for up to 3 months after treatment has been withdrawn [13]. However, the benefit has not been reproduced in all studies [11], with more favourable results with use of chondroitin sulphate combined with glucosamine [11, 14]. Although the GAIT study [11] found no significant effect of combined glucosamine and chondroitin on reducing pain in all patients with OA, the study did show that this combination treatment was effective in reducing pain in a subgroup of patients with moderate to severe pain. A recent meta-analysis [14] of the use of glucosamine and chondroitin in OA found trials to demonstrate an effect on symptoms, although this was more modest early in treatment (4 weeks).

Although there are no long-term placebo-controlled trials on the disease modification role of chondroitin, two small trials have shown potential. One trial in rabbits [15] with chemically induced unilateral knee OA showed use of chondroitin, given either orally or by intramuscular (i.m.) injection, resulted in higher cartilage proteoglycan levels, suggesting that chondroitin may have a protective effect on damaged cartilage. A further study of 119 patients examined the role of chondroitin sulphate in the progression of finger joint OA [16]. This study showed a significant decrease in the number of patients with new erosive OA finger joints, suggesting a potential role of chondroitin sulphate in protecting against progression into an erosive OA.

ANTIOXIDANTS AND VITAMINS

Antioxidants have long been thought to play a part in the treatment of arthritis through their role in the prevention of cellular damage. Antioxidants safely interact with free radicals and terminate the subsequent chain reaction before vital molecules are damaged. Free radicals are thought to have a role in the pathogenesis of OA [17], in particular through effects on cartilage and lipids [18]. Although there are several enzyme systems within the body that scavenge free radicals, the principal micronutrient (vitamin) antioxidants are vitamins A, C and E and the trace metal selenium.

VITAMIN A

Vitamin A, retinol, has been shown to have an *in vitro* effect on cartilage and bone [19]. Despite this, studies examining vitamin A in subjects with OA have not found such results. One study looking at serum and synovial fluid retinol levels in a small cohort of subjects with OA [20] found no significant difference in these parameters when compared with a control group. A further trial found vitamin A to have no effect on symptoms in subjects with OA [21], but this trial did not include a control group.

VITAMIN C

Vitamin C is thought to be important in OA through effects on cartilage via the stabilization of type II procollagen through addition of hydroxyl groups [22] and the stimulation of levels of glycosaminoglycans by acting as a sulphate carrier [23].

There have, however, been conflicting results for the role of vitamin C supplementation in OA. Vitamin C-deficient guinea pigs have been found to have reduced synthesis of collagen and proteoglycan [24], and in guinea pigs with surgically induced OA vitamin C supplementation has been to shown to reduce the incidence of new OA [25]. In contrast, vitamin C supplementation (in similar doses to those used to prevent surgically induced OA) increased the severity of OA in guinea pig models with spontaneous OA [26].

Wang *et al.* [27] found higher vitamin C intake to be associated with a reduction in tibial plateau bone area and the presence of bone marrow lesions. As both of these processes have been implicated as risk factors for OA, these results suggest a protective effect of vitamin C in OA.

The overall recommendation should be to encourage a healthy diet in order to achieve the recommended daily intake of vitamin C, but there is no convincing evidence to support supplementation above this level.

VITAMIN E

Studies have shown vitamin E to have a weaker effect on progression of knee OA compared with vitamin C, with a stronger effect in men [28]. This difference may be due to differences in solubility of the vitamins – vitamin C is water soluble and therefore able to easily enter the extracellular matrix, whereas vitamin E is fat soluble.

Randomized controlled trials have shown inconsistent results in terms of symptomatic benefit with vitamin E, with some showing an improvement in symptoms [29, 30] which has not been seen in others [31].

Trials of disease modification with vitamin E have not been promising. Wluka *et al.* [32] followed cartilage volume, as well as symptoms, in patients with knee OA over a 2-year period and found vitamin E to have no effect. There were similar findings by Wang *et al.* [27].

SELENIUM

Selenium is a component of glutathione peroxidase, which provides protection from oxidation stress. Studies looking into the role of selenium in OA have used a selenium preparation, selenium-ACE, which also contains vitamins A, C and E. There are no studies to date using selenium alone.

Hill *et al.* [33] found no significant difference in subjects with primary or secondary OA taking selenium-ACE or placebo, in either pain, stiffness or radiographic changes. A more recent study in mice with mechanically induced OA, which used a similar drug preparation, found a significantly lower incidence of OA in those mice receiving the vitamin supplementation [34].

VITAMIN D

Vitamin D is a hormone that is produced in the skin and can also be obtained from the diet. It is produced from the conversion of 7-dehydrocholesterol in the skin to cholecalciferol or ergocalciferol (vitamin D). This is then hydroxylated in the liver to weakly active 25-hydroxy-vitamin D, which is the best substance for measuring vitamin D status. This undergoes further hydroxylation into the most active form of the vitamin, 1,25-dihydroxy-vitamin D.

Vitamin D is important in bone metabolism and essential for bone health. Suboptimal levels of vitamin D can result in secondary hyperparathyroidism, which leads to increased bone turnover and increased rates of bone loss. *In vitro* studies have shown vitamin D to stimulate synthesis of proteoglycans by mature chondrocytes, and vitamin D receptors have been shown to be closely associated with sites of prevalent matrix metalloproteinase (MMP) expression in osteoarthritic cartilage [35]. Vitamin D, therefore, has important effects on both cartilage and bone, in addition to important effects on muscle function.

The Medical Research Council (MRC) Hertfordshire cohort study assessed vitamin D intake in subjects in whom serial knee radiography was performed [36]. This study found that both low intake and low serum levels of vitamin D were associated with higher osteophytes score on radiography, with no association with loss of joint space. Rate of disease progression was also higher in those with low intake or serum vitamin D levels. A similar relationship was seen in results from the Framingham Heart Study [37], which also showed an increased risk of progression of knee OA in those with lower serum levels and vitamin D intake as assessed by osteophytes growth as well as cartilage loss (Table 11.1).

The Study of Osteoporotic Fractures [38] determined the relationship of serum levels of vitamin D to incident changes of radiographic hip OA among elderly white women. This study found that those with mild and severe vitamin D deficiencies had a threefold increased risk of incident radiographic OA, in particular joint space narrowing, compared with those with higher vitamin D levels.

These results do suggest that low intake and serum levels of vitamin D are associated with incidence and progression of OA at various sites, which indicates a potential role of vitamin D as a disease-modifying drug in OA. Several trials are currently under way to formally assess its benefit in subjects with knee OA.

BONE-ACTIVE DRUGS

BISPHOSPHONATES

Localized subchondral changes, including bone marrow lesions, are important features of OA and are associated with progression of disease. Bisphosphonates are used in the treatment of osteoporosis, and have the ability to suppress bone turnover, resulting in the potential role of bisphosphonates as disease-modifying drugs in OA.

Table 11.1 Incidence and progression of osteoarthritis of the knee: independent associations with dietary intake and serum levels of vitamin D

Variable	Incidence			Progression		
	Patients (n)	Odds ratio (95% CI)	P-value	Patients (n)	Odds ratio (95% CI)	P-value
Dietary intake of vitamin D						
Lowest tertile (3–170 IU/day)	24	1.02 (0.47 to 2.20)	>0.2	25	4.05 (1.40 to 11.6)	0.009
Middle tertile (170–347 IU/day)	35	2.48 (1.40 to 11.6)	0.01	24	2.99 (1.06 to 8.49)	0.04
Highest tertile (386–1612 IU/day)	16	1	–	13	1	–
Serum levels of vitamin D						
Lowest tertile (4.9–24.0 ng/ml)	25	0.92 (0.45 to 1.87)	>0.2	33	2.89 (1.01 to 8.25)	0.05
Middle tertile (27.0–33.0 ng/ml)	25	0.90 (0.48 to 1.80)	>0.2	20	2.83 (1.02 to 7.85)	0.05
Highest tertile (36.0–79.0 ng/ml)	25	1	–	9	1	–

*Odds ratios for serum levels of vitamin D were adjusted for age, sex, body mass index, weight change, physical activity index, knee injury, and health status. Odds ratios for dietary intake of vitamin D were adjusted for these factors and for total energy intake.

Source: McAlindon TE, Felson DT, Zhang Y, Hannan MT, Aliabadi P, Weissman B *et al*. Relation of dietary intake and serum levels of vitamin D to progression of osteoarthritis of the knee among participants in the Framingham study. *Ann Intern Med* 1996; 125:353–359 [37].

The BRISK study [39] demonstrated that bisphosphonate risedronate significantly reduces WOMAC score in patients with mild to moderate medial compartment knee OA. A trend was also seen towards reduction of joint space narrowing in those taking higher doses (15 mg risedronate daily), which was also seen to reduce the markers of cartilage degradation and bone resorption.

These results were not replicated in the KOSTAR trial [40], which showed no improvement in pain or radiographic progression of OA; however, a dose-dependent reduction in the level of a cartilage degradation marker associated with progressive OA was seen in patients receiving risedronate.

These doses of risedronate (15 mg daily) have been shown to preserve vertical trabecular structure in patients with marked cartilage loss, classified as joint space narrowing of 0.6 mm or more, whereas those receiving risedronate doses of 50 mg/week were found to have increased vertical trabecular number, which maintains the structural integrity of subchondral bone in knee OA [41].

A study of another bisphosphonate, alendronate, examined elderly women with knee OA [42]. This study examined the effect of alendronate on the structural features of knee OA as assessed by magnetic resonance imaging (MRI) and radiography, and the symptoms of knee OA in elderly women. Alendronate use was associated with lower values for bone attrition as compared with that in the non-use group, as well as with significantly lower WOMAC pain scores compared with non-use.

These results suggest a role of bisphosphonates in disease modification in OA, along with an effect on severity of symptoms; however, additional studies are required to further clarify their role.

STRONTIUM

The primary indication of strontium ranelate is for the treatment of post-menopausal osteoporosis. Previous *in vivo* studies have suggested a potential role of strontium ranelate in the treatment of OA. If human normal and OA chondrocytes have either been treated or not treated with interleukin 1β (IL-1β), strontium ranelate has been shown to stimulate the synthesis of type II collagen and proteoglycan [43]. Further studies have also shown strontium ranelate to significantly decrease the levels of a cartilage degradation biomarker with high tissue specificity, urinary C-terminal telopeptides of type-II collagen (u-CTX-II), as compared with placebo [44]. These studies suggest that strontium ranelate plays a part in the progression of OA.

In the clinical setting, a recent study examined the effect of 3-year treatment with strontium ranelate on progression of spinal OA [45]. This study found that the proportion of patients with a worsening overall spinal OA score, as assessed by the presence and severity of osteophytes, disc space narrowing and sclerosis in the lumbar intervertebral spaces, was reduced by 42% in the strontium ranelate group, as compared with placebo (Figure 11.1). Significantly more patients in the strontium ranelate group experienced an improvement in back pain after 3 years than in the placebo group, but there was no significant difference in health-related quality of life.

CALCITONIN

The action of calcitonin is both in cartilage and bone turnover. The effect on cartilage has been shown *in vitro* to be anti-catabolic and anabolic, by reducing proteoglycan and type-II collagen degradation as well as stimulating synthesis [46]. A trial using oral salmon calcitonin demonstrated a significant improvement in function and biomarkers of joint metabolism in subjects with knee OA compared with placebo, but there was no significant difference in symptoms between the groups [47]. This study recruited only a small number of subjects in each group ($n = 18$), hence reducing the power of this study, but these results do suggest a potential role of calcitonin on the treatment of OA.

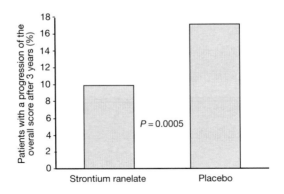

Figure 11.1 The percentage of patients with an increase in the overall score after 3 years' follow-up among the whole study population. Source: Bruyere O, Delferriere D, Roux C, Wark J D, Spector T, Devogelaer J-P *et al.* Effects of strontium ranelate on spinal osteoarthritis progression. *Ann Rheum Dis* 2008; 67:335–339 [45].

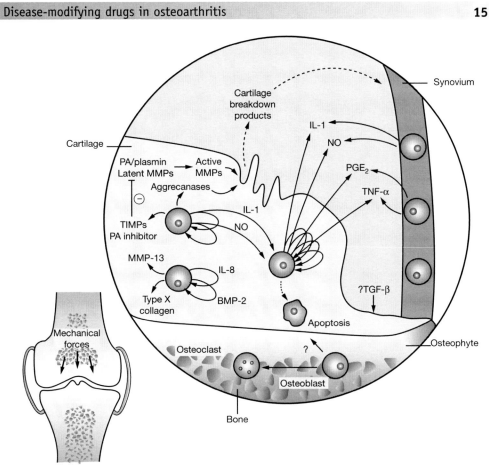

Figure 11.2 Molecular pathogenesis of osteoarthritis. Potential biomarkers and targets for disease modification are released as a result of events in cartilage, bone, and synovium. Source: Krasnokutsky S, Samuels J, Abramson SB. Osteoarthritis in 2007. *Bull NYU Hosp Jt Dis* 2007; 65:222–228 [50].

MATRIX METALLOPROTEINASE INHIBITORS

Matrix metalloproteinases degrade the major components of the extracellular matrix, as shown in Figure 11.2. MMPs are therefore important potential targets to inhibit for disease-modifying drugs in OA.

The tetracyclines, such as doxycycline, have been the subject of research in view of their action as MMP inhibitors [48]. One trial has shown doxycycline to reduce the rate of joint space narrowing in the disease knee in obese subjects with unilateral knee OA receiving treatment for 30 months [49]. This trial did not show an improvement in pain scores with doxycycline treatment, but pain levels were already low at the start of the trial.

Doxycycline has been shown to have an effect on several mechanisms involved in cartilage synthesis, including nitric oxide production, which has also been implicated as a potential disease-modifying drug in OA. This is discussed later in this chapter.

Doxycycline is generally well tolerated, but can most commonly cause gastrointestinal side-effects, such as diarrhoea and abdominal pain. Excess sun exposure should be avoided whilst on tetracyclines as they can exaggerate sunburn. Tetracyclines do cross the placenta in pregnancy, and can have toxic effects on fetal bone. There are, therefore, a few potential side-effects with doxycycline, which may suggest that doxycycline would not be the treatment of choice in OA.

DIACEREIN, AVOCADO–SOYBEAN UNSAPONIFIABLES AND EXTRACT OF ROSE-HIP

DIACEREIN

Osteoarthritis chondrocytes produce increased levels of inflammatory cytokines such as IL-1β (Figure 11.2). This results in decreased collagen synthesis and increased levels of degradative proteases, such as MMPs, and of inflammatory mediators, such as IL-8, IL-6, prostaglandin E_2 and nitric oxide (NO) [50]. Inhibition of IL-1β has important potential in the disease modification of OA.

The IL-1β inhibitor diacerein has been shown to have a beneficial effect on joint space narrowing in a 3-year study on hip OA [51], but there was no associated improvement in symptoms. This trial found diacerein to be well tolerated, with few bowel symptoms only.

A subsequent meta-analysis of diacerein in the treatment of knee and hip OA [52] demonstrated that diacerein was as effective as non-steroidal anti-inflammatory drugs (NSAIDs) in improving pain and function, but diacerein alone was seen to have persistent effects at 3 months, as well as reducing analgesic requirement. Both drugs were well tolerated, but NSAIDs are associated with more significant adverse effects than diacerein.

AVOCADO–SOYBEAN UNSAPONIFIABLES

Avocado–soybean unsaponifiables (ASUs) are extracts derived from one-third avocado oil and two-thirds soybean oil after hydrolysis. This mix has been shown, *in vitro*, to have an inhibitory effect on IL-1, and to stimulate collagen synthesis in articular chondrocyte cultures [53].

A clinical trial using 300 mg ASU daily [54] has shown ASU to be superior to placebo in patients with hip or knee OA (Figure 11.3). This was demonstrated by a significant improvement in functional and pain scores, and although there was a delayed onset of action

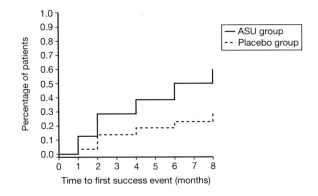

Figure 11.3 Success rate, defined as a ≥30% improvement on Lequesne's functional index and a ≥50% reduction in the level of pain by 100-mm visual analogue scale, compared with baseline. Osteoarthritis was located in the hip or knee. ASU, avocado–soybean unsaponifiables. Source: Maheu E, Mazieres B, Valat J-P, Loyau G, Le Loet X, Bourgeois P, Grouin J-M, Rozenrerg S. Symptomatic efficacy of avocado/soybean unsaponifiables in the treatment of osteoarthritis of the knee and hip. *Arthritis Rheum* 1998; 41:81–91 [54].

of ASU a prolonged effect was seen, with action persisting for 2 months after treatment discontinuation.

Further trials have also compared ASU and placebo in patients with hip or knee OA [55–57] with similar results. Two trials [55, 56] have shown improved pain and functional ability when comparing ASU and NSAID with placebo and NSAID over 3 to 6 months. These results were not reproduced in a trial including patients with hip OA only [57]. This trial demonstrated a significant reduction in loss of joint space in those patients on ASU with advanced joint space narrowing, as compared with placebo. These results suggest that ASU could have a structural effect in OA, but a larger placebo-controlled study in hip OA is required to confirm this.

EXTRACT OF ROSE-HIP

Rose-hip powder, made from the seeds and husk of fruit from a subtype of *Rosa canina*, has been evaluated in several trials for its clinical effectiveness in the treatment of OA. One 4-month RCT on the effect of 2500 mg twice daily of rose-hip powder on active and passive mobility in hip and knee OA found only improved passive hip flexion [58]. A further crossover RCT, which used the same dose of rose-hip powder, found an improvement in pain in those receiving rose-hip compared with placebo, but only when the rose-hip was given after placebo [59]. One study did show a significant improvement in pain with rose-hip powder, but this effect was only seen after 3 weeks of treatment and was not maintained at 3 months [60]. There is, therefore, conflicting evidence for the potential role of rose-hip in OA.

DISEASE-MODIFYING ANTIRHEUMATIC DRUGS

There are few studies of the use of disease-modifying antirheumatic drugs (DMARDs) in the treatment of OA, but their use has increased as erosive and inflammatory OA has been increasingly described.

HYDROXYCHLOROQUINE

One trial retrospectively reviewed the clinical records of just eight patients with erosive OA who had not responded to NSAIDs and were subsequently given hydroxychloroquine [61]. This treatment was found to be effective in 75% of the patients, with few side-effects. This is a very small study group, with other data remaining limited. A larger prospective study in the future would be useful.

OTHERS: METHOTREXATE AND SULFASALAZINE

Data regarding the use of methotrexate and sulfasalazine in OA are limited. Data with methotrexate come from a study in rabbits with experimental OA, which demonstrated methotrexate reduced cartilage damage [62]. Further data are therefore required, and at present are mainly anecdotal.

CONCLUSION

There are currently no drugs available that have been definitively proven to modify the disease process in OA. However, there a number of potentially exciting drugs with early data, such as glucosamine sulphate, strontium ranelate and vitamin D. The availability of the first proven disease-modifying drug is greatly anticipated and will change the management of OA substantially.

REFERENCES

1. Woolf AD, Pfleger B. Burden of major musculoskeletal conditions. *Bull World Health Organ* 2003; 81:646–656.
2. Felson DT, Lawrence RC, Dieppe PA, Hirsch R, Helmick CG, Jordan JM *et al.* Osteoarthritis: new insights. Part 1: the disease and its risk factors. *Ann Intern Med* 2000; 133:635–646.
3. Dieppe P. Disease modification in osteoarthritis: are drugs the answer? *Arthritis Rheum* 2005; 52:1956–1959.
4. Hannan MT, Felson DT, Pincus T. Analysis of the discordance between radiographic changes and knee pain in osteoarthritis of the knee. *J Rheumatol* 2000; 27:1513–1517.
5. Van Osch G, Uitterlinder EJ, Koevoet WLM, De Groot J, Vefhaar VAN, Weinans H. Glucosamine decreases expression of anabolic and catabolic genes in human osteoarthritic cartilage explants. *Osteoarthr Cartil* 2006; 14:963–966.
6. Altman RD, Abramson S, Bruyere O, Clegg D, Herrero-Beaumont G, Maheu E *et al.* Commentary: osteoarthritis of the knee and glucosamine. *Osteoarthr Cartil* 2006; 14:963–966.
7. Towheed TE, Maxwell L, Anastassiades TP, Shea B, Houpt J, Robinson V *et al.* Glucosamine therapy for treating osteoarthritis. *Cochrane Database Syst Rev* 2005; 2:CD002946.
8. Pavelka K, Gatterova J, Olejarova M, Machacek S, Giacovelli G, Rovati LC. Glucosamine sulfate use and delay of progression of knee osteoarthritis. A 3-year, randomized, placebo-controlled, double-blind study. *Arch Intern Med* 2002; 162:2113–2123.
9. Reginster JY, Deroisy R, Rovati LC, Lee RL, Lejeune E, Bruyere O *et al.* Long-term effects of glucosamine sulphate on osteoarthritis progression: a randomized, placebo-controlled clinical trial. *Lancet* 2001; 357:251–256.
10. Qiu GX, Weng XS, Zhang K, Zhou YX, Lou SQ, Wang YP *et al.* A multi-central, randomised, controlled clinical trial of glucosamine hydrochloride/sulphate in the treatment of knee osteoarthritis. *Zhonghua Yi Xue Za Zhi* 2005; 85:3067–3070.
11. Clegg DO, Reda DJ, Harris CL, Klein MA, O'Dell JR, Hooper MM *et al.* Glucosamine, chondroitin sulfate, and the two in combination for painful knee osteoarthritis. *N Engl J Med* 2006; 354:795–808.
12. Houpt J B, McMillan R, Wein C, Paget-Dellio S D. Effect of glucosamine hydrochloride in the treatment of pain of osteoarthritis of the knee. *J Rheumatol* 1999; 26:2423–2430.
13. Morreale P, Manopulo R, Galati M, Boccanera L, Saponati G, Bocchi L. Comparison of the anti-inflammatory efficacy of chondroitin sulfate and diclofenac sodium in patients with knee osteoarthritis. *J Rheumatol* 1996; 23:1385–1391.
14. McAlindon TE, LaValley MP, Gulin JP, Felson DT. Glucosamine and chondroitin for the treatment of osteoarthritis: a systematic quality assessment and meta-analysis. *JAMA* 2000; 283:1469–1475.
15. Uebelhart D, Thonar EJ, Zhang J, Williams JM. Protective effect of exogenous chondroitin 4,6-sulfate in the acute degradation of articular cartilage in the rabbit. *Osteoarthr Cartil* 1998; 6(Suppl.1):6–13.
16. Verbruggen G, Goemaere S, Veys EM. Chondroitin sulphate SYSMOAD (structure/disease modifying antiosteoarthritis drug) in the treatment of finger joint OA. *Osteoarthr Cartil* 1998; 6(Suppl.1):37–38.
17. Henrotin Y, Deby-Dupont G, Deby C, De Bruyn M, Lamy M, Franchimont P. Production of active oxygen species by isolated human chondrocytes. *Rheumatology* 1993; 32:562–567.
18. Tiku M L, Shah R, Allison GT. Evidence linking chondrocyte lipid peroxidation to cartilage matrix protein degradation: possible role in cartilage aging and the pathogenesis of osteoarthritis. *J Biol Chem* 2000; 275:20069–20076.
19. Fell HB, Mellanby E. The effect of hypervitaminosis A on embryonic limb-bones in vitro. *J Physiol* 1952; 116:320–349.
20. Fairney A, Patel KV, Fish DE, Seifert MH. Vitamin A in osteo- and rheumatoid arthritis. *Br J Rheumatol* 1988; 27:329–330.
21. Mahmud Z, Ali SM. Role of vitamin A and E in spondylosis. *Bangladesh Med Res Counc Bull* 1992; 18:47–59.
22. Peterkofsky B. Ascorbate requirement for hydroxylation and secretion of procollagen: relationship to inhibition of collagen synthesis in scurvy. *Am J Clin Nutr* 1991; 54:1135–1140S.
23. Schwartz ER, Adamy L. Effect of ascorbic acid on arylsulfatase activities and sulfated proteoglycan metabolism in chondrocyte cultures. *J Clin Invest* 1977; 60:96–106.
24. Peterkofsky B, Palka J, Wilson S, Takeda K, Shah V. Elevated activity of low molecular weight insulin-like growth factor binding proteins in sera of vitamin C deficient and fasted guinea pigs. *Endocrinology* 1991; 128:1769–1779.

25. Meacock SCR, Bodmer JL, Billingham MEJ. Experimental OA in guinea pigs. *J Exp Pathol* 1990; 71:279–293.
26. Kraus VB, Huebner JL, Stabler T, Flahiff CM, Setton LA, Fink C *et al.* Ascorbic acid increases the severity of spontaneous knee osteoarthritis in a guinea pig model. *Arthritis Rheum* 2004; 50:1822–1831.
27. Wang Y, Hodge AM, Wluka AE, English DR, Giles GG, O'Sullivan R *et al.* Effect of antioxidants on knee cartilage and bone in healthy, middle-aged subjects: a cross sectional study. *Arthritis Res Ther* 2007; 9:R66.
28. McAlindon TE, Jacques P, Zhang Y, Hannan MT, Aliabadi P, Weissman B *et al.* Do antioxidant micronutrients protect against the development and progression of knee osteoarthritis? *Arthritis Rheum* 1996; 39:648–656.
29. Machtey I, Ouaknine L. Tocopherol in osteoarthritis: a controlled pilot study. *J Am Geriatr Soc* 1978; 26:328–330.
30. Blakenhorn G. Clinical effectiveness of Spondyvit (vitamin E) in activated arthroses. A multicenter placebo-controlled double-blind study. *Z Orthop* 1986; 124:340–343.
31. Brand C, Snaddon J, Bailey M, Cicuttini F. Vitamin E is ineffective for symptomatic relief of knee osteoarthritis: a six month double blind, randomised, placebo controlled study. *Ann Rheum Dis* 2001; 60:946–949.
32. Wluka AE, Stuckey S, Brand C, Cicuttini FM. Supplementary vitamin E does not affect the loss of cartilage volume in knee osteoarthritis: a 2 year double blind randomised placebo controlled study. *J Rheumatol* 2002; 29:2585–2591.
33. Hill J, Bird HA. Failure of selenium-ACE to improve osteoarthritis. *Br J Rheumatol* 1990; 29:211–213.
34. Kurz B, Jost B, Schünke M. Dietary vitamins and selenium diminish the development of mechanically induced osteoarthritis and increase the expression of antioxidative enzymes in the knee joint of STR/1N mice. *Osteoarthr Cartil* 2002; 10:119–126.
35. Tetlow LC, Woolley DE. Expression of vitamin D receptors and matrix metalloproteinases in osteoarthritic cartilage and human articular chondrocytes in vitro. *Osteoarthr Cartil* 2001; 9:423–431.
36. Arden NK, Richardson A, Syddall HE, Aihie Sayer A, Dennison EM, Cooper C. Dietary vitamin D intake and radiographic knee osteoarthritis. *Osteoarthr Cartil* 2006; 14(Suppl.2):S33–S34.
37. McAlindon TE, Felson DT, Zhang Y, Hannan MT, Aliabadi P, Weissman B *et al.* Relation of dietary intake and serum levels of vitamin D to progression of osteoarthritis of the knee among participants in the Framingham study. *Ann Intern Med* 1996; 125:353–359.
38. Lane NE, Gore LR, Cummings SR, Hochberg MC, Scott JC, Williams EN *et al.* Serum vitamin D levels and incident changes of radiographic hip osteoarthritis. *Arthritis Rheum* 1999; 42:854–860.
39. Spector TD, Conaghan PG, Buckland-Wright JC, Garnero P, Cline GA, Beary JF *et al.* Effect of risedronate on joint structure and symptoms of knee osteoarthritis: results of the BRISK randomised, controlled trial. *Arthritis Res Ther* 2005; 7:R625–633.
40. Bingham CO, Buckland-Wright JC, Garnero P, Cohen SB, Dougados M, Adami S *et al.* Risedronate decreases biochemical markers of cartilage degradation but does not decrease symptoms or slow radiographic progression in patients with medial compartment osteoarthritis of the knee: results of the two-year multinational knee osteoarthritis structural arthritis study. *Arthritis Rheum* 2006; 5:3494–3507.
41. Buckland-Wright JC, Messent EA, Bingham CO, Ward RJ, Tonkin C. A 2 yr longitudinal radiographic study examining the effect of a bisphosphonate (risedronate) upon subchondral bone loss in osteoarthritic knee patients. *Rheumatology* 2007; 46:257–264.
42. Carbone LD, Nevitt MC, Wildy K, Barrow KD, Harris F, Felson F. The relationship of antiresorptive drug use to structural findings and symptoms of knee osteoarthritis. *Arthritis Rheum* 2004; 50:3516–3525.
43. Henrotin Y, Labasse A, Zheng SX, Galais P, Tsouderos Y, Crielaard JM *et al.* Strontium ranelate increases cartilage matrix formation. *J Bone Miner Res* 2001; 16:299–308.
44. Alexanderson P, Karsdal M, Qvist P, Reginster JY, Christiansen C. Strontium ranelate reduces the urinary level of cartilage degradation biomarker CTX-II in postmenopausal women. *Bone* 2007; 40:218–222.
45. Bruyere O, Delferriere D, Roux C, Wark JD, Spector T, Devogelaer J-P *et al.* Effects of strontium ranelate on spinal osteoarthritis progression. *Ann Rheum Dis* 2008; 67:335–339.
46. Karsdal MA, Tanko LB, Riis BJ, Sondergard BC, Henriksen K, Altman RD *et al.* Calcitonin is involved in cartilage homeostasis: is calcitonin a treatment for OA? *Osteoarthr Cartil* 2006; 14:617–624.

47. Manicourt DH, Azria M, Mindeholm L, Thonar EJ, Devogelaer JP *et al.* Oral salmon calcitonin reduces Lequesne's algofunctional index scores and decreases urinary and serum levels of biomarkers of joint metabolism in knee osteoarthritis. *Arthritis Rheum* 2006; 54:3205–3211.

48. Golub LM, Lee H-M, Lehrer G, Nemiroff A, McNamara TF, Kaplan R *et al.* Minocycline reduces gingival collagenolitic activity during diabetes: preliminary observations and a proposed new mechanism of action. *J Periodontal Res* 1983; 18:516–526.

49. Brandt KD, Mazzuca SA, Katz BP, Lane KA, Buckwalter KA, Yocum DE *et al.* Effects of doxycycline on progression of osteoarthritis: results of a randomized, placebo-controlled, double-blind trial. *Arthritis Rheum* 2005; 52:2015–2025.

50. Krasnokutsky S, Samuels J, Abramson SB. Osteoarthritis in 2007. *Bull NYU Hosp Jt Dis* 2007; 65:222–228.

51. Dougados M, Nguyen M, Berdah L, Mazieres B, Vignon E, Lequesne M. Evaluation of the structure-modifying effects of diacerein in hip osteoarthritis: ECHODIAH, a three-year, placebo-controlled trial. *Arthritis Rheum* 2001; 44:2539–2537.

52. Rintelen B, Neumann K, Leeb BF. A meta-analysis of controlled clinical studies with diacerein in the treatment of osteoarthritis. *Arch Intern Med* 2006; 166:1899–1906.

53. Mauviel A, Daireaux M, Hartmann DJ, Galera P, Loyau G, Pujol JP. Effets des insaponifiahles d'avocat et de soja (PIAS) sur la production de collagene par des cultures de synoviocytes, chondrocytes articulaires et fibroblastes dermiques. *Rev Rhum Mal Osteoartic* 1989; 56:207–211.

54. Maheu E, Mazieres B, Valat J-P, Loyau G, Le Loet X, Bourgeois P, Grouin J-M, Rozenrerg S. Symptomatic efficacy of avocado/soybean unsaponifiables in the treatment of osteoarthritis of the knee and hip. *Arthritis Rheum* 1998; 41:81–91.

55. Blotman F, Maheu E, Wulwik A, Caspard H, Lopez A. Efficacy and safety of avocado/soybean unsaponifiables in the treatment of symptomatic osteoarthritis of the knee and hip. A prospective, multicenter, three-month, randomized, double-blind, placebo-controlled trial. *Rev Rhum Eng Ed* 1997; 64:825–834.

56. Appelboom T, Schuermans J, Verbruggen G, Henrotin Y, Reginster JY. Symptoms modifying effect of avocado/soybean unsaponifiables (ASU) in knee osteoarthritis. A double blind, prospective, placebo-controlled study. *Scand J Rheumatol* 2001; 30:242–247.

57. Lequesne M, Maheu E, Cadet C, Dreiser RL. Structural effect of avocado/soybean unsaponifiables on joint space loss in osteoarthritis of the hip. *Arthritis Rheum* 2002; 47:50–58.

58. Warholm O, Skaar S, Hedman E, Molmen HM, Eik L. The effects of a standardized herbal remedy made from a subtype of Rosa canina in patients with osteoarthritis: a double-blind, randomised, placebo-controlled clinical trial. *Curr Ther Res* 2003; 64:21–31.

59. Rein E, Kharazmi A, Winther K. A herbal remedy, Hyben Vital (stand. powder of a subspecies of Rosa canina fruits), reduces pain and improves general wellbeing in patients with osteoarthritis – a double-blind, placebo-controlled, randomized trial. *Phytomedicine* 2004; 11:383–391.

60. Winther K, Apel K, Thamsborg G. A powder made from seeds and shells of a rose-hip subspecies (Rosa canina) reduces symptoms of knee and hip osteoarthritis: a randomized, double-blind, placebo-controlled clinical trial. *Scand J Rheumatol* 2005; 34:302–308.

61. Bryant LR, des Rosier KF, Carpenter MT. Hydroxychloroquine in the treatment of erosive osteoarthritis. *J Rheumatol* 1995; 22:1527–1531.

62. Neidel J, Schroers B, Sintermann F. The effects of high-dose methotrexate on the development of cartilage lesions in a lapine model of osteoarthrosis. *Arch Orthop Trauma Surg* 1998; 117:265–269.

12

Management of gout

Edward Roddy, Michael Doherty

INTRODUCTION

Gout is a true-crystal deposition disease caused by monosodium urate (MSU) crystal formation in and around joints. It is one of the commonest inflammatory arthritides, with a population prevalence of 0.5–2% [1–4]. The primary risk factor for the development of gout is hyperuricaemia [5, 6]. MSU crystal formation and deposition occurs as serum urate (SUA) levels rise and exceed the physiological saturation threshold of urate in body tissues (approximately 380 µmol/l). The clinical course of gout typically passes through several phases: (i) excruciatingly painful attacks of acute synovitis, most commonly affecting the first metatarsophalangeal joint (podagra); (ii) recurrent acute attacks, involving an increasing number of peripheral joints sites with intervening asymptomatic intercritical periods (interval gout); and (iii) chronic tophaceous gout characterized by clinically detectable nodular deposits of urate (tophi), joint damage and chronic symptoms.

Effective treatment for gout exists and the aim of management is cure. Recently, management guidelines have been produced by the European League Against Rheumatism (EULAR) [7] (Table 12.1) and the British Society for Rheumatology (BSR) [8]. Treatment is targeted to the clinical phase with specific therapeutic strategies, aiming firstly to relieve the pain and florid inflammation of acute gout and then secondly to lower SUA sufficiently to prevent further crystal formation and to dissolve existing crystals, thus preventing further acute attacks and the development of irreversible joint damage.

ACUTE GOUT

The treatment of acute gout aims to relieve pain rapidly by reducing inflammation and intra-articular hypertension. Non-steroidal anti-inflammatory drugs (NSAIDs), colchicine and glucocorticosteroids are the main pharmacological agents used to treat acute gout. Local application of ice-packs may also be effective.

NON-STEROIDAL ANTI-INFLAMMATORY DRUGS

One randomized controlled trial (RCT), which included 30 patients with acute gout, compared tenoxicam 40 mg daily with placebo, demonstrating 50% pain reduction at 24 hours in 67% of the tenoxicam group compared with 26% of the placebo group (number needed to treat [NNT] 3) [7, 9, 10]. Head-to-head comparisons report the efficacy of various NSAIDs for acute gout including flurbiprofen [11], indomethacin [11–14], ketoprofen [12], naproxen [15], nimesulid [14] and phenylbutazone [13, 15], although no clear evidence of superiority of one drug over

Table 12.1 European League Against Rheumatism (EULAR) recommendations for the management of gout

Optimal treatment of gout requires both non-pharmacological and pharmacological modalities and should be tailored according to:
  (i) specific risk factors (levels of serum urate, previous attacks, radiographic signs)
  (ii) clinical phase (acute/recurrent gout, intercritical gout, and chronic tophaceous gout)
  (iii) general risk factors (age, sex, obesity, alcohol consumption, urate-raising drugs, drug interactions, and co-morbidity)

Patient education and appropriate lifestyle advice regarding weight loss (if obese), diet and reduced alcohol (especially beer) are core aspects of management
Associated co-morbidity and risk factors such as hyperlipidaemia, hypertension, obesity and smoking should be addressed as an important part of the management of gout
Oral colchicine and/or NSAIDs are first-line agents for systemic treatment of acute attacks; in the absence of contraindications, an NSAID is a convenient and well-accepted option
High doses of colchicine lead to side-effects, and low doses (e.g. 0.5 mg three times daily) may be sufficient for some patients with acute gout
Intra-articular aspiration and injection of long-acting steroid is an effective and safe treatment for an acute attack
ULT is indicated in patients with recurrent acute attacks, arthropathy, tophi or radiographic changes of gout
The therapeutic goal of ULT is to promote crystal dissolution and prevent crystal formation; this is achieved by maintaining the serum uric acid below the saturation point for monosodium urate ($\leq 360\,\mu mol/l$)
Allopurinol is an appropriate long-term urate-lowering drug. It should be started at a low dose (e.g. 100 mg daily) and increased by 100 mg every 2–4 weeks if required. The dose must be adjusted in patients with renal impairment. If allopurinol toxicity occurs, options include other xanthine oxidase inhibitors, a uricosuric agent or allopurinol desensitization (the latter only in cases of mild rash)
Uricosuric agents such as probenecid and sulphinpyrazone can be used as an alternative to allopurinol in patients with normal renal function but are relatively contraindicated in patients with urolithiasis; benzbromarone can be used in patients with mild-to-moderate renal insufficiency on a named patient basis, but carries a small risk of hepatotoxicity
Prophylaxis against acute attacks during the first months of ULT can be achieved by colchicine (0.5–1 mg daily) and/or an NSAID (with gastroprotection if indicated)
When gout associates with diuretic therapy, stop the diuretic if possible; for hypertension and hyperlipidaemia consider use of losartan and fenofibrate, respectively (both have modest uricosuric effects)

NSAID, non-steroidal anti-inflammatory drug; ULT, urate-lowering therapy.

Reproduced with permission from ref. 7: the BMJ Publishing Group, Zhang *et al.*, *Ann Rheum Dis* 2006; 65:1312–1324.

another is seen. Although traditional non-selective NSAIDs are undoubtedly efficacious for acute gout, gastrointestinal toxicity is of concern and the potential risks and benefits should be considered carefully for each individual patient. Where indicated, co-prescription of a proton pump inhibitor (PPI) or use of an alternative agent such as a cyclooxygenase 2 (COX-2) selective agent or colchicine should be considered. Of currently available COX-2 selective inhibitors, there are two large double-blind multicentre RCTs comparing etoricoxib 120 mg daily with indomethacin 50 mg three times daily for acute mono/oligoarticular gout [16, 17]. Over an 8-day period, similar reductions in joint pain, tenderness and swelling were seen with etoricoxib and indomethacin in both studies. Drug-related adverse events were more frequent with indomethacin than with etoricoxib. In the second study, both gastrointestinal (7.8% vs. 18.6%) and cardiovascular (6.8% vs. 16.3%) adverse events were less frequent in the etoricoxib group [17]. However, indomethacin was one of the first NSAIDs to become available and is one of the most toxic; therefore, in the absence of evidence to show superior efficacy to any other quick-acting NSAID, it is far from the traditional NSAID of choice. A further RCT of 62 patients with acute gout compared rofecoxib 50 mg daily, diclofenac 150 mg daily and meloxicam 15 mg daily [18]. Rofecoxib has since been withdrawn by the manufacturer. Patient global assessment of response to therapy was rated good or excellent by 40% of the meloxicam group and 57% of the diclofenac group at day 3, and by 60% (meloxicam) and 81% (diclofenac) at day 8. Tolerability appeared to be similar between the groups. In these studies, COX-2-selective inhibitors appear to have at least similar efficacy to traditional non-selective NSAIDs, and etoricoxib had better gastrointestinal tolerability than indomethacin. However, although one of these trials reported fewer cardiovascular adverse events with etoricoxib than indomethacin [17], given recent concerns regarding cardiovascular side-effects of COX-2-selective inhibitors and the considerable cardiovascular co-morbidity associated with gout [1, 19], recommendations for their widespread use must be guarded.

COLCHICINE

Colchicine is a naturally occurring alkaloid derived from the meadow saffron or autumn crocus (*Colchicum autumnale*) [20]. Colchicine inhibits the phagocytic activity of polymorphonuclear leucocytes, preventing the ingestion of urate crystals and hence the release of lysosomal enzymes. It also inhibits cell-mediated immune responses by inhibiting immunoglobulin production, interleukin 1 (IL-1) production, histamine release and HLA-DR expression. A recent Cochrane review [21] identified only one RCT of colchicine for acute gout ($n = 45$) [22]. Oral colchicine produced absolute reductions of 34% for pain (NNT 3) and 30% for clinical inflammation (NNT 2) when compared with placebo [21, 22]. However, colchicine was given at an initial dose of 1 mg followed by 500-μg doses every 2 hours until relief of symptoms occurred or vomiting or diarrhoea developed. Perhaps not surprisingly, diarrhoea and/or vomiting occurred in all patients in the colchicine group. Anecdotal clinical experience suggests that such regimes are widely used in clinical practice in the UK resulting in frequent toxicity, particularly by non-specialists, encouraged by the persistence of this regime in the *British National Formulary*. Rheumatologists frequently advocate a lower-dose regime, e.g. 500 μg two to four times daily [7, 8, 23]. However, systematic research evidence of the efficacy and tolerability of lower-dose colchicine regimes for acute gout is lacking. Intravenous colchicine is no longer recommended because of severe and potentially fatal toxicity.

GLUCOCORTICOSTEROIDS

Glucocorticosteroids are a useful treatment for acute gout, particularly when NSAIDs and colchicine are contraindicated or poorly tolerated. Joint aspiration (instantly reducing intra-articular hypertension and hence severe pain) combined with intra-articular injection of long-acting glucocorticosteroid is a highly effective and safe treatment for acute gout but has not been studied in a controlled clinical trial. Intra-articular injection of triamcinolone acetonide 10 mg produced substantial pain relief within 48 hours in 19 patients with acute gout in one uncontrolled study [24]. Joint aspiration and intra-articular glucocorticosteroid injection is particularly helpful for mono-articular attacks in large joints, but is also applicable to small joints, including podagra. It also permits confirmation of MSU crystals in the synovial fluid. Systemic administration of intramuscular or oral glucocorticosteroids is commonplace, although the evidence base for their use is sparse. Intramuscular adrenocorticotropic hormone (ACTH) 40 IU or triamcinolone acetonide 60 mg appears to be at least as effective as NSAIDs [25–27]. ACTH may work by stimulating glucocorticoid release, but also has a direct anti-inflammatory effect via the melanocortin type III receptor [28]. An uncontrolled study of 13 patients with acute gout reported good responses to tapered courses of oral prednisolone following an initial dose of 20–50 mg daily [29]. Systemic glucocorticosteroids are particularly useful for severe oligo/polyarticular gout or monoarticular attacks at sites not amenable to intra-articular injection, for example the mid-foot joints, when NSAIDs/colchicine are contraindicated or poorly tolerated.

ICE-PACKS

Local application of ice is an effective treatment for acute gout. In one RCT, 19 patients were randomized either to combination therapy consisting of topical ice therapy, prednisolone 30 mg daily (6-day tapered course) and colchicine 600 µg daily or to a control group who received prednisolone and colchicine only [30]. In the treatment group, topical ice-packs were applied to the target inflamed joint for 30 minutes four times daily. Over a 1-week period, the mean reduction in pain on a 10-cm visual analogue scale was 7.75 cm in the ice-therapy group compared with 4.42 cm in the control group.

SUMMARY

First-line oral treatment for acute gout should consist of either a rapid-acting NSAID (with PPI if appropriate) or colchicine in low doses, e.g. 500 µg two to four times daily. Joint aspiration plus intra-articular injection of glucocorticosteroid is also a highly effective treatment. Systemic steroids or injection of ACTH are also effective but are recommended only when local injections are impractical, for example polyarticular attacks or monoarticular gout at poorly accessible sites, in patients who do not tolerate or have contraindications to NSAIDs or colchicine. Application of ice-packs to the affected joint is a safe, effective adjunct to pharmacological treatment.

LONG-TERM MANAGEMENT

Once the acute attack of gout has been treated, long-term management aims to lower SUA, allowing MSU crystals to dissolve, thereby preventing further acute attacks, formation of tophi and joint damage. This is best achieved by a combination of non-pharmacological and pharmacological measures, although, as discussed below, the precise indications for urate-lowering drugs remain controversial.

MODIFICATION OF ADVERSE FACTORS INCLUDING LIFESTYLE

Non-pharmacological therapy consists of modifying adverse lifestyle factors. Robust epidemiological evidence supports the independent role of excess alcohol consumption, obesity and dietary animal purine intake in the development of gout. The Health Professionals Follow-Up Study followed 47 150 men prospectively over a 12-year period observing 730 incident cases of gout. The development of gout was independently associated with alcohol consumption (relative risk [RR] 1.17 per 10 g increase in daily intake; 95% confidence interval [CI] 1.11–1.22) [31]. Beer consumption conferred the greatest degree of risk (RR 1.49 per 12-ounce serving per day; 95% CI 1.32–1.70). Consumption of meat (RR 1.41; highest vs. lowest quintile; 95% CI 1.07–1.86) and of seafood (RR 1.51; 95% CI 1.17–1.95) were also independently associated with the development of gout [32]. A graded independent association was seen between body mass index (BMI) and the risk of developing gout (BMI 21–22.9: RR 1.00; BMI 23–24.9: RR 1.31; BMI 25–29.9: RR 1.95; BMI 30–34.9: RR 2.33; BMI > 35: RR 2.97) [33]. Alcohol consumption has been shown to be a trigger of recurrent gout attacks. In an internet-based case-crossover study of 321 attacks of acute gout affecting 197 subjects, acute attacks of gout were associated with the consumption of seven alcoholic drinks within the preceding 48 hours (odds ratio [OR] 2.5; 95% CI 1.1–5.9) [34].

There have been few studies of lifestyle modification for the treatment of gout. In the Health Professionals Follow-Up Study, weight loss reduced the risk of developing gout (RR 0.61; 95% CI 0.40–0.92) [33]. In a pilot study in 13 obese men with symptomatic gout, weight loss as a result of restricted carbohydrate intake and increased proportional intake of protein and unsaturated fat reduced SUA levels and the frequency of acute attacks [35]. Uncontrolled studies demonstrate reduction in SUA following alcohol restriction and weight reduction in patients with gout [36] and following a low-purine diet in hyperuricaemic subjects [37]. Despite acknowledging the paucity of evidence, both the BSR and EULAR recommendations highlight the importance of weight loss and restriction of dietary purines and alcohol (especially beer) in the management of gout [7, 8].

Diuretic therapy is a further modifiable risk factor for some patients with gout. In both the Health Professionals Follow-Up Study (RR 1.77; 95% CI 1.42–2.20) [33] and a case–control study undertaken in the UK General Practice Research Database including 63 105 patients with gout (OR 1.72; 95% CI 1.67–1.76) [1], diuretic use was independently associated with the development of gout. Ongoing diuretic use is a risk factor for symptomatic gout. In the internet-based case-crossover study described above, the occurrence of acute gout was associated with use of any diuretic in the preceding 48 hours (OR 3.6; 95% CI 1.4–9.7) [38]. There have been no studies of diuretic cessation as a treatment strategy for gout. However, both the EULAR and BSR recommendations advise discontinuation of diuretics if possible, but acknowledge that this may not be appropriate in all patients, particularly when the diuretic is prescribed for cardiac failure rather than hypertension [7, 8]. The angiotension II receptor losartan has modest uricosuric properties [39] and hence maybe a suitable alternative to diuretics in some hypertensive patients (discussed further below).

URATE-LOWERING THERAPIES

XANTHINE OXIDASE INHIBITORS

The most commonly used group of drugs used to lower urate and treat gout in the long term are xanthine oxidase inhibitors, principally the non-specific inhibitor allopurinol,

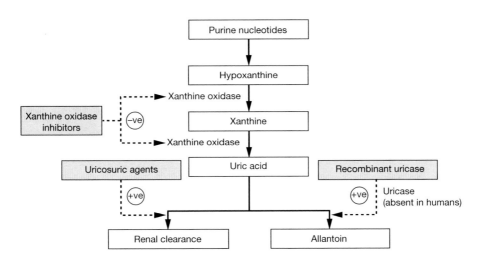

Figure 12.1 Simplified purine metabolism showing sites of action of urate-lowering agents.

which reduces uric acid production (Figure 12.1). Although placebo-controlled RCTs of allopurinol for the treatment of gout are lacking, numerous uncontrolled studies show that allopurinol produces meaningful reductions in SUA. In one open RCT, allopurinol 200 mg daily with colchicine 500 µg twice daily was compared with colchicine 500 µg twice daily alone in 59 patients with gout [40]. SUA reduction was greater in the allopurinol-treated group, although the number of acute attacks of gout was similar in both groups. The EULAR recommendations [7] describe a re-analysis of individual patient data from two uncontrolled studies [41, 42] demonstrating a dose-dependent effect of allopurinol on SUA of the order of reduction of 60 µmol/l (1 mg/dl) for every 100-mg increase in the dose of allopurinol.

Allopurinol is usually well tolerated. Infrequent side-effects include marrow suppression, derangement of liver function and rashes. Rarely, a severe life-threatening hypersensitivity reaction can occur, consisting of rash, fever, worsening renal function, eosinophilia, hepatitis and leucocytosis [43]. Such reactions are more common in patients with existing renal insufficiency. It is therefore frequently recommended that lower doses of allopurinol should be used in patients with renal failure and that dose escalation should be more cautious [7, 8, 44]. Schedules for dosing allopurinol according to creatinine clearance have been proposed (Table 12.2), based upon pharmacological studies which show inverse linear relationships between creatinine clearance and both serum oxypurinol half-life and the serum oxypurinol concentration attained from a long-term daily dose of allopurinol of 300 mg daily [43]. However, there is no firm evidence that such dosing schedules reduce the incidence of hypersensitivity reactions. In a retrospective study of 120 patients with allopurinol-treated primary gout, allopurinol-related adverse events were infrequent (including only one case of allopurinol hypersensitivity syndrome) and similar between patients receiving adjusted and non-adjusted doses [45]. Furthermore, renal dosing of allopurinol may not be sufficient to reduce SUA to target levels. A recent retrospective study of 227 patients found that the target SUA levels were achieved less frequently with adjusted dosing of allopurinol compared with higher-than-recommended doses [46]. Further studies are warranted to establish the safety and efficacy of allopurinol in patients with renal failure.

Oxypurinol and tisopurine (thiopurinol) are alternatives to allopurinol, which both exert their effect on the metabolic pathways leading to uric acid production. Oxypurinol is the active metabolite of allopurinol and has a much longer half-life [41]. The urate-lowering effect of oxypurinol is similar to allopurinol in hyperuricaemic subjects [47] and has been shown to be of benefit in patients with gout [48, 49]. Tisopurine reduces plasma and urine uric acid levels without increasing xanthine or hypoxanthine excretion, suggesting that it exerts its urate-lowering effect at the earlier stages of purine breakdown rather than through xanthine

Table 12.2 Proposed dosing schedule of allopurinol according to creatinine clearance

Creatinine clearance (ml/min)	Maintenance dose of allopurinol
0	100 mg every 3 days
10	100 mg every 2 days
20	100 mg daily
40	150 mg daily
60	200 mg daily
80	250 mg daily
100	300 mg daily
120	350 mg daily
140	400 mg daily

Reprinted from *Am J Med* 1984; 76. Hande K *et al.*, 'Severe allopurinol toxicity: description and guidelines for prevention in patients with renal insufficiency', Copyright (1984)[43] with permission from Elsevier.

oxidase inhibition [50]. However, neither drug is widely available and cross-reactivity with oxypurinol is commonplace in those who have experienced reactions to allopurinol [51].

The treatment of gout in patients who are intolerant of allopurinol can be particularly challenging. Cross-reactivity to other purine xanthine oxidase inhibitors is common. Adverse reactions to allopurinol are more frequent in the presence of renal failure, which also reduces the effectiveness, and increases renal toxicity, of uricosuric agents. Oral desensitization to allopurinol has been described, whereby allopurinol is commenced at a very low dose and then escalated very slowly every few days, increasing up to 100 mg daily over the course of a month (Table 12.3) [52, 53]. A retrospective study of 32 patients who had experienced mild cutaneous reactions with allopurinol reported successful desensitization in 75% [53]. Desensitization, however, is only recommended in patients who have had a mild cutaneous reaction to allopurinol and cannot be treated with other urate-lowering drugs.

Recently, a novel, specific, non-purine xanthine oxidase inhibitor, febuxostat, has been developed. In a multicentre, phase II, double-blind RCT which randomized 153 patients with gout and significant hyperuricaemia, no patients in the placebo group achieved a target SUA level below 6 mg/dl (360 μmol/l) at 28-day follow-up compared with 56%, 76% and 94% of the febuxostat 40 mg, 80 mg and 120 mg groups, respectively [54]. Treatment-related adverse events were similar in all groups. Subsequently, a 52-week multicentre, double-blind RCT randomized 762 subjects with gout and significant hyperuricaemia to allopurinol 300 mg or febuxostat 80 mg or 120 mg once daily [55]. Target SUA levels were reached and sustained over 3 months in 21% of the allopurinol group compared with 53% of the febuxostat 80 mg group and 62% of the 120 mg group. There were no differences in reduction in gout flares or tophus size, or adverse-event rates, including hypersensitivity reactions, between the three groups. These studies suggest that febuxostat is an effective urate-lowering agent. Although target SUA levels were reached more frequently with febuxostat than with allopurinol 300 mg daily, higher doses of allopurinol are frequently used in clinical practice. Also, in this comparative trial a significant proportion (c. 40–50%) of gout patients still did not achieve the therapeutic target on febuxostat 80 or 120 mg. Given the association of allopurinol hypersensitivity with impaired renal function, febuxostat might be of particular use in patients with renal failure. However, both of these RCTs excluded patients with significant renal dysfunction. A study of 31 non-gout subjects with differing degrees of renal function did not find any influence of renal impairment on the pharmacodynamic properties or safety profile of febuxostat 80 mg

Table 12.3 Dose regime for allopurinol desensitization

Daily dose	Days (approximate)
50 μg	1–3
100 μg	4–6
200 μg	7–9
500 μg	10–12
1 mg	13–15
5 mg	16–18
10 mg	19–21
25 mg	22–24
50 mg	25–27
100 mg	28+

For high-risk patients, a modified desensitization protocol, with initial allopurinol doses of 10 μg and 25 μg, and a dosage escalation every 5–10 days or longer, is recommended.

Reprinted from Fam *et al.* [53], *Arthritis Rheum* 2001; 44: 231–8, with permission of Wiley-Liss, Inc., a subsidiary of John Wiley & Sons, Inc.

daily [56]. However, the use of febuxostat in the presence of renal impairment, and the maximum safe doses that can be used to achieve the therapeutic target, requires further evaluation.

URICOSURIC AGENTS

Uricosuric drugs inhibit renal tubular reabsorption of urate at the renal tubular organic anion transporter (OAT) URAT 1 [57] (Figure 12.2), thereby increasing urinary urate excretion (Figure 12.1). Hence, uricosuric drugs are contraindicated in over-excretors of urate or those with a history of urolithiasis. Uricosuric agents such as sulfinpyrazone, probenecid and benzbromarone provide an alternative to xanthine oxidase inhibitors in some patients. Of these, benzbromarone is the more efficient urate-lowering agent. Other drugs, such as losartan and fenofibrate, also have uricosuric properties.

There are few controlled studies of uricosuric agents. Uncontrolled studies demonstrate effective urate-lowering potential of sulfinpyrazone [58, 59] and probenecid [60]. A small number of studies compare the relative efficacy of uricosuric drugs and allopurinol. In one study, SUA reduction was greater with allopurinol 300–600 mg daily than with probenecid 1–2 g daily or sulfinpyrazone 400 mg daily (mean SUA reduction allopurinol 4.6 mg/dl, uricosuric 3.3 mg/dl) [61]. A more recent parallel, open-label study of 86 men with chronic gout allocated over-producers of urate to allopurinol 300 mg daily and under-excretors to either allopurinol 300 mg daily or benzbromarone 100 mg daily [62]. Mean SUA reduction was 5.04 mg/dl with benzbromarone compared with 3.06 mg/dl with allopurinol. A further randomized, non-blinded study compared the efficacy of allopurinol 100–300 mg daily and benzbromarone 100–200 mg daily in 36 patients with chronic gout and impaired renal function (creatinine clearance 20–80 ml/min) [63]. Mean SUA reduction was 5.35 mg/dl with benzbromarone compared with 3.06 mg/dl with allopurinol. Few studies have evaluated the combination of uricosuric drugs with xanthine oxidase inhibitors. An early controlled study of 48 patients with gout found no difference in SUA reduction between combination therapy with allopurinol and sulfinpyrazone, and allopurinol monotherapy [64]. A recent prospective, open study treated 50 patients with gout who had previously received benzbromarone with allopurinol 200–300 mg daily for 2 months, then adding probenecid 1 g daily if target urate levels were not reached [65]. Allopurinol–probenecid combination therapy more frequently achieved target SUA levels and was similar to previous benzbromarone therapy. In summary, probenecid and sulfinpyrazone appear to be less efficacious urate-lowering agents than allopurinol, whereas benzbromarone appears to be more potent. Whereas sulfinpyrazone and

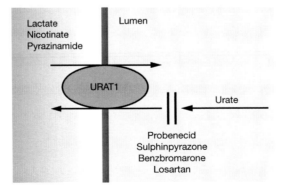

Figure 12.2 Schematic diagram showing transportation of organic anions across the renal tubular membrane and drug action at URAT1.

probenecid are not effective in patients with renal dysfunction [60], benzbromarone appears to remain effective in the presence of mild-to-moderate renal impairment [63]. However, reported cases of severe hepatotoxicity have led to the withdrawal of benzbromarone in some countries [66–73].

Losartan is an angiotensin II receptor antagonist which has mild uricosuric properties [39]. However, RCTs suggest that this effect is not generalizable to other angiotensin II receptor antagonists [74, 75]. Losartan has been shown to reduce hyperuricaemia occurring secondary to thiazide diuretics [76, 77], suggesting that it may be a suitable antihypertensive agent in patients with diuretic-induced gout. In an RCT of 304 patients with hypertension inadequately controlled by thiazides, a modest dose-dependent urate-lowering effect was seen in patients randomized to receive losartan in addition to hydrochlorothiazide compared with those receiving hydrochlorothiazide only [77]. Similarly, fenofibrate, which has modest uricosuric properties not generalizable to other fibrates, is an established treatment for hyperlipidaemia [78, 79]. Both losartan and fenofibrate appear to enhance the effect of traditional urate-lowering drugs. A 3-week open crossover study of 10 men with symptomatic gout on stable doses of allopurinol observed a 19% reduction in SUA following treatment with fenofibrate 200 mg daily, but this reversed on fenofibrate withdrawal [80]. A 2-month uncontrolled study of 52 subjects with gout receiving allopurinol 200 mg twice daily or benzbromarone 50 mg daily added fenofibrate 300 mg daily or losartan 50 mg in subjects with concomitant hypertriglyceridaemia or hypertension, respectively. Small further reductions in mean SUA levels were seen in both the fenofibrate and losartan groups [81]. Fenofibrate–losartan combination therapy may have additional urate-lowering effects [82, 83] but, to date, has not been studied in patients with gout. Fenofibrate and losartan may prove to be useful additional urate-lowering agents in patients with gout with hypertriglyceridaemia or hypertension, respectively, but further studies are required.

Vitamin C is also a novel uricosuric agent. In a 2-month double-blind RCT of 184 normal subjects, a mean reduction in SUA of 0.5 mg/dl was seen with vitamin C 500 mg daily compared with no change with placebo [84]. Further evaluation in patients with gout is required but vitamin C could prove to be a simple, safe adjunct.

URICASE

In man and the great apes, uric acid is the end-product of purine metabolism. Most other animals possess the enzyme urate oxidase (uricase), which converts uric acid to the more soluble allantoin (Figure 12.1). Following a series of parallel mutations in the Eocene period, higher mammals lost the ability to produce uricase, causing susceptibility to hyperuricaemia [85]. Man, however, is the only mammal to spontaneously develop gout. Recombinant uricase (rasburicase) is a potent intravenous urate-lowering therapy (ULT) derived from *Aspergillus flavus*, which is effective for the prevention and treatment of tumour lysis syndrome [86–88]. Initial case reports describe dramatic SUA lowering, cessation of acute attacks and reduction of tophi following the use of rasburicase for refractory gout [89, 90]. A more recent retrospective study reported the use of rasburicase 0.2 mg/kg, given either monthly for 6 months or daily for 5 days, in 10 patients with severe tophaceous gout (refractory to or intolerant of allopurinol) and established renal failure [91]. Rapid SUA lowering was seen in both groups but was not sustained in those receiving daily infusions. Reduction in tophus size was seen in two of five patients who received monthly infusions. The most frequent adverse event was gout flare, although significant hypersensitivity reactions occurred in two patients. A recombinant intravenous uricase coupled to polyethylene glycol (PEGylated uricase) has been developed with the aim of prolonging half-life and reducing antigenicity. In a recent phase I study, 24 patients with refractory gout received a single infusion of PEGylated uricase leading to significant reductions of SUA sustained at 21 days [92]. Acute gout flares were frequent, but no patients experienced a hypersensitivity reaction. Further evaluation of recombinant uricase for the treatment of gout is required.

PRINCIPLES OF URATE-LOWERING THERAPY

INDICATIONS

Several groups have attempted to define indications for the use of ULT. The EULAR [7] and BSR [8] recommendations and US quality of care indicators [44] agree that ULT should be offered to all patients with recurrent acute gout or tophaceous deposits. ULT is also recommended when there are radiographic changes of gouty arthropathy by the EULAR and US groups and in gout patients with renal insufficiency, uric acid stones or diuretic therapy which cannot be stopped by the BSR group. The precise number and frequency of acute attacks that constitutes 'recurrent' acute attacks is not defined by current research evidence, although the BSR and US groups recommend that ULT should be considered if a patient has had two or more attacks in a 1-year period. The EULAR recommendations state that opinion varies between starting ULT after the first attack (when crystal load is smaller) and waiting for attacks to become frequent and troublesome (as some patients experience only relatively infrequent attacks).

TARGET SERUM URATE LEVELS AND TITRATION OF URATE-LOWERING THERAPY

Urate-lowering therapy aims to reduce SUA below the physiological saturation threshold within serum (approximately 380 μmol/l or 6.4 mg/dl) thereby discouraging the formation of new MSU crystals and facilitating dissolution of existing crystals. There is debate as to what the target level of SUA should be. The EULAR recommendations advocate reducing urate levels to below 360 μmol/l (6 mg/dl) [7]. Two studies demonstrate less-frequent acute attacks [93, 94] and greater depletion of MSU crystals in fluid aspirated from asymptomatic knee joints [93] when SUA was lowered to below 360 μmol/l (6 mg/dl). The BSR guidelines advocate a target below 300 μmol/l (5 mg/dl), the median SUA level in men [8]. This level is well below the theoretical physiological saturation threshold of urate, although the evidence for using this cut-off is not clear. The speed ('velocity') of tophus reduction has been shown to be inversely proportional to SUA levels and was greatest at SUA levels below 240 μmol/l (4.0 mg/dl) [95]. Although optimal target SUA levels remain uncertain, it is clear that SUA levels should be reduced to well below the physiological saturation threshold of urate which lies within the 'normal range' of urate in most clinical laboratories. In order to achieve target SUA levels, it is standard practice to commence ULT at low dose and titrate the dose upwards every 2–4 weeks following sequential measurement of the SUA level until the target level is reached [7, 8].

PROPHYLAXIS AGAINST ACUTE ATTACKS

One adverse effect of ULT is the precipitation or worsening of an acute attack of gout following initiation of therapy. It is thought that urate-lowering leads to partial dissolution of MSU crystals, thus facilitating shedding of crystals into the joint space, triggering acute inflammation. A number of strategies are available to reduce this risk. Firstly, the initiation of ULT is usually delayed until at least 1–2 weeks after the acute attack has resolved [8]. However, in some patients acute attacks are so frequent that a therapeutic window of this duration is never available. A second strategy, as discussed above, is to commence ULT at low dose and slowly escalate the dose, bringing about smaller sequential reductions in urate and hence, theoretically, slower dissolution of crystals and less tendency to crystal shedding [7]. Thirdly, anti-inflammatory agents (e.g. colchicine, NSAIDs or glucocorticosteroids) are commonly co-prescribed when initiating ULT until a stable dose is reached. Two randomized double-blind placebo-controlled trials have evaluated the use of colchicine for prophylaxis in this setting. A study of 43 subjects commencing allopurinol demonstrated reduced frequency of acute attacks over a 6-month period in patients randomized to receive colchicine 600μg twice daily compared with placebo [96]. Another randomized trial of 52 patients receiving probenecid 1500 mg daily reported less-frequent acute attacks over 6 months in patients taking colchicine 500μg three times daily compared with placebo [97]. Although diarrhoea was seen more frequently in the patients randomized to colchicine in both studies, diarrhoea may resolve on reducing the frequency of colchicine to once daily [96]. A small, uncontrolled study showed a reduction in synovial fluid white-cell count following treatment with colchicine 1 mg daily for 1 month in the intercritical period [98]. Chronic colchicine use may be complicated by myopathy or myelosuppression, more commonly in the presence of renal failure [99].

There have been few studies of NSAIDs for the prophylaxis of acute attacks and no studies of glucocorticosteroids. One multicentre controlled trial which compared azapropazone, an NSAID with uricosuric properties, 600 mg twice daily with allopurinol found significantly fewer acute attacks of gout with azapropazone, even though urate reduction was similar in both groups [100]. However, toxicity, particularly upper gastrointestinal adverse events, was more common with azapropazone.

DURATION OF URATE-LOWERING THERAPY

Once commenced, ULT is usually considered to be lifelong therapy. Small observational studies report that discontinuation of ULT frequently leads to rapid rebound hyperuricaemia with eventual recurrence of acute attacks and tophi [101, 102], even after protracted maintenance of target SUA levels with successful dissolution of tophi [102]. A larger prospective study found that patients whose average SUA levels were less than 5.05 mg/dl over 5 years of ULT had the longest time to recurrence on cessation (greater than 4 years) [101]. The authors suggest that 5-year intermittent ULT, instead of lifelong ULT, could be offered to patients who achieve good SUA control; however, further intervention studies are required.

SUBOPTIMAL TREATMENT OF GOUT

The management of gout is often relatively straightforward if simple principles for acute and long-term treatment are followed. However, successive surveys have shown that management is often suboptimal. One hospital study found that NSAIDs were frequently used to treat acute gout in patients with impaired renal function [103]. Two UK primary care surveys reported that lifestyle modification advice is offered to less than half of patients [104, 105]. The latter study identified poor concordance with the EULAR management recommendations [105]. ULT was taken by only 30% of patients; 99% being prescribed allopurinol 300 mg daily or less. Target SUA levels were not achieved in the majority of patients even amongst those treated with ULT, suggesting that higher doses may be necessary. However, allopurinol dosing is not appropriately adjusted in 22–26% of patients with impaired renal function [106, 107]. The reasons for suboptimal management are not known but poor education of doctors and patients is likely to be a key factor. Although the advent of new therapeutic options is an exciting development, the management of gout would be greatly enhanced by better application of existing treatments.

NOVEL THERAPEUTIC APPROACHES: BIOLOGICAL AGENTS

Recently, there has been interest in the use of biological agents to treat gout. Anakinra, an interleukin 1 (IL-1) receptor antagonist, has received particular interest. MSU crystals are specifically detected via the NALP3 inflammasone, an intracellular receptor within monocytes. Subsequent activation of the enzyme caspase-1 activates IL-1β, initiating an inflammatory response [108, 109]. IL-1 blockade reduced MSU crystal-induced inflammation in an *in vivo* mouse model [110]. A subsequent open-label pilot study of anakinra in 10 patients with acute gout in whom NSAIDs, colchicine and glucocorticosteroids were ineffective or not tolerated, demonstrated rapid resolution in gout symptoms in all patients with complete resolution of clinical signs of inflammation within 3 days in 90% [110]. Biological agents targeting tumour necrosis factor (TNF)-α are highly efficacious for the treatment of rheumatoid arthritis, juvenile idiopathic arthritis, ankylosing spondylitis and psoriatic arthritis. Levels of TNF-α are elevated in joints affected by gout [111]. Case reports describe the treatment of chronic polyarticular tophaceous gout, refractory to NSAIDs, colchicine and glucocorticosteroids, with infliximab [112] and etanercept [113]. The role of biological agents in the treatment of gout merits further study.

CONCLUSION

Gout is a common cause of inflammatory arthritis for which effective treatment strategies (Table 12.1) and eventual cure exist. However, the treatment of gout is frequently suboptimal [103–107]. Further research should focus on optimizing use of existing treatment strategies in addition to further evaluation of novel agents such as febuxostat, recombinant uricase and biological agents.

REFERENCES

1. Mikuls TR, Farrar JT, Bilker WB *et al*. Gout epidemiology: results from the UK General Practice Research Database, 1990–1999. *Ann Rheum Dis* 2005; 64:267–272.
2. Lawrence RC, Helmick CG, Arnett FC *et al*. Estimates of the prevalence of arthritis and selected musculoskeletal disorders in the United States. *Arthritis Rheum* 1998; 41:778–799.
3. Harris CM, Lloyd DC, Lewis J. The prevalence and prophylaxis of gout in England. *J Clin Epidemiol* 1995; 48:1153–1158.
4. Wallace KL, Riedel AA, Joseph-Ridge N *et al*. Increasing prevalence of gout and hyperuricemia over 10 years among older adults in a managed care population. *J Rheumatol* 2004; 31:1582–1587.
5. Campion EW, Glynn RJ, DeLabry LO. Asymptomatic hyperuricemia. Risks and consequences in the Normative Aging Study. *Am J Med* 1987; 82:421–426.
6. Lin KC, Lin HY, Chou P. The interaction between uric acid level and other risk factors on the development of gout among asymptomatic hyperuricemic men in a prospective study. *J Rheumatol* 2000; 27:1501–1505.
7. Zhang W, Doherty M, Bardin T *et al*. EULAR evidence based recommendations for gout – Part II Management: report of a task force of the Standing Committee for International Clinical Studies Including Therapeutics (ESCISIT). *Ann Rheum Dis* 2006; 65:1312–1324.
8. Jordan KM, Cameron JS, Snaith M *et al*. British Society for Rheumatology and British Health Professionals in Rheumatology guideline for the management of gout. *Rheumatology* (Oxford) 2007; 46:1372–1374.
9. Garcia de la Torre I. A comparative, double-blind, parallel study with tenoxicam vs placebo in acute gouty arthritis. *Investigación Médica Internacional* 1987; 14:92–97.
10. Sutaria S, Katbamna R, Underwood M. Effectiveness of interventions for the treatment of acute and prevention of recurrent gout – a systematic review. *Rheumatology* (Oxford) 2006; 45:1422–1431.
11. Lomen PL, Turner LF, Lamborn KR *et al*. Flurbiprofen in the treatment of acute gout. A comparison with indomethacin. *Am J Med* 1986; 80:134–139.

12. Altman RD, Honig S, Levin JM *et al.* Ketoprofen versus indomethacin in patients with acute gouty arthritis: a multicenter, double blind comparative study. *J Rheumatol* 1988; 15:1422–1426.
13. Smyth CJ, Percy JS. Comparison of indomethacin and phenylbutazone in acute gout. *Ann Rheum Dis* 1973; 32:351–353.
14. Klumb EM, Pinheiro GRC, Ferrari A *et al.* The treatment of acute gout arthritis. Double-blind randomised comparative study between nimesulid and indomethacin. *Rev Brasil Med* 1996; 53:540–546.
15. Sturge RA, Scott JT, Hamilton EB *et al.* Multicentre trial of naproxen and phenylbutazone in acute gout. *Ann Rheum Dis* 1977; 36:80–82.
16. Schumacher HR Jr, Boice JA, Daikh DI *et al.* Randomised double blind trial of etoricoxib and indometacin in treatment of acute gouty arthritis. *BMJ* 2002; 324:1488–1492.
17. Rubin BR, Burton R, Navarra S *et al.* Efficacy and safety profile of treatment with etoricoxib 120 mg once daily compared with indomethacin 50 mg three times daily in acute gout: a randomized controlled trial. *Arthritis Rheum* 2004; 50:598–606.
18. Cheng TT, Lai HM, Chiu CK *et al.* A single-blind, randomized, controlled trial to assess the efficacy and tolerability of rofecoxib, diclofenac sodium, and meloxicam in patients with acute gouty arthritis. *Clin Ther* 2004; 26:399–406.
19. Abbott RD, Brand FN, Kannel WB *et al.* Gout and coronary heart disease: the Framingham Study. *J Clin Epidemiol* 1988; 41:237–242.
20. Cutler T. Plants from the Chelsea Physic Garden. Colchicum autumnale (meadow saffron, autumn crocus). *College Commentary* 2004; 1:38.
21. Schlesinger N, Schumacher R, Catton M *et al.* Colchicine for acute gout. *Cochrane Database Syst Rev* 2006; CD006190.
22. Ahern MJ, Reid C, Gordon TP *et al.* Does colchicine work? The results of the first controlled study in acute gout. *Aust N Z J Med* 1987; 17:301–304.
23. Morris I, Varughese G, Mattingly P. Colchicine in acute gout. *BMJ* 2003; 327:1275–1276.
24. Fernandez C, Noguera R, Gonzalez JA *et al.* Treatment of acute attacks of gout with a small dose of intraarticular triamcinolone acetonide. *J Rheumatol* 1999; 26:2285–2286.
25. Alloway JA, Moriarty MJ, Hoogland YT *et al.* Comparison of triamcinolone acetonide with indomethacin in the treatment of acute gouty arthritis. *J Rheumatol* 1993; 20:111–113.
26. Axelrod D, Preston S. Comparison of parenteral adrenocorticotropic hormone with oral indomethacin in the treatment of acute gout. *Arthritis Rheum* 1988; 31:803–805.
27. Siegel LB, Alloway JA, Nashel DJ. Comparison of adrenocorticotropic hormone and triamcinolone acetonide in the treatment of acute gouty arthritis. *J Rheumatol* 1994; 21:1325–1327.
28. Getting SJ, Christian HC, Flower RJ *et al.* Activation of melanocortin type 3 receptor as a molecular mechanism for adrenocorticotrophic hormone efficacy in gouty arthritis. *Arthritis Rheum* 2002; 46:2765–2775.
29. Groff GD, Franck WA, Raddatz DA. Systemic steroid therapy for acute gout: a clinical trial and review of the literature. *Semin Arthritis Rheum* 1990; 19:329–336.
30. Schlesinger N, Detry MA, Holland BK *et al.* Local ice therapy during bouts of acute gouty arthritis. *J Rheumatol* 2002; 29:331–334.
31. Choi HK, Atkinson K, Karlson EW *et al.* Alcohol intake and risk of incident gout in men: a prospective study. *Lancet* 2004; 363:1277–1281.
32. Choi HK, Atkinson K, Karlson EW *et al.* Purine-rich foods, dairy and protein intake, and the risk of gout in men. *N Engl J Med* 2004; 350:1093–1103.
33. Choi HK, Atkinson K, Karlson EW *et al.* Obesity, weight change, hypertension, diuretic use, and risk of gout in men: the health professionals follow-up study. *Arch Intern Med* 2005; 165:742–748.
34. Zhang Y, Woods R, Chaisson CE *et al.* Alcohol consumption as a trigger of recurrent gout attacks. *Am J Med* 2006; 119:800 e13–8.
35. Dessein PH, Shipton EA, Stanwix AE *et al.* Beneficial effects of weight loss associated with moderate calorie/carbohydrate restriction, and increased proportional intake of protein and unsaturated fat on serum urate and lipoprotein levels in gout: a pilot study. *Ann Rheum Dis* 2000; 59:539–543.
36. Gibson T, Kilbourn K, Horner I *et al.* Mechanism and treatment of hypertriglyceridaemia in gout. *Ann Rheum Dis* 1979; 38:31–35.
37. Kullich W, Ulreich A, Klein G. [Changes in uric acid and blood lipids in patients with asymptomatic hyperuricemia treated with diet therapy in a rehabilitation procedure]. *Rehabilitation* (Stuttg) 1989; 28:134–137.

38. Hunter DJ, York M, Chaisson CE *et al.* Recent diuretic use and the risk of recurrent gout attacks: the online case-crossover gout study. *J Rheumatol* 2006; 33:1341–1345.

39. Nakashima M, Umemura K. The clinical pharmacology of losartan in Japanese subjects and patients. *Blood Press Suppl* 1996; 2:62–66.

40. Gibson T, Rodgers V, Potter C *et al.* Allopurinol treatment and its effect on renal function in gout: a controlled study. *Ann Rheum Dis* 1982; 41:59–65.

41. Rundles RW, Metz EN, Silberman HR. Allopurinol in the treatment of gout. *Ann Intern Med* 1966; 64:229–258.

42. Yu TF. The effect of allopurinol in primary and secondary gout. *Arthritis Rheum* 1965; 8:905–906.

43. Hande KR, Noone RM, Stone WJ. Severe allopurinol toxicity. Description and guidelines for prevention in patients with renal insufficiency. *Am J Med* 1984; 76:47–56.

44. Mikuls TR, MacLean CH, Olivieri J *et al.* Quality of care indicators for gout management. *Arthritis Rheum* 2004; 50:937–943.

45. Vazquez-Mellado J, Morales EM, Pacheco-Tena C *et al.* Relation between adverse events associated with allopurinol and renal function in patients with gout. *Ann Rheum Dis* 2001; 60:981–983.

46. Dalbeth N, Kumar S, Stamp L *et al.* Dose adjustment of allopurinol according to creatinine clearance does not provide adequate control of hyperuricemia in patients with gout. *J Rheumatol* 2006; 33:1646–1650.

47. Walter-Sack I, de Vries JX, Ernst B *et al.* Uric acid lowering effect of oxipurinol sodium in hyperuricemic patients – therapeutic equivalence to allopurinol. *J Rheumatol* 1996; 23:498–501.

48. Earll JM, Saavedra M. Oxipurinol therapy in allopurinol-allergic patients. *Am Fam Physician* 1983; 28:147–148.

49. Rundles RW. Metabolic effects of allopurinol and allo-xanthine. *Ann Rheum Dis* 1966; 25:615–620.

50. Grahame R, Simmonds HA, Cadenhead A *et al.* Metabolic studies of thiopurinol in man and the pig. *Adv Exp Med Biol* 1974; 41:597–605.

51. Lockard O, Jr., Harmon C, Nolph K *et al.* Allergic reaction to allopurinol with cross-reactivity to oxypurinol. *Ann Intern Med* 1976; 85:333–335.

52. Fam AG, Lewtas J, Stein J *et al.* Desensitization to allopurinol in patients with gout and cutaneous reactions. *Am J Med* 1992; 93:299–302.

53. Fam AG, Dunne SM, Iazzetta J *et al.* Efficacy and safety of desensitization to allopurinol following cutaneous reactions. *Arthritis Rheum* 2001; 44:231–238.

54. Becker MA, Schumacher HR Jr, Wortmann RL *et al.* Febuxostat, a novel nonpurine selective inhibitor of xanthine oxidase: a twenty-eight-day, multicenter, phase II, randomized, double-blind, placebo-controlled, dose-response clinical trial examining safety and efficacy in patients with gout. *Arthritis Rheum* 2005; 52:916–923.

55. Becker MA, Schumacher HR, Wortmann RL *et al.* Febuxostat compared with allopurinol in patients with hyperuricemia and gout. *N Engl J Med* 2005; 353:2450–2456.

56. Mayer MD, Khosravan R, Vernillet L *et al.* Pharmacokinetics and pharmacodynamics of febuxostat, a new non-purine selective inhibitor of xanthine oxidase in subjects with renal impairment. *Am J Ther* 2005; 12:22–34.

57. Enomoto A, Kimura H, Chairoungdua A *et al.* Molecular identification of a renal urate anion exchanger that regulates blood urate levels. *Nature* 2002; 417:447–452.

58. Kuzell WC, Glover RP, Gibbs JO *et al.* Effect of sulfinpyrazone on serum uric acid in gout. A long-term study. *Geriatrics* 1964; 19:894–909.

59. Persellin RH, Schmid FR. The use of sulfinpyrazone in the treatment of gout. *JAMA* 1961; 175:971–975.

60. Bartels EC, Matossian GS. Gout: six-year follow-up on probenecid (benemid) therapy. *Arthritis Rheum* 1959; 2:193–202.

61. Scott JT. Comparison of allopurinol and probenecid. *Ann Rheum Dis* 1966; 25:623–626.

62. Perez-Ruiz F, Alonso-Ruiz A, Calabozo M *et al.* Efficacy of allopurinol and benzbromarone for the control of hyperuricaemia. A pathogenic approach to the treatment of primary chronic gout. *Ann Rheum Dis* 1998; 57:545–549.

63. Perez-Ruiz F, Calabozo M, Fernandez-Lopez MJ *et al.* Treatment of chronic gout in patients with renal function impairment. An open, randomized, actively controlled study. *J Clin Rheumatol* 1999; 5:49–55.

64. Kuzell WC, Seebach LM, Glover RP *et al.* Treatment of gout with allopurinol and sulphinpyrazone in combination and with allopurinol alone. *Ann Rheum Dis* 1966; 25:634–642.

65. Reinders MK, van Roon EN, Houtman PM *et al.* Biochemical effectiveness of allopurinol and allopurinol-probenecid in previously benzbromarone-treated gout patients. *Clin Rheumatol* 2007; 26:1459–1465.

66. Babany G, Larrey D, Pessayre D et al. Chronic active hepatitis caused by benzarone. J Hepatol 1987; 5:332–335.
67. Nakad A, Azzouzi K, Gerbaux A et al. [Hepatitis caused by benzarone: a second case]. Gastroenterol Clin Biol 1990; 14:782–784.
68. Sepulchre D, De Plaen JL, Geubel AP. [Drug-induced hepatitis due to benzarone (Fragivix): apropos of a clinical case report]. Acta Gastroenterol Belg 1990; 53:499–503.
69. van der Klauw MM, Houtman PM, Stricker BH et al. Hepatic injury caused by benzbromarone. J Hepatol 1994; 20:376–379.
70. Gehenot M, Horsmans Y, Rahier J et al. Subfulminant hepatitis requiring liver transplantation after benzarone administration. J Hepatol 1994; 20:842.
71. Wagayama H, Shiraki K, Sugimoto K et al. Fatal fulminant hepatic failure associated with benzbromarone. J Hepatol 2000; 32:874.
72. Suzuki T, Kimura M, Shinoda M et al. [A case of fulminant hepatitis, possibly caused by benzbromarone]. Nippon Shokakibyo Gakkai Zasshi 2001; 98:421–425.
73. Arai M, Yokosuka O, Fujiwara K et al. Fulminant hepatic failure associated with benzbromarone treatment: a case report. J Gastroenterol Hepatol 2002; 17:625–626.
74. Wurzner G, Gerster JC, Chiolero A et al. Comparative effects of losartan and irbesartan on serum uric acid in hypertensive patients with hyperuricaemia and gout. J Hypertens 2001; 19:1855–1860.
75. Puig JG, Mateos F, Buno A et al. Effect of eprosartan and losartan on uric acid metabolism in patients with essential hypertension. J Hypertens 1999; 17:1033–1039.
76. Shahinfar S, Simpson RL, Carides AD et al. Safety of losartan in hypertensive patients with thiazide-induced hyperuricemia. Kidney Int 1999; 56:1879–1885.
77. Soffer BA, Wright JT Jr, Pratt JH et al. Effects of losartan on a background of hydrochlorothiazide in patients with hypertension. Hypertension 1995; 26:112–117.
78. Desager JP, Hulhoven R, Harvengt C. Uricosuric effect of fenofibrate in healthy volunteers. J Clin Pharmacol 1980; 20:560–564.
79. Bastow MD, Durrington PN, Ishola M. Hypertriglyceridemia and hyperuricemia: effects of two fibric acid derivatives (bezafibrate and fenofibrate) in a double-blind, placebo-controlled trial. Metabolism 1988; 37:217–220.
80. Feher MD, Hepburn AL, Hogarth MB et al. Fenofibrate enhances urate reduction in men treated with allopurinol for hyperuricaemia and gout. Rheumatology (Oxford) 2003; 42:321–325.
81. Takahashi S, Moriwaki Y, Yamamoto T et al. Effects of combination treatment using anti-hyperuricaemic agents with fenofibrate and/or losartan on uric acid metabolism. Ann Rheum Dis 2003; 62:572–575.
82. Ka T, Inokuchi T, Tsutsumi Z et al. Effects of a fenofibrate/losartan combination on the plasma concentration and urinary excretion of purine bases. Int J Clin Pharmacol Ther 2006; 44:22–26.
83. Elisaf M, Tsimichodimos V, Bairaktari E et al. Effect of micronized fenofibrate and losartan combination on uric acid metabolism in hypertensive patients with hyperuricemia. J Cardiovasc Pharmacol 1999; 34:60–63.
84. Huang HY, Appel LJ, Choi MJ et al. The effects of vitamin C supplementation on serum concentrations of uric acid: results of a randomized controlled trial. Arthritis Rheum 2005; 52:1843–1847.
85. Oda M, Satta Y, Takenaka O et al. Loss of urate oxidase activity in hominoids and its evolutionary implications. Mol Biol Evol 2002; 19:640–653.
86. Coiffier B, Mounier N, Bologna S et al. Efficacy and safety of rasburicase (recombinant urate oxidase) for the prevention and treatment of hyperuricemia during induction chemotherapy of aggressive non-Hodgkin's lymphoma: results of the GRAAL1 (Groupe d'Etude des Lymphomes de l'Adulte Trial on Rasburicase Activity in Adult Lymphoma) study. J Clin Oncol 2003; 21:4402–4406.
87. Goldman SC, Holcenberg JS, Finklestein JZ et al. A randomized comparison between rasburicase and allopurinol in children with lymphoma or leukemia at high risk for tumor lysis. Blood 2001; 97:2998–3003.
88. Jeha S, Kantarjian H, Irwin D et al. Efficacy and safety of rasburicase, a recombinant urate oxidase (Elitek), in the management of malignancy-associated hyperuricemia in pediatric and adult patients: final results of a multicenter compassionate use trial. Leukemia 2005; 19:34–38.
89. Vogt B. Urate oxidase (rasburicase) for treatment of severe tophaceous gout. Nephrol Dial Transplant 2005; 20:431–433.
90. Moolenburgh JD, Reinders MK, Jansen TL. Rasburicase treatment in severe tophaceous gout: a novel therapeutic option. Clin Rheumatol 2006; 25:749–752.

91. Richette P, Briere C, Hoenen-Clavert V *et al.* Rasburicase for tophaceous gout not treatable with allopurinol: an exploratory study. *J Rheumatol* 2007; 34:2093–2098.
92. Sundy JS, Ganson NJ, Kelly SJ *et al.* Pharmacokinetics and pharmacodynamics of intravenous PEGylated recombinant mammalian urate oxidase in patients with refractory gout. *Arthritis Rheum* 2007; 56:1021–1028.
93. Li-Yu J, Clayburne G, Sieck M *et al.* Treatment of chronic gout. Can we determine when urate stores are depleted enough to prevent attacks of gout? *J Rheumatol* 2001; 28:577–580.
94. Shoji A, Yamanaka H, Kamatani N. A retrospective study of the relationship between serum urate level and recurrent attacks of gouty arthritis: evidence for reduction of recurrent gouty arthritis with antihyperuricemic therapy. *Arthritis Care Res* 2004; 51:321–325.
95. Perez -Ruiz F, Calabozo M, Pijoan JI *et al.* Effect of urate-lowering therapy on the velocity of size reduction of tophi in chronic gout. *Arthritis Care Res* 2002; 47:356–360.
96. Borstad GC, Bryant LR, Abel MP *et al.* Colchicine for prophylaxis of acute flares when initiating allopurinol for chronic gouty arthritis. *J Rheumatol* 2004; 31:2429–2432.
97. Paulus HE, Schlosstein LH, Godfrey RG *et al.* Prophylactic colchicine therapy of intercritical gout. A placebo-controlled study of probenecid-treated patients. *Arthritis Rheum* 1974; 17:609–614.
98. Pascual E, Castellano JA. Treatment with colchicine decreases white cell counts in synovial fluid of asymptomatic knees that contain monosodium urate crystals. *J Rheumatol* 1992; 19:600–603.
99. Wallace SL, Singer JZ, Duncan GJ *et al.* Renal function predicts colchicine toxicity: guidelines for the prophylactic use of colchicine in gout. *J Rheumatol* 1991; 18:264–269.
100. Templeton JS. Azapropazone or allopurinol in the treatment of chronic gout and/or hyperuricaemia. A preliminary report. *Br J Clin Pract* 1982; 36:353–358.
101. Perez-Ruiz F, Atxotegi J, Hernando I *et al.* Using serum urate levels to determine the period free of gouty symptoms after withdrawal of long-term urate-lowering therapy: a prospective study. *Arthritis Rheum* 2006; 55:786–790.
102. van Lieshout-Zuidema MF, Breedveld FC. Withdrawal of longterm antihyperuricemic therapy in tophaceous gout. *J Rheumatol* 1993; 20:1383–1385.
103. Petersel D, Schlesinger N. Treatment of acute gout in hospitalized patients. *J Rheumatol* 2007; 34:1566–1568.
104. Pal B, Foxall M, Dysart T *et al.* How is gout managed in primary care? A review of current practice and proposed guidelines. *Clin Rheumatol* 2000; 19:21–25.
105. Roddy E, Zhang W, Doherty M. Concordance of the management of chronic gout in a UK primary-care population with the EULAR gout recommendations. *Ann Rheum Dis* 2007; 66:1311–1315.
106. Mikuls TR, Farrar JT, Bilker WB *et al.* Suboptimal physician adherence to quality indicators for the management of gout and asymptomatic hyperuricaemia: results from the UK General Practice Research Database (GPRD). *Rheumatology* (Oxford) 2005; 44:1038–1042.
107. Singh JA, Hodges JS, Toscano JP *et al.* Quality of care for gout in the US needs improvement. *Arthritis Rheum* 2007; 57:822–829.
108. Martinon F, Petrilli V, Mayor A *et al.* Gout-associated uric acid crystals activate the NALP3 inflammasome. *Nature* 2006; 440:237–241.
109. Petrilli V, Martinon F. The inflammasome, autoinflammatory diseases, and gout. *Joint Bone Spine* 2007; 74:571–576.
110. So A, De Smedt T, Revaz S *et al.* A pilot study of IL-1 inhibition by anakinra in acute gout. *Arthritis Res Ther* 2007; 9:R28.
111. Yagnik DR, Hillyer P, Marshall D *et al.* Noninflammatory phagocytosis of monosodium urate monohydrate crystals by mouse macrophages. Implications for the control of joint inflammation in gout. *Arthritis Rheum* 2000; 43:1779–1789.
112. Fiehn C, Zeier M. Successful treatment of chronic tophaceous gout with infliximab (Remicade). *Rheumatol Int* 2006; 26:274–276.
113. Tausche AK, Richter K, Grassler A *et al.* Severe gouty arthritis refractory to anti-inflammatory drugs: treatment with anti-tumour necrosis factor alpha as a new therapeutic option. *Ann Rheum Dis* 2004; 63:1351–1352.

13

Osteoporosis

Ira Pande

INTRODUCTION

Osteoporosis is defined as a skeletal disorder characterized by decreased bone mass and microarchitectural deterioration of bone tissue, with a consequent increase in bone fragility and susceptibility to fracture [1]. The most common consequences of osteoporosis are fractures of the spine, hip, wrist and proximal humerus. Although the diagnosis of the disease relies on the quantitative assessment of bone mineral density (BMD), which is a major determinant of bone strength, the clinical significance of osteoporosis lies in fractures. Hence, osteoporosis can be detected by BMD measurement or diagnosed by the presence of osteoporosis-related fractures. The lifetime probability of a woman at the menopause suffering a fracture at any site exceeds her risk of breast cancer. It is widely recognized that osteoporosis-related morbidity is associated with significant medical and social consequences. The major source of morbidity and mortality from osteoporosis is attributed to hip fractures, with excess mortality as high as 20% in the first year. As a result, therapies that effectively prevent fractures would have a major impact on morbidity and a smaller but important impact on mortality related to osteoporosis. Currently, two classes of drugs are available for the prevention and treatment of osteoporosis: anabolic therapies, directed at increasing bone formation, and antiresorptive agents, which decrease bone turnover.

The principle of evidence-based medicine encourages clinicians to use the best available information when making decisions regarding drug management in a given situation. Randomized controlled clinical trials, systematic reviews and meta-analyses provide the highest quality of evidence. This chapter reviews drugs currently available for the management of osteoporosis, presents an update of ongoing drug trials and reviews new developments in this field that are likely to impact on how we manage our patients with osteoporosis in the future. The analysis of evidence is primarily based on recently published systematic reviews of randomized trials and or meta-analyses.

THE HORMONE REPLACEMENT THERAPY DEBATE

The risk of osteoporosis and fractures increases with age and is greater in post-menopausal women than in men of a similar age. Women lose bone rapidly following the menopause, with slower bone loss continuing into old age. The menopause is, therefore, a major risk factor for osteoporosis and fractures in women. Many studies have shown that hormone replacement therapy (HRT) is effective in reducing bone turnover, increasing bone density and reducing risk of fractures at all sites, i.e. vertebral and non-vertebral, including hip fractures. The landmark Women's Health Initiative (WHI) study [2] compared the effects of continuous combined oestrogen–progestogen with placebo in 16 608 post-menopausal women aged 50–80 years over a 5-year period. There was a significant reduction in risk of all fractures (hazard ratio [HR] 0.76, 95% confidence interval [CI] 0.69–0.85), including vertebral (HR 0.66, 95% CI 0.44–0.98) and hip (HR 0.66, 95% CI 0.45–0.98) (Table 13.1). This equates to a 34% reduction in vertebral and hip fractures and 23% reduction in other osteoporotic fractures. Meta-analysis of prospective studies published around the same time [3] also supported a protective effect of HRT against both non-vertebral and vertebral fractures. However, evidence indicates that there is attenuation of the beneficial effects of HRT soon after treatment is discontinued and the protective effect against fracture is lost 5 years or so after stopping treatment [4, 5]. Since a woman's greatest risk of fracture is later in life, use of HRT at the time of the menopause is unlikely to have a significant impact decades later. HRT also has additional extraskeletal benefits. The most important is towards oestrogen deficiency symptoms, such as hot flushes, for which it remains the drug of choice. Therefore, until recently, HRT was the gold-standard drug of choice for the prevention and treatment of post-menopausal osteoporosis.

However, evidence from prospective studies has, in recent years, changed our perceptions about some of the extraskeletal benefits of long-term HRT [6] and altered our views on the role of HRT in osteoporosis. Effects of HRT on heart disease came from the Heart Estrogen Replacement Study [7]. This was a secondary prevention trial of HRT in women with established cardiovascular disease. To the surprise of many, women on HRT had excess death related to coronary heart disease (CHD). Other adverse events related to HRT included the well-established increased risk of breast cancer by 26% and excess venous thrombo-embolism. The WHI study had also shown a 29% increase in CHD and 41% increase in stroke in women on HRT. The Million Women Study (MWS), a large UK observational study, and the results from the General Practice Research Database (GPRD) have more recently reported their findings of increased risk of endometrial and breast cancer [8, 9] associated with various forms of HRT. In light of these recent publications, in most women for whom bone protective therapy is indicated risks with long-term use of HRT far outweigh the potential benefits. Consequently, in the majority of women, HRT is no longer recommended for either the prevention or treatment of osteoporosis. Its use is currently restricted to relieve debilitating climacteric symptoms in perimenopausal women in whom

Table 13.1 Fracture risk reduction in women with post-menopausal osteoporosis: evidence from clinical trials

Drug	Vertebral	Non-vertebral	Hip
Hormone replacement therapy	✓	✓	✓
Raloxifene	✓	NA	NA
Etidronate	✓	NA	NA
Alendronate	✓	✓	✓
Risedronate	✓	✓	✓
Ibandronate	✓	NA	NA
Zoledronate	✓	✓	✓
Calcitonin	✓	NA	NT
Strontium	✓	✓	✓
Parathyroid	✓	✓	✓
Testosterone	NA	NT	NT
Calcium + vitamin D	NA	✓	✓
Vitamin D	NA	NA	NA

NA, no effect demonstrated; NT, not tested.

HRT will additionally reduce the rate of bone loss associated with the menopause. Even in this situation, it is considered good practice to use HRT at the lowest effective dose for the shortest possible time, and to review the need to continue treatment at least annually.

WHAT ABOUT SELECTIVE OESTROGEN RECEPTOR MODULATORS?

Selective oestrogen receptor modulators (SERMs) are non-hormonal agents that bind with high affinity to oestrogen receptor and exhibit oestrogen agonist effects on bone and oestrogen antagonistic effects on the endometrium and breast. The concept of SERMs was triggered by observing reduced rate of bone loss in women on tamoxifen. Raloxifene (60 mg/day) is the only SERM available for the prevention and treatment of post-menopausal osteoporosis. Effects of the drug on fracture risk reduction come primarily from the 3-year Multiple Outcome of Raloxifene Evaluation (MORE) trial, which enrolled 7705 women [10]. This showed a positive effect of raloxifene on vertebral fractures (RR 0.60 [95% CI 0.50–0.70]) with little effect on non-vertebral fractures (0.92 [95% CI 0.79–1.07]). A meta-analysis of seven published and unpublished randomized control trials that estimated the effect of raloxifene on bone density showed significant increase in BMD at the lumbar spine, combined hip and total body at all years examined, although larger effects on bone density were after 2 rather than 1 year of treatment with raloxifene [11]. Only two studies have evaluated the impact of raloxifene on fractures [10, 12]. The size of these trials and their results are very disparate, explaining why fracture results across the two trials could not be pooled. The meta-analysis, therefore, could not support any significant effects of raloxifene on non-vertebral fractures and, in particular, hip fractures (Table 13.1). This lack of efficacy meant raloxifene was effective only for vertebral fractures, and this fared badly in health economic analyses performed by the National Institute for Health and Clinical Excellence (NICE).

Raloxifene is associated with some oestrogen antagonist effects outside the skeleton. Adverse effects associated with raloxifene therapy include significant hot flushes (RR 1.46 [95% CI 1.23–1.74]) and deep venous thrombosis (RR 3.51 [95% CI 1.44, 8.56]); there is no increased risk of cardiovascular disease. The adverse events were initially reported in the MORE study and later its placebo-controlled 4-year follow-up (Continuing Outcomes Relevant to Evista [CORE]) study [13].

More recently, raloxifene has been associated with a sustained and significant decrease in the risk of breast cancer, which has been subsequently confirmed in two large cohorts, including the STAR (Study of Tamoxifen and Raloxifene) study, which showed similar breast cancer rates with raloxifene and tamoxifen in high-risk populations [14]. This has led to a new licence indication in the USA. The RUTH (Raloxifene Use for the Heart) study, performed in post-menopausal women at high risk of cardiovascular disease [15] showed no effect of raloxifene on CHD and stroke [16].

Raloxifene, therefore, has an overall favourable risk–benefit ratio and is best suited for the post-menopausal woman who is at high risk of vertebral fracture but does not have any vasomotor menopausal symptoms. It is contraindicated in women with known, or at high risk of, venous thromboembolism. Data on breast cancer reduction has the potential to make a major impact on NICE's health economic modelling, which may increase the use of this drug.

Third-generation SERMs currently in clinical development include lansofoxifene, bazedoxifene and arzoxifene. Arzoxifene is currently undergoing a phase III clinical trial.

BISPHOSPHONATES

Bisphosphonates (BPs) are naturally occurring stable analogues of pyrophosphates. The mechanism of action of these drugs is to inhibit bone resorption through their effects on osteoclast function: reduce their recruitment and activity and increase apoptosis. BPs are poorly absorbed (1–3% of the dose ingested). Food, calcium, iron, coffee, tea and orange juice all impair absorption. Clearance from plasma is quick, with about 50% excreted in urine and the remaining 50% avidly taken up by bone on active sites of bone resorption. Their half-life in bone is very prolonged. A variety of BPs have been synthesized, the potency of which depends on the length and structure of the side chain. BPs currently available for use in the management of osteoporosis include etidronate, alendronate, risedronate, ibandronate and zoledronate. All except etidronate belong to the potent second-generation amino-BPs (the side chain has an amino terminal). Ibandronate and zoledronate are the only two BPs currently available for intravenous use.

Etidronate belongs to the first-generation BPs and is the least potent of all currently available BPs for the management of osteoporosis. A Cochrane systematic review [17] looked at a total of 1248 patients from 11 studies and showed significant reductions in risk of vertebral fracture in secondary prevention trials (RR 0.53, 95% CI 0.32–0.87) at the recommended dose of 400 mg per day. No significant risk reductions were seen for non-vertebral, hip or wrist fractures, regardless of whether etidronate was used for primary or secondary prevention (Table 13.1). The level of evidence for all outcomes was therefore classified as 'silver'. Amongst the BPs, etidronate no longer remains the drug of choice for the treatment of osteoporosis.

Alendronate 70 mg once weekly and risedronate 35 mg once weekly are the most commonly used BPs. The Fracture Intervention Trial (FIT) [18], using alendronate (10 mg daily), was the first of the very large clinical trials which subsequently shaped future practice and trial design for other bone agents. In the FIT study, alendronate was shown to reduce the incidence of vertebral, wrist and hip fracture by approximately half in women with prevalent vertebral fracture. In women without prevalent fracture, there was no significant decrease in clinical fractures, although one-third of women who had osteoporosis at the hip (BMD t-score less than –2.5 SD) showed significant decrease in fracture risk. The recent Cochrane review analysed 11 trials representing 12 068 women on alendronate daily or weekly [19]. For vertebral fractures, a significant 45% RRR (relative risk reduction) was found for both primary and secondary prevention. For non-vertebral fractures, RRR was significant for secondary prevention (23%) but not for primary prevention. Similarly, a significant 53% RRR was found for secondary prevention of hip fractures but not for primary prevention. The only significance found for wrist fractures was in secondary prevention (50% RRR) (Table 13.1).

Risedronate 5 mg daily has been shown in women with prevalent vertebral fractures to reduce the incidence of vertebral and non-vertebral fractures by 40–50% and 30–36%, respectively [20, 21]. In a large population of elderly women, risedronate significantly decreased the risk of hip fractures (30%). This effect was greater in women with osteoporosis [22]. The recently published Cochrane systematic review analysed seven trials representing 14 409 women on risedronate (daily/weekly) [23]. Risk estimates for primary prevention were available only for vertebral and non-vertebral fractures and showed no statistically significant effect of the drug on fractures. For secondary prevention, a significant reduction in vertebral (39%), non-vertebral fractures (20%) and hip fractures (26%) was found (Table 13.1). The level of evidence, therefore, for both alendronate and risedronate is 'gold' in secondary prevention of osteoporotic fractures and 'silver' for primary prevention.

Although alendronate and risedronate represent a huge advance in our management of this condition, therapy with this class of drugs is not without problems. Firstly, the drugs are poorly absorbed from the gut and may cause gut dyspepsia and oesophagitis. As a consequence, they have to be taken fasting with large amounts of water and this impairs compliance. Soon after their launch, both alendronate and risedronate were introduced as weekly preparations (70 mg alendronate, 35 mg risedronate), which improved patient convenience but only marginally improved compliance to 50% at 1 year.

Modification to the basic bisphosphonate structure increased potency of the newer BPs (ibandronate, zoledronate) by increasing its binding to hydroxyapatite, thus prolonging its retention in bone. This has led to less frequent dosing and administration via intravenous route. Ibandronate given orally at a daily dose of 2.5 mg has been shown to reduce the risk of vertebral fracture by 50–60%. Its effect on non-vertebral fracture, however, has only been demonstrated in a post hoc analysis of women with osteoporosis (baseline t score below –3 SD) [24, 25] (Table 13.1). Studies with ibandronate have shown that intermittent administration, where the drug was given every 3 months, had the same effect on BMD and bone turnover markers as the daily dose [26, 27]. This trial has led to the introduction of a once-monthly 150-mg oral dose and still further development of a 3-mg intravenous bolus injection every 3 months. Introduction of monthly oral and 3-monthly intravenous ibandronate is based on non-inferiority trials whereby the new dosing schedules are equivalent or superior to daily ibandronate in increasing BMD and decreasing bone turnover markers. This has, therefore, become a very attractive option for patients who are intolerant to oral BPs or in whom oral BPs are contraindicated. It is equally attractive for patients on polypharmacy or in whom compliance is an issue.

The latest addition to the BPs is zoledronic acid. Based on a large phase III trial in over 7500 post-menopausal women, a yearly infusion of zoledronate 5 mg over 3 years has been found to significantly reduce the risk of all fractures: vertebral fractures by 75% (RR 0.25, 95% CI 0.64–0.87), hip fracture by 40% (RR 0.60, 95% CI 0.43–0.85) and non-vertebral fractures by 25% (RR 0.75, 95% CI 0.64–0.87) [28, 29] (Table 13.1). A subsequent study has since shown zoledronate to decrease the risk of fracture and its attendant mortality when given shortly after an incident hip fracture [30]. This further offers the potential of improved compliance as well as convenience for the patient.

Overall, intravenous BPs are safe. However, they have been associated with acute influenza-like syndrome within the first 72 hours after administration. This presents as fever, bone and muscle pain that improves or disappears with subsequent infusions. The underlying mechanism has been identified as being due to accumulation of mevolonate metabolites caused by inhibition of a key enzyme (farnesyl diphosphate synthase), which in turn activates gamma delta T cells, leading to an acute phase reaction. In general, symptoms are mild, transient, improve with subsequent courses and can be overcome with prophylactic paracetamol or non-steroidal anti-inflammatory agents. Trials have shown no systematic influence of intravenous BPs on renal function, although caution needs to be exerted if used in known severe renal impairment. The complication that has been associated with great publicity is the potential risk of oversuppressing bone turnover resulting in osteonecrosis of the jaw (ONJ). Although the majority of reported cases of ONJ have occurred in cancer patients receiving intravenous zoledronate and pamidronate (at higher cumulative doses than used for osteoporosis), some osteoporosis patients receiving oral BPs have also developed the condition [31, 32]. The incidence of ONJ in osteoporotic patients treated with oral and intravenous BP appears to be extremely low (1/100 000 cases), with the most common triggering factor being dental extraction [33].

All BPs have, therefore, been shown to reduce the risk of vertebral fractures (Table 13.1). Some have also been shown to reduce the risk of non-vertebral fractures, in some cases specifically hip fractures. The development of intravenous preparations and less-frequent dosage has increased the range of options available to patients and doctors to maximize efficacy and increase compliance. It will be interesting to see the relative position of the BPs in the coming years with the introduction of newer preparations and routes of administration.

CALCITONIN – DOES IT HAVE A ROLE?

Calcitonin is an endogenous polypeptide hormone that inhibits bone resorption by osteoclasts [34]. Salmon calcitonin is approximately 40–50 times more potent than human calcitonin and has hence been used in the majority of randomized controlled trials (RCTs). It is available as an injection to be administered subcutaneously and as an intranasal formulation. The latter provides 25–50% of the biological activity of the parenterally administered dose.

The largest study (PROOF; Prevent Recurrence of Osteoporotic Fractures) that assessed bone density and fracture risk in 1255 post-menopausal women with a mean age of 68 years used salmon calcitonin in three doses (100 IU, 200 IU, 400 IU) and compared it with placebo over a 5-year period [35]. Clinical vertebral fracture risk was reduced (RR 0.79, 95% CI 0.62–1.00); however, reduction in risk of non-vertebral fractures did not reach statistical significance (RR 0.80, 95% CI 0.59–1.09). There was a very high rate of dropout (59.3%) making the reliability of this study's result less secure.

The meta-analysis of 30 RCTs published soon after confirmed favourable effects on vertebral fracture risk reduction (RR 0.46, 95% CI 0.25–0.87) but non-significant RR of 0.52 (95% CI 0.22–1.23) for non-vertebral fractures [36] (Table 13.1). Of the 30 published RCTs, only four trials ($n = 1404$) that reported results for vertebral and non-vertebral fractures could be used for purposes of the above meta-analysis. There was large variability in results between the three small trials and the fourth larger trial (PROOF), with the large effect size being driven by the three smaller trials, with sample size of 45–164. The meta-analysis on the effects of calcitonin on bone density showed increases in bone density at the lumbar spine and forearm with a weighted mean difference (WMD) of 3.74 (95% CI 2.04–5.43) and 3.02 (95% CI 0.98–5.07), respectively, but not at the femoral neck. The true effect may be smaller than the pooled estimate because of the heterogeneity amongst studies with respect to sample size, calcitonin dose, route of administration and primary end-points of the studies. The pooled estimates of calcitonin's effect on BMD are somewhat lower than those for oral BPs. Given that nasal calcitonin is the more widely used preparation, has variable bioavailability and may have fewer effects than the parenteral formulation, there is considerable uncertainty concerning effects of calcitonin on bone density. The trials were poor in their reporting of adverse events and, hence, difficult to interpret.

In conclusion, although BMD increase at the lumbar spine may be modest, the questionable impact on vertebral fractures, equivocal effect on non-vertebral fractures, the drawbacks of repeated injections and the high cost of nasal formulation preclude the use of calcitonin as first-line treatment for osteoporosis. It may, however, have a role for acute pain following a spinal fracture related to its analgesic properties, which is independent of its effect on osteoclastic resorption.

STRONTIUM: IS IT A DUAL-ACTING BONE AGENT?

Strontium (Sr) ranelate is composed of two atoms of stable strontium combined with ranelic acid, which acts as carrier and dissociates after ingestion. Unlike other drugs used in the management of osteoporosis, Sr has a dual effect on bone remodelling. It has the ability to stimulate bone formation by osteoblasts, a property shared with bone-forming agents, and can inhibit bone resorption by osteoclasts, as do antiresorptive medications. The precise molecular mechanism is elusive, but, as Sr is a divalent cation, closely resembling calcium in its atomic and ionic properties, it has been hypothesized that Sr could act as an agonist of the extracellular calcium-sensing receptor that is expressed by osteoblasts in all stages of their development and could form the basis of the known anabolic effects of calcium in bone [37, 38].

One of the key elements in the cross-talk between osteoblasts and osteoclasts is the receptor activator of NF-kappaB (RANK) ligand (RANKL) and osteoprotegerin (OPG) system. The OPG–RANKL ratio is decisive for bone resorption, and a decrease in the ratio has been described in osteoporosis associated with the menopause, glucocorticosteroid use and inflammatory diseases (e.g. rheumatoid and hormone therapy for breast and prostate cancer). Strontium enhances OPG expression and downregulates RANKL expression in rats [39]. Apart from possible interference with the OPG–RANKL system, Sr interferes directly with osteoclasts by inhibiting cell differentiation and enhancing apoptosis [40, 41]. As calcium receptor (CaR) is involved in both osteoclast differentiation and apoptosis, strontium effects on osteoclast may also be CaR mediated. *In vivo* experiments in animals show increased markers of bone formation, decreased markers of bone resorption, increased bone diameter, enhanced bone mass on dual X-ray absorptiometry (DXA) and improved microarchitecture assessed by histomorphometry [42, 43].

The efficacy of Sr has been assessed in two large multicentre, randomized, double-blind, placebo-controlled trials. The Spinal Osteoporosis Therapeutic Intervention (SOTI) trial studied its effects on the risk of vertebral fracture in 1649 osteoporotic post-menopausal women aged, on average, 70 years [44]. The Treatment of Peripheral Osteoporosis (TROPOS) trial studied the effects on the risk of non-vertebral fractures in 5091 osteoporotic post-menopausal women aged 74 years (or 70 years with one risk factor for fracture) [45]. Sr reduces the risk of new vertebral fracture by 49% at 1 year, 41% at 3 years and 33% over 4 years based on intent-to-treat analysis. Non-vertebral fracture risk was reduced by an average of 15% throughout the 5-year study (RR 0.85, 95% CI 0.73–0.99). A subsequent subgroup analysis on 1977 women aged over 74 years at high risk of hip fracture revealed reduction in risk of hip fracture by 36% (RR 0.64, 95% CI 0.41–0.99) [46]. Although these results were obtained in a post hoc analysis, it is worth remembering that no other trial has been conducted so far versus placebo during 5 years with non-vertebral fracture incidence as an end-point. A preplanned pooling of data from both SOTI and TROPOS trials has demonstrated significant treatment effects in the elderly (women aged 80–100 years). In this subgroup, compared with placebo, Sr reduced the incidence of vertebral fractures by 59% after 1 year and 32% after 3 years. The reduction in non-vertebral fractures was 41% and 31% after 1 and 3 years, respectively. The 2006 Cochrane review included a total of four trials, three of which investigated the effects of Sr in a treatment population and one in a prevention population [47]. In osteoporotic, post-menopausal women a 37% reduction in vertebral fractures (two trials, $n = 5082$, RR 0.63, 95% CI 0.56–0.71) and a 14% reduction in non-vertebral fractures (two trials, $n = 6572$, RR 0.86, 95% CI 0.75–0.98) was demonstrated over a 3-year period (Table 13.1). An increase in BMD at all sites was shown. The decrease in fracture rates observed with strontium is of a similar magnitude to that described for oral bisphosphonates and was classified as 'silver' evidence. Administration of Sr resulted in increased levels of serum bone alkaline phosphatase (+8.1%) and a decrease in serum telopeptide of type I collagen (–12.2%) from the third month. These changes are moderate, but opposite and concomitant, and support the potential dual action of the drug.

Diarrhoea is a common adverse event, generally seen during the first 3 months of treatment. It was reported in the original trial and subsequently during systematic review (RR 1.38%, 95% CI 1.02–1.87). The trial data showed a slight increase in annual incidence of venous thromboembolism (VTE; 0.9% vs. 0.6%) at 3 years, and remained unchanged since the third year. This excess risk is also seen on systematic review: VTE OR 1.5; 95% CI 1.1–2.1. No underlying potential mechanism has been postulated as there is no known interaction between strontium and parameters of haemostasis. Although regulatory authorities have not considered a history of VTE as a contraindication to the use of the drug, caution should be used in patients at increased risk including those with a past history. During post-marketing surveillance, cases of hypersensitivity syndrome (i.e. drug rash with eosinophila and systemic symptoms [DRESS syndrome]) have been reported. This typically occurs 2–6 weeks after initiating therapy and presents with skin reaction, fever, systemic upset, hypereosinophilia, hepatic abnormality and renal impairment. Because of potential fatal outcome linked to the syndrome, treatment should be discontinued immediately and permanently in case of skin rash developing on the drug.

Strontium ranelate is available as a powder (2-g sachet). Strontium and ranelic acid are both eliminated unchanged, the latter excreted almost exclusively by the gut. The absorption of strontium is reduced by food, milk and dairy products. It should therefore be administered between meals, ideally taken at bedtime, preferably 2 hours after eating. No dosage adjustment is needed in relation to age or in patients with mild-to-moderate renal impairment. It is not recommended in severe renal impairement with creatinine clearance below 30 ml/min.

It is worth knowing that because of greater attenuation of X-rays by strontium, BMD measurements over-estimate actual BMD changes. In clinical practice, increase in BMD probably reflects compliance to therapy and is likely to translate to reduced fracture risk, as the SOTI and TROPOS pooled data analysis showed that the higher the increase in femoral neck BMD the lower the incidence of vertebral fracture. Another question is the persistence of the gain in BMD after stopping treatment. In SOTI, treated patients were randomized at the end of the fourth year to either placebo or Sr for the final year. In those who switched from Sr to placebo, there was a significant decrease in BMD at the spine and hip by 3.2% and 2.5%, respectively. This decrease mimics the observed increase in annual BMD during the first year of treatment; probably reflecting clearance of Sr from the bone and the change in bone remodelling induced by stopping therapy.

Based on existing evidence, Sr has a role where there is a high risk of either vertebral and/ or non-vertebral fracture, especially in the very elderly with high hip fracture risk. Caution needs to be taken in patients at risk of VTE and in the interpretation of bone densitometry measurements. The treating physician should be aware of hypersensitivity to the drug, which, although extremely rare, can be occasionally fatal.

PARATHYROID HORMONE

Parathyroid hormone (PTH) is secreted by the parathyroid glands and is critical to calcium homeostasis. Hyperparathyroidism is a well-established cause of brittle bone disease. Continuous endogenous production of parathyroid hormone causes deleterious consequences for the skeleton, particularly cortical bone, and hypercalcaemia. By contrast, intermittent exposure to low doses of PTH is shown to increase the number and activity of osteoblasts and stimulate activation frequency, leading to improvement in skeletal bone mass at both cancellous and cortical sites. There is, however, a greater increase in formation markers over resorption markers early in treatment. The intact PTH molecule has 84 amino acids. Recombinant human PTH is now available for treatment as two formulations: teriparatide (Forsteo), containing the 1–34 N-terminal fragment, and Preotact, the entire molecule (1–84).

Teriparatide (hPTH 1–34) has been studied in 1637 women (mean age 70 years) with severe osteoporosis (average number of vertebral fractures per patient was over 2) [48]. Patients received 20 µg/day teriparatide or placebo for a median 18-month period. New vertebral fractures occurred in 14% of the women in the placebo group and in 5% of the PTH group (RR 0.35, 95% CI 0.22–0.55). New non-vertebral fractures occurred in 6% of the placebo and 3% of the treated group (RR 0.47, 95% CI 0.25–0.88). The pivotal study was not powered to assess effects on hip fracture.

Preotact (hPTH 1–84) has been studied in 2532 post-menopausal women, mean age 64 years at the licensed dose of 100 µg/day for a maximum 2-year period [49]. This group had a lower baseline risk than women in the teriparatide study, as less than 20% had radiological evidence of a vertebral fracture. There was a significant (58%) reduction in risk of vertebral fracture. However, only 67.2% of patients who received at least one dose completed the study. There were no data showing effects on non-vertebral fracture. Hypercalciuria and hypercalcaemia were common. Currently, monitoring of calcium is recommended in the initial months of therapy.

Therefore, treatment with either agent has been shown to reduce the risk of vertebral fractures, whereas teriparatide also reduces the risk of non-vertebral fractures (Table 13.1). Both formulations are administered daily as subcutaneous injections. The recommended dose is based on their molecular weights; 20 µg of teriparatide (1–34) is 40% of 100 µg PTH (1–84). Duration of treatment is maximum 18 months for teriparatide and 24 months for parathyroid hormone. Beneficial effects appear to persist for up to 30 months after stopping treatment with teriparatide; these include a significant reduction in risk of vertebral fractures (at 18 months) and non-vertebral fractures (at 30 months). There are no published data of follow-up for Preotact. The most common adverse events are nausea, pain in the limbs, headache and dizziness. Transient rise in serum calcium has been observed with both agents. The change is small, clinically insignificant and does not require routine monitoring of serum calcium during therapy with teriparatide but is needed if using 1–84 parathyroid. Teriparatide is NICE approved and licensed for use in men and post-menopausal women, whereas Preotact is currently licensed for use in women only.

Both agents are contraindicated in conditions characterized by abnormally increased bone turnover such as Paget's disease, known hypercalcaemia, patients with bone metastasis, skeletal malignancy or history of radiotherapy.

In most countries PTH therapy is currently targeted to patients at high risk for fracture, driven by issues relating to the cost-effectiveness of treatment rather than to clinical effectiveness. Studies are under way to assess whether it is more appropriate for patients to receive PTH therapy as single-treatment course or if the dosing can be intermittent and cyclical, thereby prolonging the overall treatment period. Effects of pretreatment with bisphosphonates and the role for combination therapy is also being evaluated.

A recent meta-analysis [50] examined the effects of PTH alone or in combination with antiresorptive therapy on changes in BMD and fracture risk. PTH alone or in combination with antiresorptive drugs reduced vertebral [RR = 0.36, 95% CI 0.28–0.47] and non-vertebral (RR = 0.62, 95% CI 0.48–0.82) fracture risk and increased spine BMD by 6.6% (95% CI 5.2–8.1%) and hip BMD non-significantly by 1.0% (95% CI –0.1 to 2.1%) during 11–36 months of follow-up (13 trials). The gain in spine and hip BMD tended to increase with the length of the PTH treatment. No significant effect of study duration on fracture risk could be demonstrated. The major adverse events were hypercalcaemia, nausea and discomfort at the injection site. The authors were unable to draw any conclusions on the superiority of PTH plus antiresorptive drug versus antiresorptive drug or PTH alone with respect to BMD or fractures due to lack of such data.

TESTOSTERONE USE IN MEN

Androgen deficiency is a risk factor for osteoporosis. The extent to which testosterone can prevent and treat osteoporosis in men is still unclear. A recent meta-analysis of eight trials in men to estimate the effect of testosterone use in bone health [51] showed that, compared with placebo, intramuscular testosterone was associated with an 8% (95% CI 4–13%) gain in lumbar spine BMD but a non-significant gain of 4% (95% CI –2 to 9%) at the femoral neck. Transdermal testosterone had no significant impact on BMD at either site. No trials assessed the effects of testosterone on fractures (Table 13.1). Without fracture data, the available studies offer weak and indirect evidence about the efficacy of testosterone on osteoporosis prevention and treatment in men. At the time of writing, the only drugs licensed for use in men with osteoporosis are alendronate, risedronate and teriparatide.

SHOULD WE USE CALCIUM OR CALCIUM IN COMBINATION WITH VITAMIN D?

A recent meta-analysis of 29 randomized trials [52] in which either calcium or calcium with vitamin D was used to assess bone loss and fracture outcome involving 63 897 patients sheds light on this hotly debated topic (Figure 13.1). Twenty-three trials ($n = 41\,419$) assessed BMD. Pooled analysis showed significantly reduced rates of bone loss at all sites: 0.54% at the hip and 1.19% in the spine. Seventeen trials ($n = 52\,625$) that reported fracture as an outcome showed 12% reduction in fractures of all types (RR 0.88, 95% CI 0.83–0.95). The meta-analyses also showed that treatment effects were significantly better with calcium doses of 1200 mg or more and vitamin D doses of 800 IU or more. The authors concluded that calcium alone or in combination with vitamin D is effective for prevention of osteoporosis. The recommended minimum doses are 1200 mg calcium and 800 IU vitamin D. Effectiveness of calcium and vitamin D combination in reducing risk of hip and non-vertebral fractures has since been confirmed in the Cochrane review. However, no significant effect of vitamin D and calcium were seen on vertebral fractures [53, 54] (Table 13.1).

Vitamin D alone showed no statistically significant effect on hip fracture (seven trials, 18 668 patients), vertebral fracture (four trials, 5698 patients) or any new fracture (eight trials, 18 935 patients) [53, 54]. Results of an earlier comparative meta-analysis suggested superiority of vitamin D analogues (alphacalcidol and calcitriol) in preventing bone loss and spinal fractures compared with native vitamin D [55]. However, studies on alphacalcidol were small and the effects of calcitriol were based on a single trial by Tilyard [56]. The risk of hypercalcaemia associated with vitamin D analogues, particularly calcitriol, is high (RR 2.38, 95% CI 1.52–3.71). In clinical practice, therefore, based on the evidence so far, frail older people confined to institutions may sustain fewer hip and other non-vertebral fractures if given adequate calcium and vitamin D supplements. Effectiveness of vitamin D alone in fracture prevention is unclear. There is no advantage of vitamin D analogues which may additionally be associated with adverse events such as hypercalcaemia.

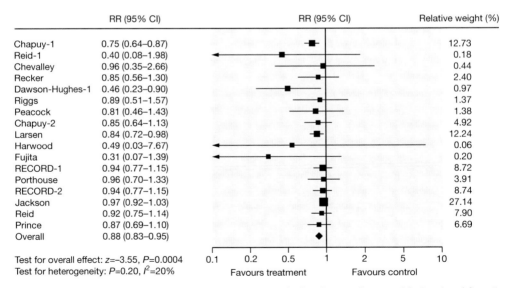

	RR (95% CI)	RR (95% CI)	Relative weight (%)
Chapuy-1	0.75 (0.64–0.87)		12.73
Reid-1	0.40 (0.08–1.98)		0.18
Chevalley	0.96 (0.35–2.66)		0.44
Recker	0.85 (0.56–1.30)		2.40
Dawson-Hughes-1	0.46 (0.23–0.90)		0.97
Riggs	0.89 (0.51–1.57)		1.37
Peacock	0.81 (0.46–1.43)		1.38
Chapuy-2	0.85 (0.64–1.13)		4.92
Larsen	0.84 (0.72–0.98)		12.24
Harwood	0.49 (0.03–7.67)		0.06
Fujita	0.31 (0.07–1.39)		0.20
RECORD-1	0.94 (0.77–1.15)		8.72
Porthouse	0.96 (0.70–1.33)		3.91
RECORD-2	0.94 (0.77–1.15)		8.74
Jackson	0.97 (0.92–1.03)		27.14
Reid	0.92 (0.75–1.14)		7.90
Prince	0.87 (0.69–1.10)		6.69
Overall	0.88 (0.83–0.95)		

Test for overall effect: $z=-3.55$, $P=0.0004$
Test for heterogeneity: $P=0.20$, $I^2=20\%$

0.1   0.2   0.5   1   2   5   10
Favours treatment   Favours control

Figure 13.1 Effect of calcium and calcium in combination with vitamin D on fracture risk. Reprinted from Tang et al., *Lancet* 2007; 370: 657–666 [52], ©2007, with permission from Elsevier.

(NEAR) FUTURE TREATMENTS TO PREVENT FRACTURES

Several safe, inexpensive and widely available drugs may act through novel or yet-to-be-determined pathways to decrease fracture risk. Ideally, these need to be tested in randomized trials with fracture as primary end-point. However, because these are inexpensive generic drugs it is unlikely that large trials will be done for want of funding. These include Vitamin B_{12}, folate, nitrates, beta-blockers and statins.

Vitamin B_{12} and folate. Decrease in folate and vitamin B_{12} leads to increase in homocysteine production. Homocystinuria, a rare genetic defect, produces premature vascular disease and severe osteoporosis. Several large prospective studies have shown that older adults with high levels of homocysteine have an increased risk of hip and other non-spine fractures. The US NHANES (United States National Health and Nutrition Examination Survey) found that women with lower vitamin B_{12} levels had lower hip BMD [57]. Thus, treatment with folate and vitamin B_{12} might reduce bone loss and fracture risk by reducing homocysteine concentrations.

Nitrates. Nitric oxide (NO) produced by NO synthetase (NOS) influences bone formation and resorption. NO mediates effects of exercise and oestrogen on bone and arteries, as NO is present in bone cells and endothelial cells. Compared with wild type, NOS knockout mice form less bone. An RCT of daily isosorbide mononitrate (ISMO) for 12 weeks in 144 post-menopausal women with osteoporosis showed favourable effects on bone turnover markers: 45.4% decrease in urine N-telopeptide (NTx) and 23.3% increase in bone-specific alkaline phosphatase (BSALP) [58]. These findings suggest that nitrates may be useful for the prevention of post-menopausal osteoporosis.

Beta-blockers. The sympathetic nervous system may control bone formation, as beta-2 receptors have been found on osteoblasts and nerves. *In vivo*, beta-blockers increase osteoblast activity, and mice treated with propranolol have increased bone density. A number of large cohort studies have shown higher hip BMD and significant hip and non-spine fracture reduction associated with use of a beta-blocker [59, 60]. However, although current use of beta-blockers was associated with a reduced risk of fracture in both the study populations, the protective effect was present only amongst patients with history of use of another antihypertensive agent. As the mechanism by which beta blockers can influence BMD is not known, larger RCTs with fracture as clinical end-points are needed.

Statins. There has also been much recent interest in the statins. These drugs are used to reduce cholesterol and have shown experimentally to induce BMP-2 and increase bone mass in rats. A variety of epidemiological studies suggest that statin users have lower rates of hip fracture than non-users, but prospective clinical trials and a recent systematic review [61] have proved difficult to demonstrate large effects on bone mass and turnover.

NOVEL TREATMENTS

New and novel treatments arising from our understanding of basic bone biology have promising potential to reduce fracture risk. Cathepsin K (Cat K) inhibitors, RANKL antibodies, sclerostin and Dickkopf-1 proteins are some of the promising agents currently in various stages of development.

Cathepsin K is the most abundant cysteine protease expressed in the osteoclast and produces hydrogen ions to acidify the area under the osteoclast which is instrumental in bone matrix degradation necessary for bone resorption. Cat K is capable of degrading several components of the bone matrix, including type I collagen. Although there are currently no approved cat K inhibitors, proof of concept for the mechanism has been established [62]. At least two Cat K inhibitors (odanacatib and balicatib) have shown reductions in bone resorption markers and increases in BMD in post-menopausal women. There is concern that Cat K inhibitors may affect skin collagen [63], and a phase III trial is under way.

Rank ligand. Identification and characterization of the OPG/RANKL/Rank system is a major addition to the list of momentous events in bone biology. Unravelling this pathway solved the longstanding question in bone biology, namely the precise mechanism by which preosteoblastic/stromal cells controlled osteoclast development to ensure that the processes of bone resorption and formation are tightly coupled to maintain skeletal integrity. Osteoclast proliferation, maturation and activity is controlled by RANKL and RANK (its receptor). Osteoprotegerin is a circulating (decoy) receptor that binds with RankL and decreases the effect of RankL. Absence of OPG and or unopposed RankL causes bone resorption (Figure 13.2). A number of cytokines and hormones have since been found to exert their effects on osteoclastogenesis by regulating osteoblastic/stromal cell production of OPG and RANKL: PTH and glucocorticosteroids (increase RANKL and decrease OPG), Vitamin D (increase RANKL), oestrogen and TGF-β (increase OPG).

Denosumab is a monoclonal antibody to RankL. The RCT on 412 post-menopausal osteoporotic women given denosumab subcutaneously every 3 or 6 months showed dramatic decrease in bone resorption, improvement in bone density at all sites and adverse events similar to placebo over 2 years with both doses of denosumab (Figure 13.3) [64]. The effects on bone markers were fully reversible with treatment discontinuation and restored with subsequent re-treatment [65]. Further studies are under way as the drug looks promising for the treatment of osteoporosis associated with the menopause, inflammatory diseases such as rheumatoid arthritis, chemotherapy for breast/prostate cancer and osteoporosis in men.

Wnts are a large family of proteins that participate in a number of cellular biological processes, such as embryogenesis, organogenesis and tumour formation. These proteins bind to membrane receptor complexes comprising a frizzled (Fz) G-protein-coupled receptor and other membrane co-receptors forming molecular groups that initiate, at least, three different intracellular signalling cascades leading to nuclear generation of transcription factors which regulate various cellular events. These events result in selective cellular differentiation, reduction or inhibition of the apoptotic mechanisms or changes in the biological behaviour of various cell lines. During the last decade, Wnt signalling has been shown to play a significant role in the control of osteoblastogenesis and bone formation. In several clinical cases, mutations have been found in the Wnt receptor complexes that are associated with changes in bone mineral density and fractures. Osteocytes secrete a protein identified as sclerostin (SOST), which blocks the membrane complex activation by Wnt, resulting in inhibition of bone formation. Dickkopf-1 (DKK-1) protein is another key regulator of the Wnt signalling pathway. Glucocorticosteroids increase DKK-1 expression, which may be

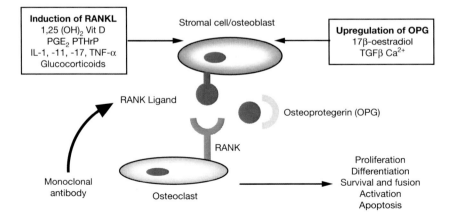

Figure 13.2 Receptor activator of NF-kappaB (RANK), RANK ligand (RANKL) and osteoprotegerin (OPG) system.

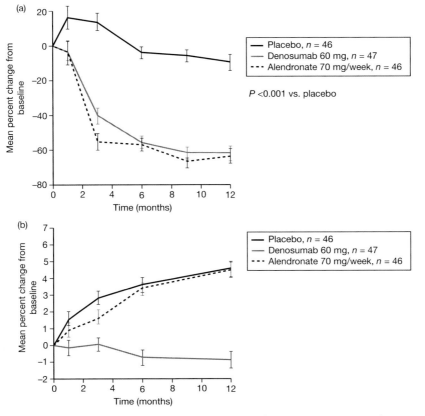

Figure 13.3 (a) Denosumab: bone-specific alkaline phosphatase. Phase II: post-menopausal women with low bone mineral density. (b) Lumbar spine bone mineral density after Denosumab. Phase II: post-menopausal women with low bone mineral density. In all of the denosumab dose cohorts (and the alendronate group), the median per cent changes in bone-specific alkaline phosphatase (BSAP) at month 12 were statistically significantly greater than in the placebo group (P<0.001). At 12 months median per cent change from baseline in BSAP was −50.2% to −72.6%, −62.8% and −19.2%, respectively, for denosumab every 3–6 months, alendronate and placebo. McClung MR *et al.* Denosumab in postmenopausal women with low bone mineral density. *N Engl J Med* 2006; 354:821–831 [64] (and supplementary appendix available at www.nejm.org).

involved in glucocorticosteroid-induced osteoporosis. Experimental evidence demonstrates that monoclonal antibodies against these two inhibitor proteins (sclerostin and DKK-1) can result in increased bone mass.

CONCLUSION

Not so long ago our therapeutic options for the management of patients with osteoporosis were limited to HRT, calcitonin injections or calcium/vitamin D. The development of bisphosphonates ushered in a new era in managing the disease. Recent development in different formulations and delivery methods has provided us the opportunity to choose a bisphosphonate that best suits the individual needs of the patient and enhances efficacy by improving compliance. The development of anabolic agents for the treatment of osteoporosis is currently an area of intense focus as, until now, drugs relied predominantly on increasing bone mass by inhibiting bone breakdown rather than stimulating bone formation. A major limitation in our search for anabolic agents had been our lack of understanding of the basic bone biology. Recent insights into the molecular mechanisms of bone formation and breakdown have led to the development of novel targeted therapies. The coming years will witness the launch of more effective and easier to use novel agents with superior bone density and fracture outcomes. An important, still unanswered, question is whether administering these drugs sequentially or in combination will provide added therapeutic advantage by exploiting the different mechanisms of action on bone, and thereby enhance effects on fracture risk. The search for the 'ideal' agent to treat osteoporosis is still on.

REFERENCES

1. Consensus Development Conference Diagnosis, prophylaxis and treatment of osteoporosis. *Am J Med* 1993; 94:646–650.
2. Rossouw JE, Anderson GL, Prentice RL *et al.* Writing Group for the Women's Health Initiative Investigators. Risks and benefits of estrogen plus progestin in healthy postmenopausal women: principal results from the Women's Health Initiative randomized controlled trial. *JAMA* 2002; 288:321–333.
3. Torgerson DJ, Bell-Syer SE. Hormone replacement therapy and prevention of nonvertebral fractures: a meta-analysis of randomized trials. *JAMA* 2001; 285:2891–2897.
4. Michaëlsson K, Baron JA, Farahmand BY *et al.* Hormone replacement therapy and risk of hip fracture: population based case–control study. The Swedish Hip Fracture Study Group. *BMJ* 1998; 316(7148):1858–1863.
5. Schneider DL, Barrett-Connor EL, Morton DJ. Timing of postmenopausal estrogen for optimal bone mineral density. The Rancho Bernardo Study. *JAMA* 1997; 277:543–547.
6. Beral V, Banks E, Reeves G. Evidence from randomised trials on the long-term effects of hormone replacement therapy. *Lancet* 2002; 360(9337):942–944.
7. Hulley S, Grady D, Bush T *et al.* Randomized trial of estrogen plus progestin for secondary prevention of coronary heart disease in postmenopausal women. Heart and Estrogen/progestin Replacement Study (HERS) Research Group. *JAMA* 1998; 280:605–613.
8. Beral V, Bull D, Reeves G; Million Women Study Collaborators. Endometrial cancer and hormone-replacement therapy in the Million Women Study. *Lancet* 2005; 365(9470):1543–1551.
9. de Vries CS, Bromley SE, Thomas H, Farmer RD. Tibolone and endometrial cancer: a cohort and nested case–control study in the UK. *Drug Saf* 2005; 28:241–249.
10. Ettinger B, Black DM, Mitlak BH *et al.* Reduction of vertebral fracture risk in postmenopausal women with osteoporosis treated with raloxifene: results from a 3-year randomized clinical trial. Multiple Outcomes of Raloxifene Evaluation (MORE) Investigators. *JAMA* 1999; 282:637–645.
11. Cranney A, Tugwell P, Zytaruk N *et al.* Osteoporosis Methodology Group and The Osteoporosis Research Advisory Group. Meta-analyses of therapies for postmenopausal osteoporosis. IV. Meta-analysis of raloxifene for the prevention and treatment of postmenopausal osteoporosis. *Endocr Rev* 2002; 23:524–528.
12. Lufkin EG, Whitaker MD, Nickelsen T *et al.* Treatment of established postmenopausal osteoporosis with raloxifene: a randomized trial. *J Bone Miner Res* 1998; 13:1747–1754.
13. Cummings SR, Eckert S, Krueger KA *et al.* The effect of raloxifene on risk of breast cancer in postmenopausal women: results from the MORE randomized trial. Multiple Outcomes of Raloxifene Evaluation. *JAMA* 1999; 281:2189–2197.
14. Vogel VG, Costantino JP, Wickerham DL *et al.* Effects of tamoxifen vs raloxifene on the risk of developing invasive breast cancer and other disease outcomes: the NSABP Study of Tamoxifen and Raloxifene (STAR) P-2 trial. *JAMA* 2006; 295:2727–2741.
15. Mosca L, Barrett-Connor E, Wenger NK *et al.* Design and methods of the Raloxifene Use for The Heart (RUTH) study. *Am J Cardiol* 2001; 88:392–395.
16. Barrett-Connor E, Mosca L, Collins P *et al.* Raloxifene Use for The Heart (RUTH) Trial Investigators. Effects of raloxifene on cardiovascular events and breast cancer in postmenopausal women. *N Engl J Med* 2006; 355:125–137.
17. Wells GA, Cranney A, Peterson J *et al.* Etidronate for the primary and secondary prevention of osteoporotic fractures in postmenopausal women. *Cochrane Database Syst Rev* 2008; (1):CD003376.
18. Black DM, Thompson DE, Bauer DC *et al.* Fracture Intervention Trial. Fracture risk reduction with alendronate in women with osteoporosis: the Fracture Intervention Trial. FIT Research Group. *J Clin Endocrinol Metab* 2000; 85:4118–4124.

19. Wells GA, Cranney A, Peterson J *et al.* Alendronate for the primary and secondary prevention of osteoporotic fractures in postmenopausal women. *Cochrane Database Syst Rev* 2008; (1):CD001155.

20. Harris ST, Watts NB, Genant HK *et al.* Effects of risedronate treatment on vertebral and nonvertebral fractures in women with postmenopausal osteoporosis: a randomized controlled trial. Vertebral Efficacy With Risedronate Therapy (VERT) Study Group. *JAMA* 1999; 282:1344–1352.

21. Reginster J, Minne HW, Sorensen OH *et al.* Randomized trial of the effects of risedronate on vertebral fractures in women with established postmenopausal osteoporosis. Vertebral Efficacy with Risedronate Therapy (VERT) Study Group. *Osteoporos Int* 2000; 11:83–91.

22. McClung MR, Geusens P, Miller PD *et al.* Hip Intervention Program Study Group. Effect of risedronate on the risk of hip fracture in elderly women. Hip Intervention Program Study Group. *N Engl J Med* 2001; 344:333–340.

23. Wells G, Cranney A, Peterson J *et al.* Risedronate for the primary and secondary prevention of osteoporotic fractures in postmenopausal women. *Cochrane Database Syst Rev* 2008; (1):CD004523.

24. Chesnut III CH, Skag A, Christiansen C *et al.* Osteoporosis Vertebral Fracture Trial in North America and Europe (BONE). Effects of oral ibandronate administered daily or intermittently on fracture risk in postmenopausal osteoporosis. *J Bone Miner Res* 2004; 19:1241–1249.

25. Delmas PD, Recker RR, Chesnut CH 3rd *et al.* Daily and intermittent oral ibandronate normalize bone turnover and provide significant reduction in vertebral fracture risk: results from the BONE study. *Osteoporos Int* 2004; 15:792–798.

26. Reginster JY, Adami S, Lakatos P *et al.* Efficacy and tolerability of once-monthly oral ibandronate in postmenopausal osteoporosis: 2 year results from the MOBILE study. *Ann Rheum Dis* 2006; 65:654–661.

27. Delmas PD, Adami S, Strugala C *et al.* Intravenous ibandronate injections in postmenopausal women with osteoporosis: one-year results from the dosing intravenous administration study. *Arthritis Rheum* 2006; 54:1838–1846.

28. Reid IR, Brown JP, Burckhardt P *et al.* Intravenous zoledronic acid in postmenopausal women with low bone mineral density. *N Engl J Med* 2002; 346:653–661.

29. Black DM, Delmas PD, Eastell R *et al.* HORIZON Pivotal Fracture Trial. Once-yearly zoledronic acid for treatment of postmenopausal osteoporosis. *N Engl J Med* 2007; 356:1809–1822.

30. Lyles KW, Colón-Emeric CS, Magaziner JS *et al.* HORIZON Recurrent Fracture Trial. Zoledronic acid and clinical fractures and mortality after hip fracture. *N Engl J Med* 2007; 357:1799–1809.

31. Woo SB, Hellstein JW, Kalmar JR. Narrative [corrected] review: bisphosphonates and osteonecrosis of the jaws. *Ann Intern Med* 2006; 144:753–761.

32. Khosla S, Burr D, Cauley J *et al.* Bisphosphonate-associated osteonecrosis of the jaw: report of a task force of the American Society for Bone and Mineral Research. *J Bone Miner Res* 2007; 22:1479–1491.

33. Mavrokokki T, Cheng A, Stein B, Goss A. Nature and frequency of bisphosphonate-associated osteonecrosis of the jaws in Australia. *J Oral Maxillofac Surg* 2007; 65:415–423.

34. Plosker GL, McTavish D. Intranasal salcatonin (salmon calcitonin). A review of its pharmacological properties and role in the management of postmenopausal osteoporosis. *Drugs Aging* 1996; 8:378–400.

35. Chesnut CH 3rd, Silverman S, Andriano K *et al.* A randomized trial of nasal spray salmon calcitonin in postmenopausal women with established osteoporosis: the prevent recurrence of osteoporotic fractures study. PROOF Study Group. *Am J Med* 2000; 109:267–276.

36. Cranney A, Tugwell P, Zytaruk N *et al.* Osteoporosis Methodology Group and The Osteoporosis Research Advisory Group. Meta-analyses of therapies for postmenopausal osteoporosis. VI. Meta-analysis of calcitonin for the treatment of postmenopausal osteoporosis. *Endocr Rev* 2002; 23:540–551.

37. Dvorak MM, Siddiqua A, Ward DT *et al.* Physiological changes in extracellular calcium concentration directly control osteoblast function in the absence of calciotropic hormones. *Proc Natl Acad Sci USA* 2004; 101:5140–5145.

38. Chattopadhyay N, Quinn SJ, Kifor O *et al.* The calcium-sensing receptor (CaR) is involved in strontium ranelate-induced osteoblast proliferation. *Biochem Pharmacol* 2007; 74:438–447.

39. Marie PJ. Strontium ranelate: a novel mode of action optimizing bone formation and resorption. *Osteoporos Int* 2005; 16(Suppl. 1):S7–10.

40. Takahashi N, Sasaki T, Tsouderos Y, Suda T. S12911–2 inhibits osteoclastic bone resorption in vitro. *J Bone Miner Res* 2003; 18:1082–1087.

41. Mentaverri R, Yano S, Chattopadhyay N *et al.* The calcium sensing receptor is directly involved in both osteoclast differentiation and apoptosis. *FASEB J* 2006; 20:2562–2564.

42. Ammann P, Shen V, Robin B *et al.* Strontium ranelate improves bone resistance by increasing bone mass and improving architecture in intact female rats. *J Bone Miner Res* 2004; 19:2012–2020.

43. Arlot ME, Jiang Y, Genant HK *et al.* Histomorphometric and microCT analysis of bone biopsies from postmenopausal osteoporotic women treated with strontium ranelate. *J Bone Miner Res* 2008; 23:215–222.

44. Meunier PJ, Roux C, Seeman E *et al.* The effects of strontium ranelate on the risk of vertebral fracture in women with postmenopausal osteoporosis. *N Engl J Med* 2004; 350:459–468.

45. Reginster JY, Seeman E, De Vernejoul MC *et al.* Strontium ranelate reduces the risk of nonvertebral fractures in postmenopausal women with osteoporosis: Treatment of Peripheral Osteoporosis (TROPOS) study. *J Clin Endocrinol Metab* 2005; 90:2816–2822.

46. Seeman E, Vellas B, Benhamou C *et al.* Strontium ranelate reduces the risk of vertebral and nonvertebral fractures in women eighty years of age and older. *J Bone Miner Res* 2006; 21:1113–1120.

47. O'Donnell S, Cranney A, Wells GA *et al.* Strontium ranelate for preventing and treating postmenopausal osteoporosis. *Cochrane Database Syst Rev* 2006; (4):CD005326.

48. Neer RM, Arnaud CD, Zanchetta JR *et al.* Effect of parathyroid hormone (1–34) on fractures and bone mineral density in postmenopausal women with osteoporosis. *N Engl J Med* 2001; 344:1434–1441.

49. Greenspan SL, Bone HG, Ettinger MP *et al.* Treatment of Osteoporosis with Parathyroid Hormone Study Group. Effect of recombinant human parathyroid hormone (1–84) on vertebral fracture and bone mineral density in postmenopausal women with osteoporosis: a randomized trial. *Ann Intern Med* 2007; 146:326–339.

50. Vestergaard P, Jorgensen NR, Mosekilde L *et al.* Effects of parathyroid hormone alone or in combination with antiresorptive therapy on bone mineral density and fracture risk – a meta-analysis. *Osteoporos Int* 2007; 18:45–57.

51. Tracz MJ, Sideras K, Boloña ER *et al.* Testosterone use in men and its effects on bone health. A systematic review and meta-analysis of randomized placebo-controlled trials. *J Clin Endocrinol Metab* 2006; 91:2011–2016.

52. Tang BM, Eslick GD, Nowson C *et al.* Use of calcium or calcium in combination with vitamin D supplementation to prevent fractures and bone loss in people aged 50 years and older: a meta-analysis. *Lancet* 2007; 370(9588):657–666.

53. Avenell A, Handoll HH. Nutritional supplementation for hip fracture aftercare in older people. *Cochrane Database Syst Rev* 2006; (4):CD001880.

54. Avenell A, Gillespie WJ, Gillespie LD, O'Connell DL. Vitamin D and vitamin D analogues for preventing fractures associated with involutional and post-menopausal osteoporosis. *Cochrane Database Syst Rev* 2005; (3):CD000227.

55. Richy F, Ethgen O, Bruyere O, Reginster JY. Efficacy of alphacalcidol and calcitriol in primary and corticosteroid-induced osteoporosis: a meta-analysis of their effects on bone mineral density and fracture rate. *Osteoporos Int* 2004; 15:301–310.

56. Tilyard MW, Spears GF, Thomson J, Dovey S. Treatment of postmenopausal osteoporosis with calcitriol or calcium. *N Engl J Med* 1992; 326:357–362.

57. Morris MS, Jacques PF, Selhub J. Relation between homocysteine and B-vitamin status indicators and bone mineral density in older Americans. *Bone* 2005; 37:234–242.

58. Jamal SA, Cummings SR, Hawker GA. Isosorbide mononitrate increases bone formation and decreases bone resorption in postmenopausal women: a randomized trial. *J Bone Miner Res* 2004; 19:1512–1517.

59. Schlienger RG, Kraenzlin ME, Jick SS, Meier CR. Use of beta-blockers and risk of fractures. *JAMA* 2004; 292:1326–1332.

60. de Vries F, Pouwels S, Bracke M *et al.* Use of beta-2 agonists and risk of hip/femur fracture: a population-based case–control study. *Pharmacoepidemiol Drug Saf* 2007; 16:612–619.

61. Toh S, Hernández-Díaz S. Statins and fracture risk. A systematic review. *Pharmacoepidemiol Drug Saf* 2007; 16:627–640.

62. Stoch SA, Wagner JA. Cathepsin K inhibitors: a novel target for osteoporosis therapy. *Clin Pharmacol Ther* 2008; 83:172–176.

63. Peroni A, Zini A, Braga V *et al.* Drug-induced morphea: report of a case induced by balicatib and review of the literature. *J Am Acad Dermatol* 2008; 59:125–129.

64. McClung MR, Leweicki M, Cohen SB *et al.* Denosumab in postmenopausal women with low bone mineral density. *N Engl J Med* 2006; 354:821–831.

65. Miller PD, Bolognese MA, Lewiecki EM *et al.* for the Amg 162 Bone Loss Study Group. Effect of denosumab on bone density and turnover in postmenopausal women with low bone mass after long-term continued, discontinued, and restarting of therapy: a randomized blinded phase 2 clinical trial. *Bone* 2008; 43:222–229.

Abbreviations

AASV	antineutrophil cytoplasmic antibody-associated vasculitis
ABCA4	ATP-binding cassette type A
ACCP	American College of Chest Physicians
ACE	angiotensin-converting enzyme
aCL	anticardiolipin
ACR	American College of Rheumatology
ACTH	adrenocorticotropic hormone
AHSRC	autologous haematopoietic stem cell rescue
AIM	Abatacept in Inadequate Responders to Methotrexate
AMP	adenosine monophosphate
ANA	antinuclear antibody
ANCA	antineutrophil cytoplasmic antibody
APASS	Antiphospholipid Antibody Stroke Study
aPL	antiphospholipid
APRIL	a proliferation-inducing ligand
APS	antiphospholipid syndrome
AS	ankylosing spondylitis
ASAS	Assessment in Ankylosing Spondylitis working group
ASPIRE	Active-Controlled Study of Patients Receiving Infliximab for Treatment of Rheumatoid Arthritis of Early Onset
ASSIST	American Scleroderma Stem Cell versus Immune Suppression Trial
ASSURE	Abatacept Study of Safety in Use with other RA Therapies
ASTIS	Autologous Stem Cell Transplantation International Scleroderma
ASU	avocado–soybean unsaponifiable
ATG	antithymocyte globulin
ATIC	5-aminoimidazole-4-carboxamide-ribonucleotide transformylase
ATTAIN	Abatacept Trial in Treatment of Anti-TNF Inadequate Responders
AZA	azathioprine
BAFF	B-cell activating factor
BAFF-R	B-cell activating factor receptor
BASDAI	Bath Ankylosing Spondylitis Disease Activity Index
BASFI	Bath Ankylosing Spondylitis Functional Index
BASMI	Bath Ankylosing Spondylitis Metrology Index
BASRI	Bath Ankylosing Spondylitis Radiology Index
BCMA	B-cell maturation protein
BeSt	Behandel Strategieën
BILAG	British Isles Lupus Assessment Group
BLyS	B-lymphocyte stimulator protein
BMD	bone mineral density
BMI	body mass index
bp	basepair
BP	biphosphonate

BSA	body surface area
BSALP	bone-specific alkaline phosphatase
BSR	British Society for Rheumatology
CAMERA	computer-assisted management of early RA
CAPS	catastrophic antiphospholipid syndrome
CaR	calcium receptor
CAU	chronic anterior uveitis
CCP	cyclic citrullinated peptide
CD	Crohn's disease
CHARISMA	Chugai Humanized Anti-human Recombinant Interleukin-Six Monoclonal Antibody
CHD	coronary heart disease
CHOP	cyclophosphamide, doxorubicin, vincristine and prednisone
CI	confidence interval
CIMESTRA	Ciclosporin–Methotrexate Steroid Treatment in Rheumatoid Arthritis
CNV	copy number variant
COBRA	Combination Therapy in Early Rheumatoid Arthritis
COMET	Combination of Methotrxate and Etanercept
CORE	Continuing Outcomes Relevant to Evista
COX	cyclooxygenase
CRP	C-reactive protein
CSA	ciclosporin A
CSS	Churg–Strauss syndrome
CT	computed tomography
CYC	cyclophosphamide
DANCER	Dose-ranging Assessment: International Clinical Evaluation of Rituximab in Rheumatoid Arthritis
DcSSc	diffuse cutaneous systemic sclerosis
DAS	disease activity score
DHODH	dihydroorotate dehydrogenase
DIP	distal interphalangeal
DISTOL	Digital Ischemic Lesions in Scleroderma Treated with Oral Treprostinil Dithanolamine
DKK-1	Dickkopf-1
DLQI	Dermatology Life Quality Index
DMARD	disease-modifying antirheumatic drug
DMOAD	disease-modifying osteoarthritis drug
DRESS	drug rash with eosinophila and systemic symptoms
DXA	dual X-ray absorptiometry
EBMT	European Group for Blood and Marrow Transplantation
EMG	electromyography
ERA	enthesitis-related arthritis
ESC	European Society of Cardiology
ESR	erythrocyte sedimentation rate
ETN	etanercept
EULAR	European League Against Rheumatism
EUVAS	European Vasculitis Study Group
FAST	Fibrosing Alveolitis in Scleroderma Trial
FDA	Food and Drug Administration
FIN-RACo	Finnish Rheumatoid Arthritis Combination Therapy
FIT	Fracture Intervention Trial
FVC	forced vital capacity
Fz	frizzled
GAIT	Glucosamine/Chondroitin Arthritis Intervention Trial
GI	gastrointestinal
GO-REVEAL	Golumimab – Randomized Evaluation of Safety and Efficacy in Subjects with Psoriatic Arthritis using a Human Anti-TNF Monoclonal Antibody
GPRD	General Practice Research Database
GRAPPA	Group for Research and Assessment of Psoriasis and Psoriatic Arthritis
HAQ	Health Assessment Questionnaire
HCQ	hydroxychloroquine
HLA	human leucocyte antigen
HR	hazard ratio

HRCT	high-resolution computed tomography
HRQoL	health-related quality of life
HRT	hormone replacement therapy
HSCT	haematopoietic stem cell transplantation
IA	intra-articular
IBD	inflammatory bowel disease
IBP	inflammatory back pain
IFN	interferon
Ig	immunoglobulin
IL	interleukin
ILAR	International League of Associations for Rheumatology
i.m.	intramuscular
IMPACT	Infliximab Multinational Psoriatic Arthritis Controlled Trials
INR	international normalized ratio
ISMO	isosorbide mononitrate
i.v.	intravenous
IVF	*in vitro* fertilization
IVIg	intravenous immunoglobulin
IVMP	intravenous pulses of methylprednisolone
JCA	juvenile chronic arthritis
JIA	juvenile idiopathic arthritis
JPsA	juvenile psoriatic arthritis
JRA	juvenile rheumatoid arthritis
LA	lupus anticoagulant
LcSSc	limited cutaneous systemic sclerosis
LDL	low-density lipoprotein
LFA-3	lymphocyte function antigen 3
LFL	leflunomide
LGL	large granular lymphocyte
LMW	low molecular weight
MAS	macrophage activation syndrome
MASCOT	Management of Atrial Fibrillation Suppression in Atrial Fibrillation/Heart Failure Comorbidity Therapy
MASES	Maastricht Ankylosing Spondylitis Enthesitis Score
MDT	multidisciplinary team
MEI	Mander Enthesitis Index
MHC	major histocompatibility complex
MITAX	Myositis Intention To Treat Index
MMF	mycophenolate mofetil
MMP	matrix metalloproteinase
MORE	Multiple Outcome of Raloxifene Evaluation
MP	methylprednisolone
MPA	microscopic polyangiitis
MRC	Medical Research Council
MRI	magnetic resonance imaging
MRP	multidrug resistance protein
MRSS	modified Rodnan skin score
mSASSS	modified Stoke Ankylosing Spondylitis Spinal Score
MSU	monosodium urate
MTX	methotrexate
MWS	Million Women Study
MYOACT	Myositis Disease Activity Assessment
NAT2	N-acetyltransferase 2
NHS	National Health Service
NICE	National Institute for Health and Clinical Excellence
NIH	National Institutes of Health
NNT	number needed to treat
NO	nitric oxide
NOS	nitric oxide synthase
NSAID	non-steroidal anti-inflammatory drug
nsNSAID	non-selective non-steroidal anti-inflammatory drug

nt-proBNP	N-terminal probrain natriuretic peptide
OA	osteoarthritis
OAT	organic anion transporter
ONJ	osteonecrosis of the jaw
OPG	osteoprotegerin
OR	odds ratio
PAH	pulmonary arterial hypertension
PASI	psoriasis area and severity index
PDE	phosphodiesterase
PDGF	platelet-derived growth factor
PE	phosphatidylethanolamine
PEG	polyethylene glycol
PFC	physical function component
PPI	proton pump inhibitor
PRESTA	Psoriasis Randomized Etanercept Study in Subjects with Psoriatic Arthritis
PROMPT	Probable Rheumatoid Arthritis: Methotrexate Versus Placebo Treatment
PROOF	Prevent Recurrence of Osteoporotic Fractures
PS	phosphatidylserine
PsA	psoriatic arthritis
PsARC	Psoriatic Arthritis Response Criterion
PsSpA	psoriatic spondyloarthritides
PTH	parathyroid hormone
PVR	pulmonary vascular resistance
QALY	quality-adjusted life year
QoL	quality of life
RA	rheumatoid arthritis
RADIATE	Rheumatoid Arthritis Study in Anti-TNF Failures
RANK	receptor activator of NF-kappaB
RANKL	receptor activator of NF-kappaB ligand
RCT	randomized controlled trial
REFLEX	Randomised Evaluation of Long-term Efficacy of Rituximab in Rheumatoid Arthritis
ReSpA	reactive spondyloarthritides
RF	rheumatoid factor
RFC	reduced folate carrier
rG-CSF	recombinant granulocyte colony-stimulating factor
RR	relative risk
RRR	relative risk reduction
RTX	rituximab
RUTH	Raloxifene Use for the Heart
SASSS	Stoke Ankylosing Spondylitis Spinal Score
s.c.	subcutaneous
SCOT	Scleroderma: Cyclophosphamide or Transplantation
SD	standard deviation
SE	shared epitope
SERM	selective oestrogen receptor modulator
SLAM	systemic lupus activity measure
SLE	systemic lupus erythematosus
SLEDAI	systemic lupus erythematosus disease activity index
SLS	Scleroderma Lung Study
SNAC	sodium N-(8[2-hydroxybenzoyl]amino)caprylate
SNP	single nucleotide polymorphism
SOJIA	systemic-onset juvenile idiopathic arthritis
SOTI	Spinal Osteoporosis Therapeutic Intervention
SpA	spondyloarthritides
SpAIBD	spondyloarthritides associated with inflammatory bowel disease
Sr	strontium ranelate
SRC	scleroderma renal crisis
SSc	systemic sclerosis
SSZ	sulfasalazine
STAR	Study of Tamoxifen and Raloxifene
SUA	serum urate

TACI	transmembrane activator and calcium-modulating cyclophilin ligand interactor
TGF	transforming growth factor
THF	tetrahydrofolate
TICORA	tight control in RA
TNF	tumour necrosis factor
TOWARD	Tocilizumab in Combination With traditional DMARD therapy
TPMT	thiopurine methyltransferase
TROPOS	Treatment of Peripheral Osteoporosis
TSS	total Sharp scores
UA	undifferentiated arthritis
UC	ulcerative colitis
u-CTX-II	urinary C-terminal telopeptides of type-II collagen
UIA	undifferentiated inflammatory arthritis
ULT	urate-lowering therapy
US NHANES	United States National Health and Nutrition Examination Survey
VAS	visual analogue scale
VNTR	variable numbers of tandem repeats
VTE	venous thromboembolism
WARSS	Warfarin Aspirin Recurrent Stroke Study
WG	Wegener's granulomatosis
WHI	Women's Health Initiative
WHO	World Health Organization
WMD	weighted mean difference

Index

A

abatacept 10, 26, 27, 35, 40
  pharmacogenetic studies 54
  in psoriatic arthritis, peripheral joint disease 78
  in rheumatoid arthritis
    clinical studies 40–2
    current use 43–4
    safety issues 42–3
  in SLE 111
ABCB1 gene, pharmacogenetic studies 57, 58
abetimus sodium 111
ACE gene polymorphism 130
ACE inhibitors, in systemic sclerosis 135
adalimumab 23–4, 26
  in ankylosing spondylitis 92–3
  in early rheumatoid arthritis 6, 7
  in inflammatory bowel disease 93
  pharmacogenetic studies 54, 60
  in psoriatic arthritis
    axial disease 78
    dactylitis 79
    peripheral joint disease 76–7
ADEPT (Adalimumab Effectiveness in Psoriatic
  Arthritis Trial) 76
adrenocorticotrophic hormone (ACTH), in acute
  gout 165
AIM (Abatacept in Inadequate Responders to
  Methotrexate) trial 41–2
alcohol consumption, and gout 166, 167
alefacept, in psoriatic arthritis, peripheral joint
  disease 77
alendronate
  in osteoarthritis 155
  in osteoporosis 180, 182
allopurinol 167–8
  desensitization 169
  dosing schedule 168
  EULAR recommendations 164
  see also urate-lowering therapy
alphacalcidol, in osteoporosis 188

AMBITION study (tocilizumab) 27–8
AMG 714 45–6
AMPD1 (adenosine monophosphate deaminase)
  gene, pharmacogenetic studies 56, 58
amyloidosis 29
anakinra 25, 26, 44–5
  in ankylosing spondylitis 93
  in gout 173–4
  pharmacogenetic studies 54
  in psoriatic arthritis
    axial disease 78
    peripheral joint disease 77
ankylosing spondylitis (AS) 85
  anakinra 93
  anti-TNF agents 92–3
    ASAS working group recommendations 94–5
    cost-effectiveness 93
  assessment 86
    ASAS working group core sets 87
    disease activity 87–8
    enthesitis 89
    fatigue 89
    imaging 89–90
    laboratory tests 90
    measurement domains 87
    peripheral joint involvement 89
    physical function 88
    treatment response 90–1
  DMARDs 91–2
  management 85–6
  non-steroidal anti-inflammatory drugs 91
  treatment principles 91
anterior scleritis, in rheumatoid arthritis 29
anti-β2-glycoprotein 1 antibodies 117
  in coronary artery disease 122
anti-CADM-140 antibody 142
anticardiolipin (aCL) antibodies 117
  in coronary artery disease 122
anti-CCP antibodies 59
anti-CD20 monoclonal antibody *see* rituximab

anti-CD22 monoclonal antibody *see* epratuzumab

anti-CD40 ligand monoclonal antibodies, in SLE 111

anticentromere antibodies 130

anticoagulation, antiphospholipid syndrome 119–20
  effect on headaches 120–1
  in pregnancy 121–2

anti-EL antibody 142

anti-fibrillarin antibodies 130

antifibrotic therapies, systemic sclerosis 133–4

anti-IL-6 monoclonal antibody *see* tocilizumab

anti-IL-10 monoclonal antibody, in SLE 110

anti-interferons, in SLE 110

anti-Jo-1 antibody 142

anti-KS antibody 142

anti-Ku antibody 142

antimalarials, in psoriatic arthritis 75

anti-Mi2 antibody 142

anti-MJ antibody 142

anti-nRNP antibodies 130

anti-OJ antibody 142

anti-OM-Scl antibody 142

antioxidants, in osteoarthritis 153–4

antiphospholipid syndrome (APS) 117, 124
  accelerated atheroma 122
  clinical features 118
  headache and memory loss 120–1
  heparin 122
  intravenous immunoglobulin 123
  oral heparins 122
  pregnancy 121–2, 123
  presentation 119
  primary prevention of thrombosis 118
  rituximab 123–4
  self-testing of INR 123
  thrombosis, secondary prevention 119–20
  thrombosis rates 120
  warfarin alternatives 122

anti-p155 antibody 142

anti-PL-7 antibody 142

anti-PL-12 antibody 142

anti-pm-scl antibodies 130

anti-PMS antibody 142

anti-RNA polymerase antibodies 130

anti-SRP antibody 142

anti-thymocyte globulin, in systemic sclerosis 131

anti-TNF agents 23–4, 26, 35
  in ankylosing spondylitis 92–3
  in early rheumatoid arthritis 6, 11
  in gout 174
  in inflammatory bowel disease 93
  in inflammatory myositis 144
  pharmacogenetics 60–1, 62–3
  in psoriatic arthritis
    axial disease 78
    dactylitis 79
    enthesitis 78–9

peripheral joint disease 75–7
  use of a second agent 77
  in SLE 110
  see also adalimumab; etanercept; golimumab;
    infliximab

anti-topoisomerase-1 antibodies 130

anti-U1RNP antibody 142

anti-YRS antibody 142

anti-Zo antibody 142

APASS (Antiphospholipid Antibody Stroke
  Study) 119

APRIL 109

arzoxifene 181

ASAS (Assessment in Ankylosing Spondylitis)
  working group 86
  recommendation for anti-TNF therapy 94–5
  response criteria 90–1

ASAS/EULAR recommendations for AS
  management 86

ASPIRE (Active-Controlled Study of Patients
  Receiving Infliximab for Treatment of
  Rheumatoid Arthritis of Early Onset) trial 6, 7

aspirin in antiphospholipid syndrome 118
  during pregnancy 121

Aspreva Lupus Management Study 102–3

ASSIST (American Scleroderma Stem Cell versus
  Immune Suppression Trial) 132

ASSURE (Abatacept Study of Safety in Use with
  other RA Therapies) 42–3

ASTIS (Autologous Stem Cell Transplantation
  International Scleroderma) trial 131

atacicept, in SLE 109

atherosclerosis, in antiphospholipid syndrome 122

ATIC gene, pharmacogenetic studies 54, 56, 58

ATTAIN (Abatacept Trial in Treatment of Anti-TNF
  Inadequate Responders) trial 41, 42, 43

autoimmune disease risk, anti-TNF therapy 24

avocado–soyabean unsaponifiables (ASUs), in
  osteoarthritis 158–9

axial involvement, psoriatic arthritis 72
  biological therapy 78

azapropazone, in gout prophylaxis 173

azathioprine 19, 23
  in inflammatory myositis 143, 144
  pharmacogenetic studies 54
  in psoriatic arthritis 75

B

B-7–CD-28 interaction 40

B cells, role in rheumatoid arthritis 35–6

balicatib 189

BASDAI (Bath Ankylosing Spondylitis Disease
  Activity Index) 87–8, 89

BASFI (Bath Ankylosing Spondylitis Functional
  Index) 88

BASMI (Bath Ankylosing Spondylitis Metrology Index) 88
BASRI (Bath Ankylosing Spondylitis Radiology Index) 88, 89
bazedoxifene 181
belimumab 40
    in SLE 109
benzbromarone 170–1
BeSt trial 8–9
beta-blockers, in osteoporosis 189
betamethasone, intra-articular, in rheumatoid arthritis 4
BG9588 111
biological therapy 26, 35
    abatacept 27, 40
        current use in rheumatoid arthritis 43–4
        safety issues 42–3
        studies in rheumatoid arthritis 40–2
    anakinra 25, 44–5
    belimumab 40
    in early rheumatoid arthritis 5–6, 7
    in gout 173–4
    interleukin 15 blockade 45–6
    pharmacogenetics 60–1, 62–3
    in psoriatic arthritis
        axial disease 78
        dactylitis 79
        enthesitis 78–9
        peripheral joint disease 75–8
    rituximab 25, 27, 36
        current use in RA 39
        duration of benefit 39
        safety issues 38–9
        studies in rheumatoid arthritis 36–8
    T-cell targeted 44
    tocilizumab 27–8, 45
    see also anti-TNF agents
bisphosphonates
    in ankylosing spondylitis 92
    in osteoarthritis 154–5
    in osteoporosis 181–3
        fracture risk reduction 180
BLISS-52, BLISS-76 studies 109
BLyS (B lymphocyte stimulator protein) 109
body mass index (BMI), relationship to gout risk 166
bone erosions, rheumatoid arthritis 1
bone mineral density (BMD) 179
    effect of strontium ranelate 186
bone remodelling, effect of strontium ranelate 184–5
bosentan
    in SSc-associated digital ulceration 136
    in SSc-associated pulmonary hypertension 135
breast cancer, preventive action of raloxifene 181
BRISK study (The British Study of Risedronate in Structure and Symptoms of Knee OA) 155

C
C-reactive protein, in assessment of ankylosing spondylitis 90
calcitonin
    in osteoarthritis 156
    in osteoporosis 180, 183–4
calcitriol, in osteoporosis 188
calcium intake, glucocorticosteroid therapy 22
calcium supplements, in osteoporosis 180, 188
CAMERA (Computer-Assisted Management of Early Rheumatoid Arthritis) trial 3
Campath-1H 44
candidate genes, drug response variation 53
carbon monoxide diffusion capacity 132
CAT-192 133–4
catastrophic antiphospholipid syndrome (CAPS) 123
cathepsin K inhibitors 189
CD4+ T cells, role in inflammatory arthritis 44
CD20 25, 36
CHARISMA (Chugai Humanized Anti-human Recombinant Interleukin-Six Monoclonal Antibody) study 27, 45
chloroquine, in psoriatic arthritis 75
chondroitin 152
CHOP (cyclophosphamide, doxorubicin, vincristine and prednisone) 36
ciclosporin 19, 23
    in combination therapy 21
    in inflammatory myositis 143
    pharmacogenetic studies 54
    in psoriatic arthritis 73, 74
CIMESTRA (Ciclosporin–Methotrexate Steroid treatment in Rheumatoid Arthritis) study 4
co-stimulation 40
co-stimulatory blockers see abatacept
COBRA (Combination Therapy in Early Rheumatoid Arthritis) trial 4, 22
COL1A2 gene polymorphism 130
colchicine 165
    EULAR recommendations 164
    in initiation of urate-lowering therapy 172–3
combination therapy, DMARDs 4–5, 21–2
COMET (Combination of Methotrexate and Etanercept) study 6, 7
complement blockade, in SLE 111–12
congestive heart failure, avoidance of anti-TNF therapy 24
copy number variants (CNVs) 52–3
CORE (Continuing Outcomes Relevant to Evista) study 181
COX-2-selective inhibitors, in acute gout 164–5
creatine supplements, in inflammatory myositis 145, 146
Crohn's disease, anti-TNF agents 93
CTGF promoter polymorphism 130

CTLA4Ig (cytotoxic T lymphocyte-associated protein
　　4 IgG1) *see* abatacept
CXCR2 gene polymorphism 130
cyclophosphamide 23
　　in inflammatory myositis 143
　　in systemic sclerosis 131–2
　　　　fibrotic lung disease 132–3

D

dactylitis, psoriatic arthritis 72
　　biological therapy 79
DANCER (Dose-ranging Assessment: International
　　Clinical Evaluation of Rituximab in RA)
　　study 25, 37, 39
demyelinating disease risk, anti-TNF therapy 24
denosumab 190, 191
dermatomyositis 139, 147
　　clinical presentation 140
　　diagnostic criteria 140
　　epidemiology 140
　　extramuscular manifestations 141
　　muscle biopsy 141
　　outcomes 146–7
　　relationship to malignancy 146–7
　　rituximab 145
　　tumour necrosis factor inhibitors 144
　　see also inflammatory myositis
DHFR (dihydrofolate reductase) gene,
　　pharmacogenetic studies 56, 58
diacerein, in osteoarthritis 158
Dickkopf-1 (DKK-1) protein 190–1
diclofenac, in acute gout 165
dietary modification, gout 166–7
diffuse cutaneous SSc (DcSSc)
　　diagnosis 130
　　immunosuppressive therapy 131–2
digital ulceration, management in systemic
　　sclerosis 136
disease activity, measurement in ankylosing
　　spondylitis 87–8
disease modification, rituximab 38
disease-modifying anti-rheumatic drugs
　　(DMARD) 11, 18, 19, 51
　　in ankylosing spondylitis 91–2
　　combination therapy 4–5, 21–2
　　in early rheumatoid arthritis 4
　　　　achieving tight control 2–3
　　　　rationale 2
　　gold 20–1
　　hydroxychloroquine 18, 20
　　leflunomide 20
　　methotrexate 18
　　　　pharmacogenetics 55–60
　　in osteoarthritis 159
　　pharmacogenetics 54–5, 61
　　in psoriatic arthritis 73–5

sulfasalazine 20
disease-modifying osteoarthritis drugs
　　(DMOADs) 151
　　see also osteoarthritis
DISTOL-1 (Digital Ischemic Lesions in Scleroderma
　　Treated with Oral Treprostinil Dithanolamine)
　　study 136
diuretic therapy, gout 164, 167
doxycycline, in osteoarthritis 157–8
DR4/DR1 positivity 59
DRESS syndrome, strontium ranelate 185
drug response variation
　　genetic studies 53
　　influencing factors 61
　　see also pharmacogenetics
dual X-ray absorptiometry (DXA) 185

E

early therapy, rheumatoid arthritis 10–11, 17
　　biological therapy 5–6
　　combination therapy 4–5
　　comparison of treatment options 8–10
　　disease-modifying anti-rheumatic drugs 4
　　glucocorticoids 3–4
　　induction with biologicals and maintenance with
　　　　conventional DMARDs 6
　　methotrexate efficacy 58
　　rationale 1–2
　　tight control 2–3
eculizumab, in SLE 111–12
edratide 111
efalizumab, in psoriatic peripheral joint disease 77
electromyography 141
endothelin receptor antagonists
　　in SSc-associated digital ulceration 136
　　in SSc-associated pulmonary hypertension 135
enthesitis
　　assessment in ankylosing spondylitis (AS) 89
　　in psoriatic arthritis 72
　　　　biological therapy 78–9
episcleritis, in rheumatoid arthritis 29
epratuzumab, in SLE 105
ERA (Early Rheumatoid Arthritis) trial 6, 7
erythrocyte sedimentation rate (ESR), in assessment
　　of ankylosing spondylitis 90
etanercept 23–4, 26
　　in ankylosing spondylitis 92–3
　　in early rheumatoid arthritis 6, 7, 8
　　in gout 174
　　in inflammatory bowel disease 93
　　in inflammatory myositis 144
　　pharmacogenetic studies 54, 60–1, 62–3
　　in psoriatic arthritis
　　　　axial disease 78
　　　　dactylitis 79
　　　　enthesitis 78

peripheral joint disease 76
etidronate, in osteoporosis 180, 182
etoricoxib, in acute gout 164, 165
ETRA gene polymorphism 130
European League Against Rheumatism (EULAR),
    recommendations for management of gout 164
exercise, in inflammatory myositis 145, 146
extra-articular complications, rheumatoid
    arthritis 28–9
eye complications, rheumatoid arthritis 29

F
FAST (Fibrosing Alveolitis in Scleroderma Trial) 132
fatigue, assessment in ankylosing spondylitis
    (AS) 89
Fcγ receptor polymorphisms, pharmacogenetic
    studies 60, 63
febuxostat 169–70
Felty's syndrome 29
fenofibrate, uricosuric properties 171
fibrillin-1 gene polymorphism 130
fibrotic lung disease, systemic sclerosis (SSc) 132–3
FIN-RACo (Finnish Rheumatoid Arthritis-
    Combination Therapy) study 4, 21
FIT (Fracture Intervention Trial) 182
folate, in osteoporosis 189
folic acid, administration with methotrexate 18
fondaparinux 122
FPGS (folylpoly-glutamate synthetase) gene,
    pharmacogenetic studies 57, 58
Framingham Heart Study, on vitamin D 154

G
GAIT (Glucosamine/Chondroitin Arthritis
    Intervention Trial) 152
gastrointestinal involvement, systemic sclerosis 133
genetic testing, clinical and economic value 64
genome-wide studies, drug response variation 53
GGH (γ-glutamyl hydrolase) gene, pharmacogenetic
    studies 57, 59
glucocorticosteroids
    in acute gout 165–6
    effect on DKK-1 expression 190–1
    in inflammatory myositis 143
    in psoriatic arthritis 73
    in rheumatoid arthritis 19, 22–3
        early therapy 3–4
    side-effects 4
glucosamine 151–2
glutathione peroxidase 154
GO-REVEAL (Golimumab-Randomized Evaluation
    of Safety and Efficacy in Subjects with Psoriatic
    Arthritis using a Human Anti-TNF Monoclonal
    Antibody) study 77, 78
GPRD (General Practice Research Database) 180
gold therapy 19, 20–1

in psoriatic arthritis 73, 75
golimumab, in psoriatic arthritis
    enthesitis 78
    peripheral joint disease 77
gout 163
    acute 166
        colchicine 165
        glucocorticosteroids 165–6
        ice-packs 166
        non-steroidal anti-inflammatory drugs 163–5
    biological agents 173–4
    EULAR recommendations 164
    long-term management 166
        diuretic discontinuation 167
        lifestyle modification 166–7
        uricase 171
        uricosuric agents 170–1
        xanthine oxidase inhibitors 167–70
    suboptimal treatment 173
    urate-lowering therapy
        indications 172
        prophylaxis against acute attacks 172–3
        target levels 172

H
headache, in antiphospholipid syndrome 120–1
Health Professionals Follow-Up Study, gout
    risk 167
Heart Estrogen Replacement Study 180
heparin
    oral 122
    value in antiphospholipid syndrome 122
high-resolution CT, appearances of fibrotic lung
    disease 132
HLA B27 85, 90
HLA (human leucocyte antigen) genes,
    pharmacogenetic studies 59, 60, 63
homocysteine levels, relationship to
    osteoporosis 189
hormone replacement therapy (HRT), in
    osteoporosis prevention 179–81
Hughes syndrome see antiphospholipid syndrome
HuMax-CD20 39
hydroxychloroquine 18, 19, 20
    in combination therapy 4, 5, 21
    in osteoarthritis 159
    pharmacogenetic studies 54
hyperparathyroidism 186
hyperuricaemia 163
    see also gout

I
ibandronate 183
    fracture risk reduction 180
ibuprofen, in psoriatic arthritis 72
ice-packs, in acute gout 166

IDEC-131 111
IL-1β inhibition, in osteoarthritis 158
IL-10 gene polymorphism 130
imatinib mesylate 134
immunoablation
    in SLE 112
    in systemic sclerosis 131–2
immunosuppressive therapy
    in inflammatory myositis 143–4
    in systemic sclerosis 130–2
    see also azathioprine; ciclosporin;
        cyclophosphamide; methotrexate;
        mycophenolate mofetil
IMPACT (Infliximab Multinational Psoriatic Arthritis
    Controlled Trials) 1 and 2 76, 78, 79
inclusion-body myositis 139
    clinical presentation 140
    drug treatment 145
    muscle biopsy 141
    see also inflammatory myositis
indomethacin
    in acute gout 164–5
    in psoriatic arthritis 72
infection risk
    abatacept 43
    anti-TNF agents 24
    rituximab 38–9
    tocilizumab 45
inflammation, role in systemic sclerosis 130–1, 132
inflammatory bowel disease, anti-TNF agents 93
inflammatory myositis 139, 147
    autoantibodies 141–2
    classification 139
    clinical assessment 142
    clinical presentation 140
    creatine supplements 145, 146
    diagnostic criteria 140
    epidemiology 140
    exercise 145–6
    extramuscular manifestations 141
    imaging 142
    investigations 141
    outcomes 146–7
    relationship to malignancy 146–7
    treatments
        glucocorticoids 143
        immunosuppressants 143–4
        of inclusion-body myositis 145
        intravenous immunoglobulins 143, 144
        rituximab 145
        tumour necrosis factor inhibitors 144
infliximab 23–4, 26
    in ankylosing spondylitis 92–3
    in early rheumatoid arthritis 6, 7, 8–9
    in gout 174
    in inflammatory bowel disease 93

in inflammatory myositis 144
pharmacogenetic studies 54, 60–1, 62–3
in prevention of rheumatoid arthritis 10
in psoriatic arthritis
    axial disease 78
    dactylitis 79
    enthesitis 78–9
    peripheral joint disease 75–6
in SLE 110
INR (international normalized ratio), self-testing in
    antiphospholipid syndrome 123
interleukin 1 blockade 25, 26, 44–5
    see also anakinra
interleukin 1 gene, pharmacogenetic studies 54, 63
interleukin 1 receptor antagonist, pharmacogenetic
    studies 63
interleukin 6 blockade (tocilizumab) 27–8, 45
interleukin 10, pharmacogenetic studies 60, 63
interleukin 15 blockade 45–6
interstitial lung disease, rheumatoid arthritis 29
intra-articular steroids
    in gout 164, 165
    in psoriatic arthritis 73
    in rheumatoid arthritis 4, 23
intravenous immunoglobulin (IVIg)
    in antiphospholipid syndrome 123
    in inflammatory myositis 143, 144
isosorbide mononitrate, in osteoporosis 189
ITPA (inosine triphosphatase) gene,
    pharmacogenetic studies 57, 58

J

joint aspiration, in gout 165

K

keliximab 44
KL-6 132
KOSTAR trial (risedronate) 155

L

lansofoxifene 181
large granular lymphocyte (LGL) syndrome 29
leflunomide 4, 19, 20
    in ankylosing spondylitis 92
    in combination therapy 22
    pharmacogenetic studies 54
    in psoriatic arthritis 74–5
leucapheresis, in inflammatory myositis 143
leucopenia, in rheumatoid arthritis 29
lifestyle modification, gout 164, 166–7
limited cutaneous systemic sclerosis (LcSSc) 129–30
liver toxicity, methotrexate 74
losartan, uricosuric properties 171
low-density lipoprotein (LDL) oxidation 122

low molecular weight heparin, in antiphospholipid
    syndrome
    effect on headaches 121
    in pregnancy 121
lupus anticoagulant (LA) 117
lupus nephritis
    mycophenolate mofetil 101–3
    rituximab 104–5
lymphoablation, in systemic sclerosis 131
lymphocyte function antigen 3 (LFA-3) *see* alefacept
lymphoma risk, anti-TNF therapy 24
LymphoStat-B (belimumab) 40
lymphotoxin α (LTA), pharmacogenetic studies 63

M

Maastricht Ankylosing Spondylitis Enthesitis Score
    (MASES) 89
magnetic resonance imaging (MRI), in assessment of
    ankylosing spondylitis 89
malignancy risk, anti-TNF therapy 24
Mander Enthesitis Index (MEI) 89
MASCOT (Methotrexate and Sulfasalazine
    Combination Therapy) study 5
MCP-1 gene polymorphism 130
meat consumption, and gout 166
meloxicam, in acute gout 165
memory loss, in antiphospholipid syndrome 121
menopause, osteoporosis risk 179–80
methotrexate 18
    in ankylosing spondylitis 91–2
    in combination therapy 3–4, 4–5, 6, 8, 21–2
    in early RA 4, 7, 8–9
        CAMERA trial 3
    in inflammatory myositis 143
    in osteoarthritis 159
    pharmacogenetics 54, 55–60
    in prevention of rheumatoid arthritis 10
    in psoriatic arthritis 73–4
    in systemic sclerosis 131
methylprednisolone
    administration prior to rituximab 39
    combination with methotrexate in early
        rheumatoid arthritis 3–4
migraine, in antiphospholipid syndrome 120–1
Million Women Study (MWS) 180
MITAX (Myositis Intention To Treat Index) 142
MORE (Multiple Outcome of Raloxifene Evaluation)
    trial 181
mSASSS (modified Stoke Ankylosing Spondylitis
    Spinal Score) 88, 89
MTHFD1 (methylene tetrahydrofolate
    dehydrogenase) gene, pharmacogenetic
    studies 56, 58
MTHFR (methylene tetrahydrofolate reductase
    gene), pharmacogenetic studies 55, 56, 58

MTR (5-methyltetrahydrofolate-homocysteine
    methyltransferase) gene, pharmacogenetic
    studies 56, 58, 59
MTRR (5-methyltetrahydrofolate-homocysteine
    methyltransferase reductase) gene,
    pharmacogenetic studies 57, 58, 59
muscle biopsy 141
muscle enzymes 141
    mycophenolate mofetil
    in inflammatory myositis 143
    in lupus nephritis 101–3
    in systemic sclerosis 131
        in fibrotic lung disease 133
myeloablation, in systemic sclerosis 131, 132
MYOACT (Myositis Disease Activity Assessment)
    scale 142
myositis-associated autoantibodies 141, 142
myositis-specific autoantibodies 141, 142

N

necrotizing scleritis 29
nimesulide, in psoriatic arthritis 72
nitrates, in osteoporosis 189
non-steroidal anti-inflammatory drugs (NSAIDs)
    in acute gout 163–5
    in ankylosing spondylitis 91
    in gout prophylaxis 173
    in psoriatic arthritis 72

O

ocrelizumab 39
odanacatib 189
ofatumumab 39
OPTION study (Tocilizumab Pivotal Trial in
    Methotrexate Inadequate Responders) 28
osteoarthritis 151
    antioxidants and vitamins 153–4, 155
    avocado–soyabean unsaponifiables (ASUs) 158–9
    bisphosphonates 154–5
    calcitonin 156
    diacerein 158
    disease-modifying anti-rheumatic drugs 159
    glucosamine and chondroitin 151–2
    matrix metalloproteinase inhibitors 157–8
    molecular pathogenesis 157
    rose-hip extract 159
    strontium ranelate 156
osteoporosis 179, 191–2
    bisphosphonates 181–3
    calcitonin 183–4
    calcium supplementation 188
    cathepsin K inhibitors 189
    denosumab 190, 191
    future treatments 189
    hormone replacement therapy 179–81

parathyroid hormone 186–7
  in rheumatoid arthritis 29
  selective estrogen receptor modulators 181
  strontium 184–6
  testosterone 187
  vitamin D 188
  Wnt signalling 190–1
osteoprotogerin 190
  OPG-RANKL ratio 184–5
oxypurinol 168

P

pamidronate 183
  in ankylosing spondylitis 92
parallel triple therapy, early rheumatoid arthritis 5
parathyroid hormone, in osteoporosis 180, 186–7
patient information 64
patient profiling 64
PEGylated uricase 171
D-penicillamine, in systemic sclerosis 133
pericarditis, rheumatic 29
peripheral joint involvement, assessment in
  ankylosing spondylitis 89
personalized therapy 64
pharmacogenetics 52–3
  future clinical implications 64–5
  in rheumatoid arthritis 54–5
    biological agents 60–1, 62–3
    future research perspectives 61, 64
    methotrexate 55–60
phophodiesterase (PDE)-5 antagonists
  in SSc-associated digital ulceration 136
  in SSc-associated pulmonary hypertension 135
physical function, assessment in ankylosing
  spondylitis 88
plasma exchange, in inflammatory myositis 143
pleural effusions, in rheumatoid arthritis 29
polymyositis 139, 147
  clinical presentation 140
  diagnostic criteria 140
  epidemiology 140
  muscle biopsy 141
  outcomes 146–7
  relationship to malignancy 146–7
  rituximab 145
  tumour necrosis factor inhibitors 144
  see also inflammatory myositis
preclinical stage, rheumatoid arthritis 1–2
prednisolone, in acute gout 165–6
pregnancy, antiphospholipid syndrome 121–2, 123
PREMIER trial 6, 7
Preotact 186–7
PRESTA (Psoriasis Randomized Etanercept Study in
  Subjects with Psoriatic Arthritis) 76
probenecid, in gout 164, 170
  in initiation of urate-lowering therapy 172–3

PROMPT (Probable Rheumatoid Arthritis:
  Methotrexate versus Placebo Treatment)
  study 10
PROOF (Prevent Recurrence Of Osteopathic
  Fractures) study 184
PsARC (Psoriatic Arthritis Response Criterion) 75,
  76–7
psoriatic arthritis (PsA) 71
  clinical features 72
  core outcome domains 72
  treatment strategies 71
    biological agents 75–9, 93
    DMARDs 73–5
    glucocorticoids 73
    non-steroidal anti-inflammatory drugs 72
PTPN22 gene polymorphism 130
pulmonary arterial hypertension, systemic sclerosis-
  associated 134–5
purine metabolism 167

R

R620W gene polymorphism 130
RADIATE study (Rheumatoid Arthritis Study in
  Anti-TNF Failures) 28
radiography, in assessment of ankylosing
  spondylitis 89–90
raloxifene 181
  fracture risk reduction 180
RANKL (receptor activator of NF-kappaB
  ligand) 184–5, 190
recombinant uricase (rasburicase) 171
  site of action 167
REFLEX (A Randomised Evaluation of Long-term
  Efficacy of Rituximab in RA) study 25, 37–8, 39
RFC (reduced folate carrier) gene, pharmacogenetic
  studies 57, 58
rheumatoid arthritis (RA) 1
  azathioprine 23
  biological agents 26
    abatacept 27, 40–4
    AMG 714 45–6
    anakinra 25, 44
    anti-TNF agents 23–4
    belimumab 40
    rituximab 25, 27, 36–9
    T-cell targeted therapies 44
    tocilizumab 27–8, 45
  ciclosporin A 23
  cyclophosphamide 23
  early therapy 10–11, 17
    biological therapy 5–6
    combination therapy 4–5
    comparison of treatment options 8–10
    glucocorticosteroids 3–4
    induction with biologicals and maintenance
      with conventional DMARDs 6

methotrexate efficacy 58
   rationale 1–2
   tight control 2–3
extra-articular disease manifestations 28–9
glucocorticosteroids 22–3
monitoring disease activity 3
pharmacogenetics 54–5
   biological agents 60–1, 62–3
   future research perspectives 61, 64
   methotrexate 55–60
prevention 10
role of B cells 35–6
stepwise treatment approach 51, 52
tight control 17–18
treatment response 51
see also disease-modifying anti-rheumatic drugs
   (DMARD)
risedronate
   in osteoarthritis 155
   in osteoporosis 180, 182
rituximab (RTX) 10, 25, 26, 27, 35, 36
   in antiphospholipid syndrome 123–4
   current use in RA 39
   disease modification 38
   duration of benefit 39
   in inflammatory myositis 145
   pharmacogenetic studies 54
   in psoriatic arthritis, peripheral joint
      disease 77–8
   safety issues 38–9
   in SLE 103–5
      clinical studies 106–8
   studies in rheumatoid arthritis 36–8
rofecoxib, in acute gout 165
rose-hip extract, in osteoarthritis 159
RUTH (Raloxefine Use for the Heart) study 181

S

safety issues
   abatacept 42–3
   rituximab 38–9
SASSS (Stoke Ankylosing Spondylitis Spinal
   Score) 89
scl-70 antibodies 130
scleritis, in rheumatoid arthritis 29
scleroderma renal crisis 135
sclerostin 190
SCOT (Scleroderma: Cyclophosphamide or
   Transplantation) trial 132
seafood consumption, and gout 166
selective estrogen receptor modulators (SERMS) 181
selenium, in osteoarthritis 154
shared epitope (SE) hypothesis 59
SHMT1 (serine hydroxymethyltransferase) gene,
   pharmacogenetic studies 56, 58, 59
side-effects
   of abatacept 43

of allopurinol 168
of ciclosporin 74
of gold therapy 21
of hydroxychloroquine 19
of intravenous bisphosphonates 183
of leflunomide 20, 75
of methotrexate 18, 74
   pharmacogenetic studies 58–9
of parathyroid hormone 187
of raloxifene 181
of rituximab 38–9, 104, 106–8
of strontium ranelate 185
of sulfasalazine 20
of tocilizumab 28, 45
sildenafil in SSc
   in digital ulceration 136
   in pulmonary hypertension 135
single nucleotide polymorphisms (SNPs) 52
   genome-wide analysis 53
sitaxsentan 135
Sjögren's syndrome 29
SLS (Scleroderma Lung Study) 132
SOTI (Spinal Osteoporosis Therapeutic
   Intervention) trial 185
SPARC gene polymorphism 130
spondyloarthritides 85
STAR (Study of Tamoxifen and Raloxifene)
   study 181
statins, in osteoporosis 189
step-down approach, DMARD therapy 21
step-up therapy, rheumatoid arthritis 5, 21
stepwise treatment approach, rheumatoid
   arthritis 51, 52
STEREO trial (adalimumab) 77
steroids *see* glucocorticosteroids
strontium ranelate
   in osteoarthritis 156
   in osteoporosis 180, 184–6
Study of Osteoporotic fractures 154
sulfasalazine 4, 19, 20
   in ankylosing spondylitis 91
   combination therapy 5, 21, 22
   in osteoarthritis 159
   pharmacogenetic studies 54
   in psoriatic arthritis 74
sulfinpyrazone 170
   in gout 164
systemic lupus erythematosus (SLE) 101, 112
   abetimus sodium 111
   ACR classification 102
   anticytokine therapy 110
   B-cell depletion therapy
      epratuzumab 105
      rituximab 103–5, 106–8
   B-cell survival factor inhibitors 109
   complement blockade 111–12
   edratide 111
   immunoablation 112

mycophenolate mofetil 101–3
T-cell targeting 110–11
targeted therapeutic approaches 103
systemic sclerosis (SSc) 129, 136
    antifibrotic therapies 133–4
    diffuse disease 130
    fibrotic lung disease, immunosuppression 132–3
    gastrointestinal involvement 133
    genetic associations 130
    immunosuppressive therapy 130–2
    limited disease 129–30
    pathogenesis 129
    pulmonary arterial hypertension 134–5
    scleroderma renal crisis 135

T

T-cell targeted therapies 44
T-cells, role in rheumatoid arthritis 40
tadalafil, in SSc-associated pulmonary
    hypertension 135
teriparatide 186, 187
testosterone, in osteoporosis 180, 187
tetracyclines, in osteoarthritis 157–8
TGF-β, role in systemic sclerosis 130, 133–4
thalidomide, in ankylosing spondylitis 92
thrombocytopenia, effect of rituximab in APS 123–4
thrombosis, antiphospholipid syndrome, primary
    prevention 118
TICORA (Tight Control for Rheumatoid Arthritis)
    study 2–3, 18
tisopurine 168
tocilizumab 10, 26, 27–8, 45
    in SLE 110
TOWARD study (Tocilizumab in Combination With
    traditional DMARD therapy) 28
treatment response, assessment in ankylosing
    spondylitis 90–1
treprostinil
    in SSc-associated digital ulceration 136
    in SSc-associated pulmonary hypertension 134–5
triamcinolone acetonide, in acute gout 165
TROPOS (Treatment of Peripheral Osteoporosis)
    trial 185
TSER (thymidylate synthetase enhancer region)
    gene, pharmacogenetic studies 56, 58, 59
tuberculosis risk, anti-TNF agents 24
tumour necrosis factor alpha (TNF-α) 5–6
    role in SLE 110
    TNF-863A gene polymorphism 130
    TNF-α gene, pharmacogenetic studies 54, 60, 62
    see also anti-TNF agents
TYMS gene, pharmacogenetic studies 56

U

ulcerative colitis, anti-TNF agents 93
ultrasonography, in assessment of ankylosing
    spondylitis 90
URAT1 170
urate-lowering therapy
    duration 173
    indications 172
    prophylaxis against acute attacks 172–3
    target levels 172
uricase (urate oxidase) 171
    site of action 167
    see also urate-lowering therapy
uricosuric agents 170–1
    EULAR recommendations 164
    site of action 167
    see also urate-lowering therapy
ustekinumab, in psoriatic arthritis, peripheral joint
    disease 78

V

variable numbers of tandem repeats (VNTR) 53
vasculitis, in rheumatoid arthritis 29
verdenafil, in SSc-associated pulmonary
    hypertension 135
vitamin A, in osteoarthritis 153
vitamin B$_{12}$, in osteoporosis 189
vitamin C
    in osteoarthritis 153
    uricosuric properties 171
vitamin D
    in osteoarthritis 154, 155
    in osteoporosis 180, 188
    supplementation in glucocorticosteroid
        therapy 23
vitamin E, in osteoarthritis 153

W

warfarin in antiphospholipid syndrome 119–20
    during pregnancy 122
weight reduction, effect on gout risk 167
WHI (Women's Health Initiative) study 180
window of opportunity, early rheumatoid
    arthritis 2
Wnt signalling, role in bone formation 190

X

xanthine oxidase inhibitors 167–70
    see also urate-lowering therapy

Z

zoledronate 183
    fracture risk reduction 180